Clinical Applications of Dental Materials

Clinical Applications of Dental Materials

Editor: Gerard Keith

AMERICAN
MEDICAL PUBLISHERS
www.americanmedicalpublishers.com

AMERICAN
MEDICAL PUBLISHERS
www.americanmedicalpublishers.com

Cataloging-in-Publication Data

Clinical applications of dental materials / edited by Gerard Keith.
p. cm.
Includes bibliographical references and index.
ISBN 978-1-63927-653-0
1. Dental materials. 2. Dental instruments and apparatus. 3. Dental technology.
4. Prosthodontics. I. Keith, Gerard.
RK652.5 .C55 2023
617.695--dc23

American Medical Publishers,
41 Flatbush Avenue,
1st Floor, New York,
NY 11217, USA

ISBN 978-1-63927-653-0 (Hardback)

Contents

Preface

Dental materials are special products designed for usage in dentistry. Various types of dental materials are used in dentistry and characteristics of these materials vary based on their intended purpose. Generally utilized dental materials include temporary dressings, cements, impression materials, lining materials and restorative materials. Temporary dressings are interim materials used as dental fillings, which are not meant to last long and have therapeutic properties, such as zinc oxide eugenol. Common usage of temporary dressing is done in root canal procedure, which is completed in more than one appointment. Dental cements are utilized majorly for indirect restorations, like binding crowns to the natural surface of the tooth. Materials that are used generally as dental cements include zinc oxide cement, zinc polycarboxylate cement, zinc phosphate cement, resin-based cement, glass ionomer cement, and copper-based cement. Impression materials are used for obtaining negative imprints of soft tissues and teeth, which are used for casting positive representation. This book unravels the recent studies on dental materials. It will help new researchers by foregrounding their knowledge on the clinical applications of dental materials.

This book has been the outcome of endless efforts put in by authors and researchers on various issues and topics within the field. The book is a comprehensive collection of significant researches that are addressed in a variety of chapters. It will surely enhance the knowledge of the field among readers across the globe.

It gives us an immense pleasure to thank our researchers and authors for their efforts to submit their piece of writing before the deadlines. Finally in the end, I would like to thank my family and colleagues who have been a great source of inspiration and support.

Editor

1

The Effect of Selected Dental Materials Used in Conservative Dentistry, Endodontics, Surgery and Orthodontics as Well as during the Periodontal Treatment on the Redox Balance in the Oral Cavity

Izabela Zieniewska [1,*], Mateusz Maciejczyk [2] and Anna Zalewska [3,*]

1 Doctoral Studies, Medical University of Bialystok, 24a M. Sklodowskiej-Curie Street, 15-274 Bialystok, Poland
2 Department of Hygiene, Epidemiology and Ergonomics, Medical University of Bialystok, 15-022 Bialystok, Poland; mat.maciejczyk@gmail.com
3 Experimental Dentistry Laboratory, Medical University of Bialystok, 24a M. Sklodowskiej-Curie Street, 15-274 Bialystok, Poland
* Correspondence: izazieniewska@gmail.com (I.Z.); azalewska426@gmail.com (A.Z.)

Abstract: Oxidative stress (OS) is a redox homeostasis disorder that results in oxidation of cell components and thus disturbs cell metabolism. OS is induced by numerous internal as well as external factors. According to recent studies, dental treatment may also be one of them. The aim of our work was to assess the effect of dental treatment on the redox balance of the oral cavity. We reviewed literature available in PubMed, Medline, and Scopus databases, including the results from 2010 to 2020. Publications were searched according to the keywords: oxidative stress and dental monomers; oxidative stress and amalgam; oxidative stress and periodontitis, oxidative stress and braces, oxidative stress and titanium; oxidative stress and dental implants, oxidative stress and endodontics treatment, oxidative stress and dental treatment; and oxidative stress and dental composite. It was found that dental treatment with the use of composites, amalgams, glass-ionomers, materials for root canal filling/rinsing, orthodontic braces (made of various metal alloys), titanium implants, or whitening agents can disturb oral redox homeostasis by affecting the antioxidant barrier and increasing oxidative damage to salivary proteins, lipids, and DNA. Abnormal saliva secretion/composition was also observed in dental patients in the course of OS. It is suggested that the addition of antioxidants to dental materials or antioxidant therapy applied during dental treatment could protect the patient against harmful effects of OS in the oral cavity.

Keywords: amalgam; antioxidants; dental resin composites; composites resins; endodontics treatment; glass-ionomer; orthodontics appliances; oxidative stress; periodontal treatment; redox balance; titanium implants; whitening

---

1. Introduction

Oxidative stress (OS) is defined as an imbalance between the production of oxygen (ROS) and nitrogen (RNS) free radicals and their neutralization by compounds called antioxidants [1]. Interestingly, ROS also act as signaling molecules involved in cell growth, proliferation and survival [2]. ROS/RNS are formed under the influence of external factors, such as ionizing radiation, ultraviolet radiation or ultrasound, as well as produced endogenously [3]. The main non-enzymatic, endogenous source of ROS/RNS in a cell is the mitochondrial respiratory chain. There are also enzymatic sources of ROS/RNS, including: xanthine oxidase (XO), cyclooxygenases (COX), lipoxygenases, myeloperoxidases (MPO), cytochrome P450 monooxygenase, uncoupled nitric oxide synthase (NOS), peroxidases and NADPH oxidase (NOX) [2]. The excess of ROS/RNS leads to the damage of cellular components such as proteins, lipids and nucleic acids as well as to cell death through apoptosis and necrosis [4,5].

Proteins are the main molecules attacked by ROS [6]. Highly reactive radicals cause multi-area damage to the protein side chain and backbone. Less reactive species demonstrate greater selectivity and damage smaller areas. Oxidation of proteins may cause increased hydrophilicity of the protein side chains, fragmentation of the side chains as well as the backbone, aggregation through covalent crosslinking or hydrophobic interactions, and protein conformation [7].

During protein peroxidation, cysteine and—to a lesser extent—methionine residues are oxidized. Usually hydrogen atoms are detached from the C-H or S-H bonds by the radical [7]. The separation of a hydrogen atom from carbon leads to the formation of a stabilized carbon-centered radical, which then reacts with other carbon-centered radicals or with O_2 [8]. These reactions result in protein backbone fragmentation [8].

The side chains of amino acids are also subject to oxidative damage [9]. This mechanism usually leads to the formation of carbon-centered radicals. The amino acid side chains that contain sulfur are the most exposed to the oxidation process. Free amino acids are much less frequently damaged than the side chains, probably due to the fact that there are fewer of them than the side chains [7].

Lipid oxidation occurs in the presence of numerous oxidants, including peroxynitrite, hypochlorite, lipoxygenases, cyclooxygenase, cytochrome P450, and singlet oxygen [10]. Unsaturated lipids are particularly susceptible to oxidation. Under the influence of radical oxidants such as peroxyl radicals, lipid hydroperoxides are produced [11,12].

DNA oxidation usually results in breaks in the DNA thread, modification of bases and rupture of phosphodiester bonds. The consequence of these processes is oxidative damage to DNA. The marker of oxidative damage to nucleic acids is mainly 8-hydroxy-2′-deoxyguanosine (8-OHdG). Increased concentration of 8-OHdG was observed in the course of several systemic diseases caused by oxidative stress, such as cancer or diabetes. The formation of 8-OHdG is triggered by the product in the C8 position of the deoxyguanosine imidazole ring [11].

A special role in maintaining the redox balance is played by enzymatic and non-enzymatic antioxidant systems which protect cells against harmful effects of ROS [13,14]. Antioxidants, when present in low concentrations compared to the content of the oxidized substrate, are intended to inhibit the oxidation of this substrate [15]. The ROS/RNS neutralization process occurs in one or two stages. In the latter case, ROS/RNS are transformed into weak radicals that interact with another weak radical, leading to the formation of an inactive molecule. The most important enzymatic systems include: superoxide dismutase (SOD), catalase (CAT) and glutathione peroxidase (GPx), while the main non-enzymatic antioxidants are, inter alia: the glutathione system, albumins, lactoferrin, ascorbic acid (AS), uric acid and melatonin [16,17].

The oral cavity is the initial part of the digestive tract, a vital place due to the structures it contains, and further sections of the digestive system. It is a place exposed to numerous external factors inducing ROS/RNS production and OS development. Excessive production of ROS/RNS also occurs during the intake of food, drinks, and stimulants or as a result of dental treatment [18]. The cause of redox imbalance in the oral cavity may be pathological changes such as caries, gingivitis, periodontitis, pre-cancerous conditions and cancer, inflammation, and fungal infections [18]. Interestingly, more and more reports show that these diseases and their treatment disturbs the oral redox equilibrium. Evidence showed that the performed dental procedures, such as filling cavities, endodontic, periodontic, orthodontic, and surgical treatment, may increase the production of ROS/RNS, and thus the development of OS. Of course, it should be emphasized that the ROS/RNS generated during dental treatment also positively affects the oral cavity. They promote wound healing, stimulate the immune response, and facilitate the elimination of bacteria [18].

The aim of our study was a literature review of reports on the impact of dental, periodontal, orthodontic, and surgical treatment (in terms of titanium fixation and implants) on redox balance.

2. Materials and Methods

2.1. Search Strategy

A literature review was conducted from 2010 to July 2020. We used the databases of PubMed, Medline and Scopus, and analyzed only international literature in English. Publications were searched according to the entered key words: oxidative stress and dental monomers; oxidative stress and amalgam; oxidative stress and periodontitis, oxidative stress and braces, oxidative stress, and titanium; oxidative stress and dental implants, oxidative stress and endodontics treatment, oxidative stress and dental treatment; oxidative stress and dental composite.

2.2. Inclusion Criteria

Only the works meeting the following criteria were included in this paper:

1. Works on redox disorders related to dental treatment, dental fillings, dental monomers, endodontic treatment, titanium implants, treatment of periodontal diseases, whitening.
2. Results obtained from experiments participated by human subjects, as well as experimental works.
3. Publications in English only.
4. Clinical trials on a group of at least five individuals.

2.3. Exclusion Criteria

1. Works written in languages other than English.
2. Clinical trials on a group of fewer than five individuals.
3. Meta-analyzes.
4. Publications on the redox balance in the treatment of neurocranial diseases and cancer.
5. Publications referring to prosthetic treatment and treatment of functional disorders of the masticatory organ.
6. Case studies.
7. Among the publications based on human material we excluded those that covered subjects with systemic diseases.

3. Data Extraction

The titles and abstracts resulting from this search strategy were evaluated independently by two researchers (I. Z., A. Z). In case of doubt, the given publication was included or excluded after reading its entire text. Cohen's kappa coefficient (κ) was used to measure interexaminer reliability ($\kappa = 0.89$). Each work was initially checked in the scope of its title, then abstract and the full text. When the studies met the inclusion criteria, they were included in this publication.

All works were evaluated in terms of methodology. Every publication had the following variables distinguished: authors, year of publication, study design, size of the study group, inclusion and exclusion criteria, duration of the study and study results.

4. Results

Out of approximately 27,600 publications, 37 were identified as meeting the inclusion and exclusion criteria. The literature review revealed 27,621 works from the MEDLINE (PubMed) library, of which 27,006 were excluded due to their title. A total of 412 summaries were read, 149 of which met the inclusion and exclusion criteria. Of the qualified articles, 112 proved irrelevant to the topic of our review. Therefore, 37 works were eventually included herein (Figure 1).

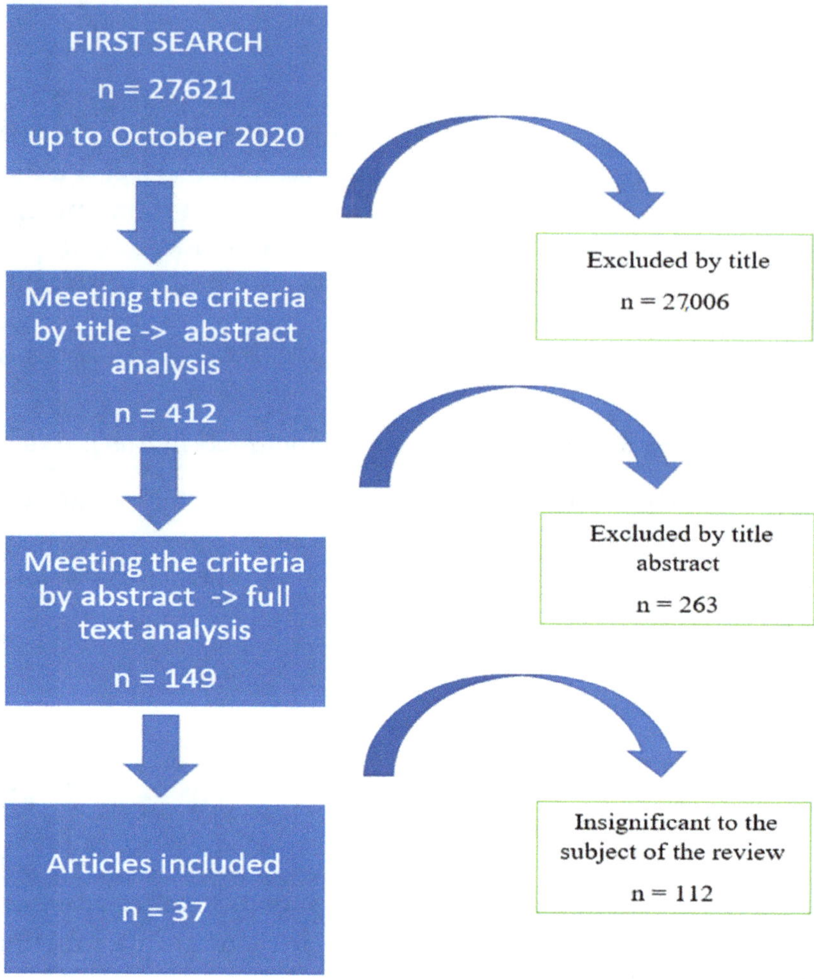

Figure 1. Flow chart of research methodology.

Research included the study are presented in Table 1.

Table 1. Research included in the study.

Experimental Model	Endpoints	References
	Amalgam	
Human gingival fibroblast cells (HGFCs) exposed to microhybrid resin-based composite, compomer resin, glass-ionomer cement and amalgam alloy for 7 and 21 days	The levels of total oxidant status (TOS) in the study groups (i.e., samples with the following materials: microhybrid resin-based composite, compomer resin, glass-ionomer cement and amalgam alloy; shaped as a 2-mm-thick disk with a diameter of 10 mm; exposed to light with the wavelength of 430–480 nm and intensity of 1200 mW/cm^2) were significantly higher in freshly prepared samples compared to the control. After 7 and 21 days, TOS level in the amalgam sample was considerably lower than at the beginning of the study. The highest level of total antioxidant capacity (TAC) was observed after 7 days in the filling with glass-ionomer cement (which prevented TOS increase). In all studied groups, TAC level after 7 days was different than at the initial stage of the study.	[19]
Unstimulated saliva of 48 generally healthy children aged 6–10 (24 males, 24 females) with two class II dental composite or amalgam restorations and the control (caries-free) group	The saliva of patients with composite fillings had significantly higher TAC compared to patients with amalgam fillings as well as caries-free subjects. However, TAC in patients with amalgam restorations was also significantly higher compared to the caries-free control. Patients with composite fillings also demonstrated decreased salivary levels of Ca^{2+} ions.	[20]
Saliva from 60 generally healthy subjects aged 15–40 with class I restorations of: amalgam (20 participants), composite (20 subjects) and glass-ionomer (20 patients), collected before the filling as well as 24 h and 7 and 14 days after the filling	Malondialdehyde (MDA) level in the saliva of patients with an amalgam filling was found to be higher than in patients with a composite or glass-ionomer filling. Significant differences were also observed between MDA concentrations on day 7 and 14, and after 24 h and 7 days in patients with composite fillings. There were no differences in MDA levels before treatment and 7 days after, or before and 14 days after the treatment. In the case of glass-ionomer, a significant difference was found only between 24 h and 7 days after the treatment.	[21]

Table 1. *Cont.*

Experimental Model	Endpoints	References
Urine collected from 106 generally healthy children aged 5–15.5 years with amalgam fillings	It was shown that in children with amalgam filling, there was a reduced excretion of 8-hydroxy-2-deoxyguanosine (8-OHdG) in the urine. It was also shown that the level of NAG in the urine of children with amalgam fillings was significantly higher compared to children without such fillings and was positively correlated with the level of MDA in the urine. There was no correlation between the concentration of 8-OHdG and malondialdehyde (MDA) in the urine of amalgam-filled children. The mercury (Hg) level was also significantly higher in children with amalgam fillings compared to children without amalgam fillings; however, no relationship was found between the Hg level and the number of fillings.	[22]
Hair samples collected from 42 generally healthy women (mean age 44 years) with amalgam fillings applied at least 10 years earlier	An increased activity of SOD-1 and an increase in GSH concentration in the hair of women with amalgam fillings as compared to women without such fillings were observed. A positive correlation was also shown between the concentration of aluminum (Al) and the concentration of GSH, and between the level of mercury (Hg) and the activity of SOD-1.	[23]
Blood collected from 41 generally healthy patients (17–23 years old), which used amalgam (19) and dental resin composite (22) fillings	A significant increase in the level of malondialdehyde (MDA) was observed 24 h after placing amalgam and composite filling. There were no changes in the concentration of 8-OHdG in women 24 h after the placement of the amalgam filling. The 8-OHdG level increased 24 h after placing the dental resin composite filling.	[24]
	Dental Resin Composites—monomers	
Human dental pulp cells (hDPCs) exposed to dental monomers (1 mM HEMA, 5 mM MMA and 1 mM TEGDMA) without and in the presence of 10 mM NAC for 24, 48, 72 and 96 h	In response to 6 h of exposure to dental monomers: 2-hydroxyethyl methacrylate (HEMA), triethylene glycol dimethacrylate (TEGDMA) and methyl methacrylate (MMA), there was a significant increase in ROS production in hDPCs compared to the control group without dental monomers. The addition of N-acetyl cysteine (NAC) decreased ROS production in the monomer-treated group. The presence of monomers also GSH level, which was observed for NAC as well, but to a lesser extent. No significant differences in the content of GSSG (oxidized disulfide) were observed for HEMA and MMA monomers, and a slight GSSG decrease was noted for TEGDMA (triethylene glycol dimethacrylate). In the case of dental monomers, MDA level increased, and after adding NAC—MDA level dropped almost to its level observed in the control group. Moreover, SOD activity decreased in the presence of all dental monomers, which was not observed after the addition of NAC. After 24 h of cell exposure to monomers, CAT activity increased significantly, and decreased after the use of NAC.	[25]
Human dental pulp cells isolated form third molars, exposed to dental monomers (bisphenol-A-glycidyl Methacrylate, Bis-GMA; urethane dimethacrylate, UDMA; and triethylene glycol dimethacrylate, TEGDMA) at concentrations of 10, 30, 100, 300 μm for 48 h	The level of free radicals was measured after 48 h of monomer action by means of 2′,7′-dichlorodihydrofluorescein diacetate (DCF) fluorescent dye, and it was observed that Bis-GMA and UDMA, at high concentrations (30, 100), induced a significant increase in oxidative stress, while the TEGDMA monomer did not trigger OS at any concentration. All monomers reduced the level of GSH.	[26]
Smulow-Glickman (S-G) human gingival epithelial cells and pulp fibroblasts (HPF) exposed to HEMA at the concentrations of 0.01–10 mm for 24 h	Higher HEMA concentrations (1, 2.5, 5, 10) caused a significant increase in the level of intracellular ROS in cells exposed to the monomer.	[27]
Gingival fibroblasts obtained during the extraction of premolars for orthodontic reasons, exposed to TEGDMA at a concentration of 0.6 mM and 1 mM for 15 min to 6 h	15-min exposure to TEGDMA significantly reduced the concentration of intracellular GSH compared to cells not exposed to this monomer. It was also demonstrated that TEGDMA-induced time-dependent increase of thiobarbituric acid reactive substances (TBARS), which indicates increased lipid peroxidation.	[28]
Human dental pulp stem cells (isolated from third molars) exposed to monomer HEMA (at a concentration of 2 mM) and AC (at 50 $\mu g \cdot mL^{-1}$) for 24 h	2-hydroxyethyl methacrylate (HEMA) increased the level of reactive oxygen species (ROS), pro-inflammatory mediators such as nuclear factor-κB (NF-kB) and inflammatory cytokines such as interleukin. In the presence of vitamin C, these changes were less noticeable. This indicates a protective effect of vitamin C on the dental pulp cells.	[29]
Human gingival fibroblasts (HGFs) treated with a relatively low level of 2-hydroxyethyl methacrylate (HEMA) for 0, 24 and 96 h	After 24 and 96 h of HGF exposure to the HEMA monomer (3 $mmol \cdot L^{-1}$), it was observed that ROS levels increased 8 and 11 times compared to the control not exposed to the monomer.	[30]
Primary human gingival fibroblasts (HGFs) and immortalized oral keratinocyte cell line OKF6/TERT2 treated with 2-hydroxyethyl methacrylate (HEMA) at a concentration of 0.5–10 mM	Significantly induced transcription of genes related to defense against oxidative stress was demonstrated for: nuclear factor erythroid 2-related factor 2 (Nrf2), heme oxygenase (HO-1), quinone dehydrogenase 1 (NQO1), superoxide dismutase 1 (SOD1) in both cell types exposed to the HEMA monomer. The transcription of nuclear factor kappa-light-chain-enhancer of activated B cells (NF-κB) and interleukin-6 (IL-6) was repressed in both cell types, while the transcription of tumor necrosis factor α (TNF-α) and interleukin-8 (IL-8) was repressed only in OKF6/TERT-2 cells.	[31]

Table 1. *Cont.*

Experimental Model	Endpoints	References
Primary human dental pulp cells (hDPCs) obtained from healthy patients aged 18–25, during the extraction of healthy third molars, exposed to 1 mM 2-hydroxyethyl methacrylate (HEMA) for 18 and 12 h	It was demonstrated that the expression of NFE2L2 (nuclear factor, erythroid 2 like 2) and HMOX1 (heme oxygenase (decycling) 1) genes encoding the proteins: Nrf2 (nuclear factor erythroid 2-related factor 2) and HO-1 (heme oxygenase 1) in the HEMA-exposed group increased compared to the group not exposed to HEMA.	[32]
Human gingival fibroblasts (HGFs) exposed to 2-hydroxyethyl methacrylate (HEMA) and triethylene glycol dimethacrylate (TEGDMA) at a concentration of 3 mM for 24, 48 and 72 h	It was demonstrated that exposure to HEMA caused autophagy and apoptosis in each of the analyzed periods of time. No signs of autophagia were observed in TEGDMA-exposed cells	[33]
	Dental Resin Composites—Cross-linked samples	
Human dental pulp cells exposed to methacrylate-based dental resin composite, including triethylene glycol dimethacrylate and composites free of 2-hydroxyethyl methacrylate and silorane-based composite (5 mm in diameter and 2 mm high) cured with light (780 mW/cm^2) for 40 s in the presence of dental polymers (reduction of free radical polymerization) and absence of polyester film	Flow cytometry showed increased ROS production in cells exposed to dental resin composite materials. A positive correlation was observed between ROS production and cell survival in groups not covered with polyester film. TEGDMA increases ROS production.	[34]
Human dental pulp cells (isolated from third molars) exposed to dental material dental resin composite s for 48 h with IGF-1 i TGF-b	Insulin-like growth factor (IGF-1) and transforming growth factor beta (TGF-β) increased cystine capture, resulting in elevated levels of cellular glutathione in a group of cells exposed to dental resin composite (Flow Line, 9.5 +/− 0.4 mg and Durafill VS, 10.0 +/− 0.4 mg). This provided increased protection against OS effect triggered by dental resin composite.	[35]
Human pulp cells obtained from impacted third molars, exposed to cured bonding agents (Clearfil SE Bond, CB; Prime & Bond 2.1, PB; and Single Bond, SB) at a concentration of 10 µL for 2 days	Dentine bonding agents decrease the level of GSH, which might be the reason for the cytotoxicity of resins. Cytotoxicity decreased when N-acetyl-L-cysteine (NAC) was added to the sample.	[36]
Saliva collected from 52 patients (32 women and 20 men) who had been treated with Filtek Z250 dental resin composite fillings, before the filling and 1 h, 1 day, 7 and 30 days after the filling	Patients with dental resin composite fillings demonstrated a significantly increased MDA level compared to subjects without fillings, but there were no statistical differences between the studied time periods. There was also a significant decrease in SOD activity 7 days after the filling compared to the controls. No significant differences were noted in SOD values between day 7 and 30 in patients with dental resin composite fillings.	[37]
	Composite resins	
Human gingival fibroblasts (HGFs) exposed to composite resin (consisting of 45% 2-hydroxyethyl methacrylate—HEMA and 55% bisphenol A-glycidyl dimethacrylate—Bis-GMA) at concentrations of up to 0.25 mM	It was demonstrated that the expression of 8-hydroxyguanine in DNA–hydrolase I, the main enzyme for repairing 8-oxoG damage in composite resin-exposed cells, was elevated compared to cells not exposed to monomers.	[38]
Mouse fibroblast cells (NIH/3T3) exposed to camphorquinone (CQ), CQ and diphenyleneiodonium hexafluorophosphate (DPI), CQ and ethyl 4-dimethylamino benzoate (EDAB), and CQ, EDAB and DPI, with EDAB in high and low concentration, for 10 and 20 s	Increased activity of SOD was observed after 10 s of polymerization vs 20 s in NIH/3T3.	[39]
	Orthodontic braces	
L929 mouse fibroblast cell line exposed to six types of orthodontic archiwires (stainless steel, nickel-titanium, copper-nickel-titanium, rhodium-coated nickel-titanium, cobalt-chromium Blue Elgiloy, titanium-molybdenum) in 1-cm-long pieces (1 mL saliva per 0.2 g of the wire)	It was demonstrated that a standard nickel-titanium orthodontic archiwire generates the strongest oxidative stress, while stainless steel and titanium-molybdenum wire triggers the lowest OS in a mouse fibroblast cell culture.	[40]

Table 1. *Cont.*

Experimental Model	Endpoints	References
L929 mouse fibroblast cell line exposed to three conventional (stainless steel, monocrystalline sapphire ceramics, polyurethane) and four self-ligating brackets (stainless steel body with a nickel-titanium clip, aluminum oxide ceramics with a cobalt-chromium clip, aluminum oxide ceramics with a nickel-cobalt clip coated with rhodium, polycarbonate-stainless steel brackets) made of different materials	The assessment of 8-hydroxy-29-deoxyguanosine (8-OHdG) in DNA of L929 murine fibroblast cell line demonstrated that the lowest OS is triggered by a conventional sapphire ceramic bracket. Full metal conventional and self-ligating brackets and conventional polyurethane brackets showed higher OS compared to cells not exposed to these brackets. The highest OS is caused by full metal and polyurethane brackets.	[41]
Saliva of 23 patients aged 12–16 enrolled in the study (12 female, 11 male subjects), treated with multibracket self-ligating vestibular orthodontic appliances	During the first 10 weeks of treatment with multibracket self-ligating vestibular orthodontic appliances, no statistically significant changes in the salivary antioxidant test (SAT) were observed.	[42]
Unstimulated saliva and gingival fluid of 50 generally healthy patients (27 females and 23 males) aged 13–20, treated with permanent brackets, collected before the treatment as well as in the 1st and 6th month of the treatment	There was no increase in oxidative damage (8-OHdG, MDA) in the saliva and gingival fluid of patients treated with permanent brackets compared to pre-treatment results.	[43]
Unstimulated (UWS) and stimulated (SWS) saliva of 37 generally healthy subjects treated with permanent orthodontic brackets, collected immediately after the fitting of the brackets as well as 1 week and 24 weeks after the fitting	There was a significant increase in thiobarbituric acid reactive substance (TBARS) in UWS and SWS one week after braces were fitted. The measured values returned to their initial state 24 weeks after the beginning of the treatment. There were no significant differences between the levels of SOD1, CAT, UA and Px activity in UWS 1 week and 24 weeks after the start of treatment. SOD1 activity was found to be significantly lower in SWS, and Px activity was considerably higher 1 week after the placement of the brackets compared to the values before the treatment and 24 weeks after its commencement. The total antioxidant status (TAS) in UWS and SWS was also found to be considerably lower 24 weeks after the start of the treatment compared to the values before the treatment as well as 1 week after its start. The highest oxidative stress index (OSI) values were observed 1 week after the treatment. 24 weeks after the treatment these values were identical to pre-treatment results.	[44]
	Fixations and dental implants	
Human dental pulp stem cells (DPSC) and murine pre- osteoblast (MC3T3-E1) cells exposed to zirconium and titanium oxide for 24 h	Intracellular oxidation of 5-(and -6)-chloromethyl-2′,7′-dichlorodihydrofluorescein diacetate and acetyl ester (CM-H2DCFDA), a ROS indicator dye, demonstrated relatively higher average ROS levels in both types of cells exposed to zirconium compared to titanium.	[45]
Periosteum of 30 patients (8 women and 22 men) with bilateral fractures of the mandible, treated with Ti6Al4V titanium alloy	The periosteum of patients treated with titanium implants showed significantly higher concentrations of the biomarkers of nitrosative (S-nitrosothiols, peroxynitrite, nitrotyrosine) and oxidative stress (malondialdehyde, protein carbonyls, dityrosine, kynurenine and N-formylkynurenine) compared to the control without titanium fixations. Osteosynthesis patients also demonstrated increased antioxidant protection expressed in elevated levels of reduced glutathione (↑GSH) and glutathione reductase (↑GR). The periosteum of patients with titanium fixations revealed a considerable decrease in the activity of mitochondrial complex I (−77.8%) and CS (citrate synthase) (−166.7%) compared to the control. There were no statistically significant differences in the activity of complex II and cytochrome C oxidase (COX) between patients after osteosynthesis as compared to healthy controls. In the periosteum of osteosynthesis patients, the production of hydrogen peroxide as well as the rate of ROS production were also significantly increased. Titanium implants caused oxidative/nitrosative stress and mitochondrial dysfunction. Moreover, a positive correlation between ROS production rate and GSH concentration was observed, which may suggest increased antioxidant defense in patients after osteosynthesis.	[46]
Whole saliva of patients aged 43–57 with peri-implantitis and five titanium implants (collected from five patients) that were rejected up to 6 months after their implantation (3 from the mandible, 2 from the maxilla); oxidative stress parameters	In the course of peri-implantitis, a significant increase was observed in AGE compared to the control. In the saliva of peri-implantitis patients the level of OS was higher than in healthy individuals.	[47]

Table 1. *Cont.*

Experimental Model	Endpoints	References
Periosteum of 32 patients operated on due to class III dentofacial deformities (21 women and 11 men aged 20–30), who had had titanium implants inserted and then removed 12–30 months after the implantation	Decreased activity of superoxide dismutase-1 (SOD1) (↓37%) and tryptophan level (↓34%) as well as significantly higher content of advanced oxidation protein products (AOPP) (↑25%), total oxidant status (TOS) (↑80%) and oxidative stress index (OSI) (↑101%) were observed in the maxillary periosteum of osteotomized patients compared to the controls. The mandibular periosteum demonstrated a significant decrease in SOD-1 activity (↓55%), total oxidant status (TAC) (↓58.6%), advanced glycation end products (AGE) (↓60%) and N-formylkynurenine (↓34%), and considerably increased content of AOPP (↑38%), malondialdehyde (MDA) (↑29%), 4-hydroxynonenal (4-HNE) (↑114%), TOS (↑99%) and OSI (↑381%) compared to the controls. Further weakening of the redox economy and increased ROS production were demonstrated in the mandibular periosteum compared to the maxillary periosteum.	[48]
Periosteum of 29 patients (aged 19–29) treated with titanium implants (due to a bilateral mandibular shaft fracture) that were removed 3–5 months after the procedure	The periosteum of patients after osteosynthesis showed significantly higher activity of NADPH and xanthine oxidase, and increased rate of free radical production compared to the control. The periosteum of patients after osteosynthesis also demonstrated a considerable increase in the levels of inflammation markers: interleukin 1 (IL-1), interleukin 6 (IL-6), tumor necrosis factor α (TNF-α), transforming growth factor β (TGF-β) and β-glucuronidase (GLU) as well as markers of apoptosis (Bax, Bax/Bcl-2), caspase-3 (CAS-3) and nitric oxide (NO) compared to the control. Titanium implants increased the production of proinflammatory cytokines and oxygen free radicals. A positive correlation between titanium content and CAS-3 activity was also demonstrated.	[49]
Periosteum, plasma, and erythrocytes collected from 31 generally healthy subjects aged 21–29 (11 women and 20 men) with bilateral mandibular fractures treated with titanium miniplates (Ti4Al4V)	Decreased CAT activity in the mandibular periosteum and its increase in erythrocytes of patients with mandibular fracture treated with titanium miniplates were demonstrated compared to the subjects not exposed to titanium implants. SOD activity and UA concentration were significantly higher in both plasma and periosteum of fracture patients compared to healthy individuals. No differences were found in GPx activity between the studied groups. There was an increase in TAC, FRAP, TOS, AGE, AOPP, 4-HNE and a decrease in OSI level in the maxillary periosteum of patients with fracture compared to healthy subjects. There were no significant differences in plasma TAC, TOS, OSI, FRAP AGE, AOPP, 4-HNE and 8-OHdG levels between patients with a fracture and healthy subjects. A positive correlation was observed between TAC concentration in the mandibular periosteum and plasma UA level in patients with a mandibular fracture. A positive correlation was also found between TOS concentration in the periosteum and CAT activity in erythrocytes, and between 8-OHdG level in the periosteum and GPx activity in erythrocytes.	[50]
	Periodontology	
Male adult Wistar rats (2 months of age) with periodontitis, subjected to antimicrobial photodynamic therapy (aPDT)	PDT was shown to increase ROS formation as well as boost the antioxidant response.	[51]
Whole saliva of patients aged 43–57 with peri-implantitis and 5 titanium implants (collected from five patients), which were rejected up to 6 months after their implantation (3 from the mandible, 2 from the maxilla)	In patients with peri-implantitis, the western blot technique revealed a significant increase in AGE compared to healthy controls. By means of TBARS assays, a higher level of OS was also observed in the saliva of peri-implantitis patients compared to healthy subjects.	[47]
Sixteen patients with chronic periodontitis (CP), undergoing non-surgical periodontal therapy alone as well as non-surgical therapy accompanied by antibiotic therapy of Amoxicillin + Metronidazole, 500 mg each, 3 times daily, for 7 days	It was demonstrated that after 3 months OS levels decreased from very high to average during antibiotic therapy, as shown by reduced derivatives of reactive oxygen metabolites (d-ROMs) (from 491.83 ± 134.85 U CARR to 375.58 ± 126.06 U CARR) and reduced glutathione (GSH) (from 48.73 ± 33.89 µmol/L to 46.46 ± 21.59 µmol/L) in plasma.	[52]
Nineteen patients with chronic periodontitis (average age: 46.8 years) examined before the therapy (scaling and root planing) as well as 1 and 2 months after the therapy.	Non-surgical treatment of periodontitis reduced plasma ROM levels compared to pre-treatment levels.	[53]
Tissues and saliva of 10 patients with peri-implantitis and 10 with chronic periodontitis, aged 40–60	In both the saliva and tissues of patients with peri-implantitis and chronic periodontitis, AGE levels more than doubled compared to healthy individuals. A strong positive correlation was also observed between ROS and AGE in the examined patients.	[54]

Table 1. *Cont.*

Experimental Model	Endpoints	References
Peri-implant crevicular fluid (PICF) collected from 31 patients	The concentration of MDA, SOD and TAC in peri-implant crevicular fluid did not differ from that in healthy subjects. However, there was a positive correlation between periodontal pocket depth (PPD) around the implant and MDA and TAC levels.	[55]
	Whitening	
Human primary periodontal ligament fibroblasts (hPDLFs) and Ca9-22 human gingival epithelial cells treated with stable aqueous ozone ultrafine bubble water (OUFBW; ozone concentration: 2.5 ppm) or UV-inactivated OUFBW	OUFBW (30 min of incubation) stimulated ROS production in both cell lines, thus activating the MAPK pathway. OUFBW triggered the activation of c-Fos, a major component of the transcription factor activator protein 1 (AP-1), and also nuclear factor erythroid 2 (NF-E2)-related factor 2 (Nrf2), which demonstrated high sensitivity to oxidative stress.	[56]
One-hundred thirteen patients (60 people using Crest® 3D Whitestrips® premium plus, 10% hydrogen peroxide, 53 subjects in the control group). Oral epithelial cells and saliva samples were collected at the beginning of the study and 30 days later from the control group, and immediately before whitening as well as 15 and 30 days after the completion of the whitening procedure	After the whitening procedure, an elevated level of 8-OHdG in saliva and a positive correlation between oxidative stress produced by hydrogen peroxide and micronuclei were found.	[57]

5. Amalgam

The choice of filling materials is constantly increasing. Despite the dynamic development of cosmetic fillings, amalgam is still commonly used, which is due to its durability as well as low price, immediate availability and ease of use [22].

The influence of amalgam, both on the oral cavity and the entire body, has been discussed for a long time. The harmful effects of amalgam fillings are related to mercury contained in them. Studies demonstrated that mercury interferes with the metabolism of porphyrins which actively participate in numerous metabolic processes, including cellular respiration. The disruption of porphyrin metabolism may result in metabolic diseases, cancer or blood disorders, i.e., anemia or porphyrias [22,23]. Organic mercury, found in the form of methylmercury (MeHg), is considered particularly harmful [23]. Initial oxidative damage caused by MeHg in living organisms occurs as a result of its reaction with thiol (-SH) and/or selenol (-SeH) groups from endogenous molecules, leading to the formation of a very stable complex of type RSHgCH3 or RSeHgCH3 [58]. In proteins and enzymes containing thiol or selenol groups, the formation of S-Hg or Se-Hg bonds leads to the impairment of a given protein function [58–62] or entails the production of protein deposits rich in cysteine residues [63,64]. As mentioned above, due to high reactivity of MeHg to thiols and selenols, mercury occurs in living organisms in a form associated with these groups. In the human body, thiols are more common than selenols [65]; they can be found not only in compounds of low molecular weight (mainly cysteine and reduced glutathione), but also in proteins, whereas selenol groups are present only in a limited group of selenoproteins [66–68]. Considering the fact that both thiol and selenol groups are critical for the catalytic activity of numerous enzymes involved in antioxidant mechanisms and that MeHg reduces the activity of, inter alia, such enzymes (i.e., glucose-6- phosphate dehydrogenase [69], creatine kinase [60], glutathione reductase [70], glutathione peroxidase [59,71], thioredoxin reductase [10,72] there are grounds to postulate that this interaction disturbs the redox balance and results in increased production of ROS and RNS. However, studies by Cabaña-Muñoz et al. [23] revealed a significant boost in the activity of superoxide dismutase 1 (SOD-1) as well as reduced glutathione (GSH) concentration in hair samples collected from women who had amalgam fillings inserted 15 years prior to the study. According to the authors, stimulation of enzymatic antioxidant systems results from MeHg-induced elevated hydrogen peroxide (H_2O_2) concentration. It was shown that MeHg influences the mitochondrial electron transport chain (mainly at the level of complex II–III), which accelerates the formation of H_2O_2 [73]. The observed increased levels of the antioxidant barrier components as well as a positive correlation between mercury concentration and SOD-1 activity may suggest compensatory mechanisms to the chronic presence of mercury in women, aimed at counteracting Hg toxicity in individuals with amalgam fillings [23].

The results of the test for oxidative stress markers in subjects with amalgam fillings are contradictory, which is due to the test methods used, study material and the time that passed between the placement of a filling and the sampling. Al-Saleh et al. [22] observed abnormal concentrations of 8-hydroxy-D-guanosine (8-OHdG) and malondialdehyde (MDA) in the urine of children with amalgam fillings (no time passed from the filling insertion to the sampling was provided), and only 8-OHdG concentration was significantly correlated with the mercury content in the urine of these children. Mercury concentration in urine showed a clear dose-effect relationship with 8-OHdG level, mainly caused by long-term exposure to low Hg concentrations. The authors believe that oxidative damage to DNA of children is a result of exposure to Hg both from amalgam fillings and other sources. What is more, they argue that the presence of amalgam fillings does not exacerbate oxidative damage to DNA, but reduces the body's ability to repair it, leading to a reduction in DNA repair products secreted into the urine compared to children without amalgam fillings. Studies indicated that 8-OHdG concentration in urine is not only a marker of oxidative modifications of the genetic material, but also reflects the efficiency of corrective mechanisms [74–76]. Interestingly, only the MDA concentration in urine was significantly correlated with the activity of urinary N-acetyl-β-D-glucosaminidase (NAG). It is worth mentioning that urinary NAG is used as a marker of renal tubular damage, especially in an environmental exposure to Hg [77]. The multiple regression model also demonstrated a statistically significant interaction between urinary Hg and MDA concentrations. This relationship suggests that exposure to Hg from amalgam fillings may result in renal tubular damage through oxidative stress (OS). In contrast, studies by Yildiz et al. [24] showed increased concentration of lipid peroxidation products (MDA) and no changes in the concentrations of oxidative markers of DNA damage in the plasma of patients 24 h after the placement of amalgam fillings. No correlation with Hg concentration was observed, which was consistent with the results of Daokar et al. [21]. These authors demonstrated a significant increase in MDA concentration in the saliva of patients who had had amalgam fillings inserted 2 weeks earlier.

In the study of Celik et al. [19] amalgam exhibited cytotoxic effect toward the HGF cell line, resulting in higher cell mortality and significantly higher total oxidant status (TOS) in freshly prepared samples compared to samples taken after 7 and 21 days. According to these authors, the decrease in cytotoxicity and TOS over time was caused by a considerable drop in the release of metal ions as the material hardened. Interestingly, amalgam had no significant effect on TOS and total antioxidant capacity (TAC) values compared to the control group. However, samples taken on day 7 and 21 demonstrated a considerably higher TAC compared to fresh samples. However, higher salivary TAC was observed in female and male children with two dental amalgam restorations (the time from the placement of the fillings to the collection of samples was not provided) compared to children who were caries-free and did not have any restorations [20]. Interestingly, females had higher TAC compared to males, which the authors claimed to be caused by hormonal changes typical of early adolescence and indicated more efficient antioxidant systems in girls in response to the increasing level of ROS.

In summary, mercury in amalgams is responsible for the redox imbalance in the system. MeHg modifies the mitochondrial electron transport chain function, which accelerates the formation of H_2O_2 [73]. A strengthening of the antioxidant barrier may suggest compensatory mechanisms to the chronic presence of mercury.

6. Glass-Ionomer Cement

Little is known about glass- ionomer-induced oxidative stress. It was demonstrated that metal ions released from glass- ionomer fillings are not toxic to cells and do not induce ROS formation, whereas polyacrylic acid [19] and fluorine ions released during the first phase of GI filling [19,78] have cytotoxic effects. During the first seven days, ROS production enhances, increasing TAC levels.

The observed increase in TAC is an adaptive reaction of the cells that effectively prevents OS development, shifting the redox balance towards antioxidant reactions [19]. After 21 days, the level of TAC in the cell culture exposed to glass-ionomer filling did not differ from the control culture level, which most likely indicated that glass-ionomer filling was no longer cytotoxic to cells, and it was a sign of achieving redox balance.

7. Dental Resin Composites

In the present paragraph, we want to point out that we do not separate the cytotoxic effect of monomers from the potential toxic effect of dental resin composites once they were properly cross-linked. We take into account such differentiation in Table 1.

Dental resin composite materials are currently the most commonly applied materials for tooth reconstruction in conservative dentistry. In recent years, significant development in the dental materials of this group was observed. They are used especially for esthetic restorations in the front and back sections. It was documented that each resin-based material releases certain amounts of its components into the saliva. The most common of them are bisphenol-A-glycidyl methacrylate (Bis-GMA), urethane dimethacrylate (UDMA), triethylene glycol dimethacrylate (TEGDMA) and 2-hydroxyethyl methacrylate (HEMA). It is believed that HEMA is released in the largest amount from composite materials, and Bis-GMA—in the smallest, which is related to the size of the molecules as well as molecular weight of these monomers [79].

It is known that monomers released from composites contribute to genetic changes at the cellular level, and show cytotoxic effects [80]. It is generally believed that the cytotoxicity of these monomers might be ranked in the decreasing order: Bis-GMA, UDMA, TEGDMA and HEMA [79]. Moreover, studies showed that OS is responsible for monomer cytotoxicity [25,34], whereas silorane-based dental resin composites Hermes III, free of TEGDMA, HEMA and other monomers, does not lead to significant ROS/RNS production, and its cytotoxicity towards pulp cells is low compared to TEGDMA and HEMA-based dental resin composites [34].

A wide range of studies demonstrated that increased ROS/RNS production in resin-exposed cells occurs parallel and simultaneously to the depletion of reduced glutathione resources [27,28,46]. The glutathione system is the most important cellular detoxification mechanism against ROS activity [81]. GSH is a tripeptide (–glutamylcysteinylglycine) with a molecular weight of 307 kDa. GSH enables the removal of free radicals from the body either directly or through the reactions catalyzed by glutathione peroxidase and other peroxidases, thus neutralizing hydrogen peroxide as well as nitrogen peroxides [82]. GSH reacts with electrophiles, creating less reactive conjugates. Interestingly, decreased concentration of GSH in human dental pulp cells (HDPCs) exposed to resin-based composites is not accompanied by increased level of oxidized glutathione (GSSG), which indicates that reduced amount of GSH resources does not result from its oxidation [25]. Studies have shown that carbonyl groups of methacrylates, adjacent to the double carbon-carbon bond, act as electron withdrawing groups. Consequently, carbon in the beta position of the double bond, as a positive charge, can react with nucleophilic centers of amine or thiol groups in small molecules such as GSH in the Michael-type addition reaction [25]. Indeed, Samuelsen et al. [83] observed spontaneous formation of a complex between HEMA and GSH. They concluded that exposure to HEMA leads to a drop in cellular GSH level, probably due to the formation of a complex with HEMA. Nocca et al. [84] found that the kinetics of the formation of GSH-methacrylate adducts depended on the reaction environment. The rate of adduct formation was different when the reaction occurred in human fibroblasts or erythrocytes than when the reaction environment was a mixture of methacrylates and GSH, which suggests that the reaction is strongly correlated with glutathione S-transferase. Studies by Schneider et al. [26] proved that the drop of GSH concentration in pulp cells caused by TEGDMA after 2 h from exposure was comparable to the decrease in GSH concentration caused by Bis-GMA and UDMA after 48 h. Interestingly, the TEGDMA-induced decrease in GSH concentration was a reversible process, and after the exposure to Bis-GMA and UDMA the treatment further decreased. Evidence showed that Bis-GMA and UDMA significantly reduce cystine uptake, while TEGDMA has the opposite effect. The so-called system x_c^- is responsible for the transport of cystine into dental pulp cells in which it is transformed into cysteine that is used for the production of GSH [35]. According to the authors, this explains the observed phenomenon of oxidative stress in the pulp cells exposed to Bis-GMA and UDMA, and its absence in the cells treated with TEGDMA. GSH directs the expression of enzymatic antioxidants that are exposed in cells to monomers, including HEMA. It was demonstrated that HEMA reduces the activity of glutathione peroxidase GPx1/2, but in the presence of L-buthionine sulfoximine (BSO), which inhibits GSH synthesis, this reduction is more intense. Moreover, significantly elevated ROS generation as well as increased catalase (CAT) activity are observed [36,85]. It is noteworthy that the inhibition of GSH synthesis by BSO in cells not treated with monomers boosts GPx1 activity as a result of increased H_2O_2 concentration due to GSH reduction. However, it seems that in cells not treated with monomers the concentration of H_2O_2 is low, because no increase in CAT concentration was observed. It was proven that GPx1/2 regulates lower H_2O_2 level, whereas CAT expression is induced by higher H_2O_2 concentrations observed in HEMA-treated cells [85].

Interestingly, the use of polyester film which reduces the occurrence of oxygen-inhibited free radical polymerization of dental polymers, results in increased monomer conversion and inhibited ROS production in pulp cells exposed to monomers [34].

According to Diomede et al. [29], a significant, spontaneously irreversible increase in ROS concentration in HDPSCs treated with HEMA after 24 h of exposure is not connected with GSH depletion, but results from mitochondrial dysfunction. Confocal microscopy of cells exposed to HEMA indicates 1000 times higher signal from ROS-sensitive indicator in the mitochondrial area compared to control cells. These differences are most likely due to HEMA-induced dysfunction of the respiratory chain dysregulating the oxidative phosphorylation process. The results of Diomede et al. [29] are consistent with the work of Jiao et al. [25,32] who observed morphological disorders of mitochondria, including their elongation and cristae derangements, depolarization of mitochondrial membranes, reduction of oxidative phosphorylation rate in cells exposed to HEMA and decrease of ATP production. Interestingly, mitochondrial dysfunction induced by monomers exacerbates ROS-induced damage to the dental pulp cells through bioenergetic failure and the internal mitochondrial apoptosis pathway [25,86]. The mitochondrial chain, located in the internal mitochondrial membrane, consists of four enzymatic complexes transporting electrons (CI-CIV) and the ATP synthase enzyme. [87]. It is still unknown which of the complexes is damaged in the course of exposure to monomers. A recent study showed CI as the most important toxicity target of TEGDMA [88]. However, in HEMA-exposed cells, the suppression of all four complexes, either by nuclear-encoded mitochondria or mtDNA-encoded transcription, was observed [89]. These discrepancies are certainly due to the method of mitochondrial isolation as well as the type of resin monomer used. It was demonstrated that although both monomers exhibit a similar toxicity mechanism, cells react differently to various resins by differential induction of the cell death (e.g., only HEMA induces autophagy in human gingival fibroblasts) [33]. Jiao et al. [25] demonstrated that NAC reduces monomer-induced oxidative stress in human pulp cells. Styllou et al. [90] found that the addition of NAC to human fibroblasts exposed to TEGDMA and HEMA significantly minimizes double strand breaks and restores cell nucleus integrity. The authors believe that the protective effect of NAC results from the ability of this molecule to neutralize ROS and replenish GSH deficiencies as well as from the direct reaction of NAC with methacrylate groups of monomers in the Michael addition. The presence of ascorbic acid (AS) counteracts the oxidative effects of HEMA, restoring ROS concentration to the level observed in the control group. AS seems to mimic the effect of NAC, because both molecules neutralize HEMA-induced ROS growth in the cytosol, with only AS being able to completely prevent excessive ROS production in mitochondria [29].

Cells have numerous mechanisms to counteract OS. One of them is the activation of the transcription factor: nuclear factor erythroid 2-related factor 2 (Nrf2)-dependent signaling pathway. Under equilibrium conditions, redox Nrf2 is synthesized and quickly degraded. In a situation of increased ROS production, Nrf2 is stabilized and transferred to the cell nucleus in which it activates the transcription of numerous genes by binding the promoter to antioxidant responsive elements (ARE) [91].

The most important genes activated by Nrf2 include heme oxygenase (HO-1), NAD(P)H quinone dehydrogenase 1 (NQO1) and superoxide dismutase 1 (SOD1). These enzymes play an important role in regulating the redox balance and counteracting monomer toxicity. Durante et al. [92] and Gozzelino et al. [93] believe that antioxidant bilirubin, resulting from the catalytic activity of HO-1, is an essential next link in strengthening the antioxidant barrier when exposed to monomers, and directly balance the cellular redox environment. The stimulation of Nrf2 signaling cascade was observed in HEMA-exposed RAW264.7 mouse macrophages [85,94], human fibroblasts [30,31] and the immortalized human oral keratinocyte cell line (OKF6/TERT-2) [31]. Interestingly, in the latter cell line it was noted that Nrf2 has a potential to enhance its own transcription through a positive feedback loop. Perduns et al. [31] observed that even "non-toxic" HEMA concentrations (0.5 mM) induce the expression of genes of antioxidant enzymes HO-1, NQO1 and SOD1 in human fibroblast and keratinocyte cells. Ramezani et al. [20] showed that dental resin composites significantly enhanced total antioxidant capacity (TAC) in saliva, as TAC level was higher than that of amalgam fillings [31]. Celik et al. [19] obtained increased TAC in gingival fibroblasts (HGFCs) after 7 days of exposure to dental resin composites as well as weakening of the antioxidant barrier on day 21, which was caused by a rapid boost of ROS production from unbound and non-polymerized monomers. The level of HEMA higher than 5 mM enhances ROS production to such an extent that we can observe the occurrence of ROS-induced gene expression disorders associated with inflammation (NF- κB, TNF-α, IL-6, IL-8) and remodeling of the extracellular matrix (COL1A, COL4A, metalloproteinase 9—MMP-9, tissue inhibitor of metalloproteinase 1—TIMP1) [19]. Indeed, studies have revealed that monomer-induced OS acts as a signal for the activation of the pathways controlling cell survival and death, although the exact mechanism of this phenomenon is unknown. It was observed that HEMA significantly increases the number of cells in late phase of apoptosis and necrosis [85]. An additional supply of cysteine, an amino acid essential for the synthesis of GSH by 2-oxothiazolidine-4-carboxylate (OTC), considerably reduces the number of apoptotic and necrotic cells. These observations suggest that HEMA-induced cell death is due to, inter alia, GSH deficiency [85]. These observations are consistent with the study by Lee et al. [95] in which the authors observed increased cell survival after the supplementation of 10 mM NAC. NAC activates GSH reductase, which leads to an increase in GSH concentration.

Yildiz et al. [24] showed that Bis-GMA and TEGDMA, and Jiao et al. [32]—that HEMA and TEGDMA significantly increase MDA concentration in human dental pulp cells. It is noteworthy that the measurement of MDA content at various times after the placement of the dental resin composites revealed its linear increase with the time passed from the material application [37]. Daokar et al. [21] observed that the salivary MDA concentration two weeks after the placement of dental resin composites, the authors did not demonstrate any differences in salivary MDA concentration after the placement of composite and glass-ionomer fillings. In another study, which evaluated TEGDMA and Bis-GMA in dental pulp cells, the increase of 8-OHdG post-application content was noted, and ROS production was correlated with DNA oxidation [24]. Interestingly, the concentration of 8-OHdG was significantly higher in samples after the application of the dental resin composites compared to the amalgam filling group. These observations prove that monomers cause higher oxidation and transformation of the genetic material of dental pulp cells compared to amalgam fillings. It was shown that resin monomers, such as HEMA, lead to the formation of double strand breaks [96–98]. Anteisson et al. [99] demonstrated that HEMA-induced genome damage results in the stimulation of ataxia telangiectasia mutated (ATM) gene and other cell cycle checkpoints, which leads to the activation of kinase signaling networks that impede the progression of the cell cycle and simultaneously activate DNA repair pathways. Similarly, Blasiak et al. [38] found that resin monomers increase the expression of 8-hydroxyguanine in DNA—hydrolase 1, the main enzyme for repairing 8-oxoG damage by trimming alkalis.

The adverse effects of dental resin composites can be attributed to monomers' presence and the influence of the composite once they were properly cross-linked. Glutathione depletion is responsible for GMA, HEMA, TEGDMA-induced OS. Moreover, HEMA and TEGDMA were shown to disrupt the mitochondrial respiratory chain's functioning and disrupt the oxidative phosphorylation process, which contributes to the exacerbation of ROS-induced apoptosis to the dental pulp cells. Interestingly, although dental resin composites increase TAC higher than amalgam fillings, unfortunately, monomers cause higher oxidation and transformation of dental pulp cells' genetic material than amalgam fillings.

8. Composite Resins

Low-viscosity resins are commonly used in restorative dentistry as binding agents connecting dental materials with dental tissue. The inclusion of iodine salts in dental bonding systems was found to be very interesting because they can act as catalysts, reducing activation energy. Due to their ionic nature, they participate in the polymerization of hydrophilic monomers and thus increase the polymerization reaction capacity and percentage of monomer conversion rate. Ferrúa et al. [60] found higher activity of superoxide dismutase (SOD) in 10 s of polymerization vs 20 s, which indicates a slight response of mouse fibroblast cells (NIH/3T3), most probably connected with increased monomer release in the initial phase of polymerization. Significant reduction of lipid peroxidation and oxidation of disulfide groups, after incorporation of iodine salts into bonding systems, was—according to the authors—associated with the inhibition of ROS producing enzymes and proved their protective action towards cell membranes.

Initiators are an essential component of light-hardened composites and dental adhesives. Currently, visible-light photoinitiators, such as phenylbis(2,4,6-trimethylbenzoyl) phosphine oxide (BAPO) and diphenyl(2,4,6-trimethylbenzoyl) phosphine oxide (TPO), are used. Both of these photoinitiators belong to the group of Norrish type I photoinitiators and unlike camphorquinone (CQ) they do not generate ROS. Popal et al. [100] found that both BAPO and TPO used in micromole concentrations do not increase ROS/RNS production in human keratinocytes and V79 fibroblasts during 90 min of exposure. Interestingly, the concentration of ROS/RNS in cells treated with the said photoinitiators was lower compared to the control cells. It is probable that aromatic and phosphine oxide groups serve as electron donors that compete with the fluorescent dye $DCFH_2$ used in the ROS detection method. In the absence of significant changes in ROS/RNS concentration, the alterations in mRNA expression of enzymatic antioxidants in the keratinocyte culture exposed to BAPO and, to a lesser extent, to TPO prove that these cells may be subjected to OS. Within 24 h, BAPO induced a significant increase in HO-1 mRNA and quinone oxidoreductase (NQO1), and TPO only triggered a significant increase in HO-1 mRNA. Yoshino et al. [101] found that long-term irradiation of the human aortic smooth muscle cells (ACBR1716) with blue light (from a quartz-tungsten-halogen lamp) induced the production of H_2O_2 and hydroxy radical ($HO^{\cdot}$). As a result, increased peroxidation of lipid membrane as well as MDA production were observed. They also proved that treatment with NAC could reduce ROS production and cytotoxicity induced by blue light irradiation. Oktay et al. [102] observed markedly increased TOS in the absence of significant changes in TAS level in rat aorta cells irradiated with blue light (400–520 nm, 1200 mV/cm^2) vs not irradiated cells. Based on the results of these studies, it is difficult to assess whether the rat aorta cells were subjected to OS or whether the antioxidant barrier was efficient enough to balance the emerging ROS/RNS.

Although BAPO and TPO show a dose-dependent cytotoxic effect, unlike CQ, they do not increase the intracellular production of ROS /RNS. Interestingly, dental resin curing blue light alone induces increased peroxidation of membrane lipids.

9. Endodontic Treatment

The complicated morphology of the root canal system of teeth makes instrumentation challenging. One of the most important elements of root canal treatment is the use of irrigating solutions which are designed to neutralize microorganisms as well as dissolve and remove tissue residues, including the smear layer. These solutions come into direct contact with periapical tissues, particularly in teeth with periapical lesions in which the identification of the anatomical apex is difficult, and the physiological opening is virtually non-existent due to periapical microresorption. The most commonly used rinsing solutions include the main ones: sodium hypochlorite (NaOCl) and chlorhexidine (CHX) as well as auxiliary solutions: ethylenediaminetetraacetic acid (EDTA) and citric acid. Botton et al. [103] observed that 2% CHX and 6% citric acid did not cause lipid peroxidation, regardless of the exposure time of human peripheral blood mononuclear cells (PBMCs). The 72-h exposure of PBMCs to both 1% and 2.5% NaOCl resulted in increased lipid peroxidation, which suggests that prolonged contact of the cells with the rinsing solution may result in OS and, consequently, disturbed integrity of cell membranes due to the destruction of the lipid bilayer [104]. The solution of 17% EDTA boosted the process of lipid peroxidation only after 24 h of exposure of the cells, which was not maintained after 72 h (Botton et al. [103]), co Saghiri et al. [104] is the adaptation of cells to environmental conditions. The genetic material appears to be more susceptible to the damaging effects of the rinsing agents, as increased oxidative DNA modifications were observed after both 24 and 72 h of exposure of PBMCs to all the flushing solutions. A similar genotoxic effect was observed by evaluating combinations of major rinsing solutions with auxiliaries after both 24 and 72 h of exposure. Soares et al. [105] observed no DNA damage due to NaOCl (1.25%, 2.5%, 5%), 17% EDTA or citric acid (10.5% and 21%); however, the exposure time in their study was only 3 h.

The effectiveness of the described disinfectants is supported by the so-called photodynamic antibacterial chemotherapy (PACT). PACT uses a light source of the narrow-band wavelength that activates rinsing chemicals [106]. A by-product of this reaction are oxygen free radicals such as ozone and H_2O_2, which on the one hand, help to eliminate infections in the root canal but, on the other, may contribute to cell death.

The final stage of endodontic treatment is filling the canal system. Different materials are chosen depending on whether the roots of primary or permanent teeth are filled. However, the filling materials should not exhibit any cytotoxic effect, but should have antibacterial properties in order to prevent reinfection. In the study by Pires et al. [107] iodoform-based pastes used to fill the root canals of deciduous teeth induced a significant increase in ROS already after 24-h exposure of PBMC cells. Interestingly, after 72 h of exposure to iodoform preparations, further significant increase in ROS concentration in the said cells was not accompanied by intensified lipid peroxidation, which—according to the authors—was due to an efficient antioxidant barrier capable of restoring the redox balance. It should be noted that pastes containing chlorhexidine induced significantly higher ROS production compared to iodoform pastes with neomycin sulfate + bacitracin as well as rifamycin SV sodium + 21 prednisolone acetate. According to Barbin et al. [108], redox imbalance induced by CHX was related to parachloroaniline and ROS-byproducts of the 2% CHX aqueous solution. Parachloroaniline has a high potential to cause oxidative DNA damage [81]. Calcium hydroxide-based pastes triggered the highest ROS increase after 24 h of exposure. After 72 h, only the paste with zinc oxide induced further significant increase in ROS production in the PBMC culture. In the TBARS assay, calcium hydroxide pastes demonstrated a similar increase in lipid peroxidation within 24 h, whereas no calcium hydroxide paste caused oxidative damage to the lipids after 72 h of exposure. All calcium hydroxide pastes and just one of the iodoform pastes (CHX) showed the ability to induce oxidative DNA damage, regardless of the exposure time.

Among the materials applied in endodontics to treat permanent dentition, root canal sealers are sealing materials in most methods based on the use of gutta-percha for canal filling. The most common include AH-Plus pastes (Paste A: bisphenol-A, bisphenol-F, calcium tungstate, zirconium dioxide, silicon monoxide, ferric oxide; Paste B: dibezyl diamine, aminoadamantane, tricyclodecane diamine, calcium tungstate, zirconium dioxide, silicon monoxide, silicone oil), MTA-Fillapex (base paste: salicylate resin, natural resin, calcium tungstate, silica nanoparticles, dyes; catalyst paste: diluted resin, mineral trioxide aggregate, silica nanoparticles, dyes) and materials applied in regenerative endodontics: MTA-Angelus (SiO_2, K_2O, Al_2O_3, Na_2O, Fe_2O_3, SO_3, CaO, Bi_2O_3, MgO and insoluble deposits of CaO, KSO_4, $NaSO_4$ and crystalline silica), Biodentine (tricalcium silicate, zirconium dioxide, calcium carbonate, calcium chloride, polymer) and BioRoot (tricalcium silicate, zirconium dioxide, calcium chloride, polymer). The results of the study by Victoria-Escandell et al. [109] demonstrated that

MTA-Angelus did not induce OS w HDPSCs after 24 h of incubation, while AH-Plus and MTA-Fillapex increased protein carbonyl concentration, which is consistent with the results of Kim et al. [110]. Chang et al. [111] demonstrated that MTA-Angelus is capable of increasing ROS production, but the simultaneously activated antioxidant barrier is strong enough to maintain the redox balance. In HDPSC cells treated with AH-Plus and MTA-Fillapex for 24 h, both CAT and SOD were down-regulated compared to the control and MTA-Angelus-treated cells [109]. Under the conditions of low ROS production, which—according to the authors—occurs during the exposure to MTA-Angelus, cells can respond by activating Nrf2 expression and then the target genes of antioxidant enzymes, e.g., CAT or SOD. In the state of OS that occurs in case of AH-Plus and MTA-Fillapex, the Nrf2 pathway is suppressed and the activity of antioxidant enzymes is decreased. No significant differences were observed in the gene expression of CAT, SOD, glutathione synthase in the human dental pulp cells treated with Biodentine and BioRoot [112]. The authors did not examine oxidative stress markers; therefore, it is difficult to assess the occurrence and possible severity of OS.

Most endodontic materials generate increased amounts of ROS, leading to the development of the OS. However, it should be emphasized that biocompatible materials used in the form of sealers seem to be the most favorable from the point of view of redox balance.

10. Orthodontic Braces

Treatment with braces is becoming more and more popular all over the world. Fixed braces are made of various steel alloys, titanium or Ni-Ti. It was demonstrated that some metals included in the alloys of which braces are made (such as iron, chromium, copper, vanadium) are directly responsible for increased ROS production [60,61], while such metals as cadmium, mercury, nickel or lead generate ROS via the indirect mechanism [60]. Interestingly, nickel increases the activity of intracellular lactate dehydrogenase, which disturbs the redox balance and stimulates apoptosis in human oral epithelium cells [113]. Moreover, it is suspected that titanium elements of dental braces are deprived of their superficial layer of titanium oxide as a result of mechanical friction during treatment, which leads to corrosion and the release of metallic particles into the oral cavity environment. The significance of this phenomenon for the redox balance is explained below. The available research results concerning the influence of orthodontic braces on the oral redox balance are contradictory and, unfortunately, limited to only several scientific studies. Özcan et al. [43] suggest that orthodontic treatment, including the use of braces, does not increase the oxidative damage observed in the saliva and gingival fluid. Kovac et al. [61] observed that both ROS and the ratio of ROS to antioxidants in the blood clearly increased within a short period of time after the fitting of braces (24 h) compared to the control group. These levels normalized 7 days after the beginning of orthodontic treatment. Buczko et al. [44] found significantly elevated levels of TBARS and TOS in the unstimulated and stimulated saliva one week after orthodontic treatment (nickel-chromium archwires) and no OS biomarkers in the saliva of orthodontically treated patients within 24 weeks of wearing dental braces. This initial severity of OS is associated with intensified nickel release, as confirmed by a positive correlation between nickel and TOS concentrations in both unstimulated and stimulated saliva in week 1 of the use of braces. In the 24th week, the salivary nickel concentration was comparable to its content before orthodontic treatment. The authors emphasize that the treated patients maintained perfect oral hygiene and showed no gingivitis. Oral hygiene and periodontal health are crucial for the salivary redox balance. Similar results were obtained by Portelli et al. [42], with measurements taken before as well as 5 and 10 weeks after the start of treatment. The researchers claimed that multi-bracket archwires with vestibular appliances do not induce OS during the first 10 weeks of treatment, which is associated with the fact that this type of braces reduces the forces exerted on the teeth and allows for good oral hygiene. On the other hand, the results of Spalj et al. [40] revealed that nickel-titanium standard braces generated the strongest, while stainless steel and titanium-molybdenum ones the least intensive OS in the L929 mouse fibroblast cell line. The use of copper-nickel-titanium and rhodium-coated nickel-titanium orthodontic appliances resulted in increased production of 8-OHdG, which was lower; however, than in the case of standard nickel-titanium archwires. Cobalt-chromium archwires triggered moderate 8-OHdG production, which was most probably connected with the suppression of mitochondrial activity in the aforementioned cell line. Similar results were obtained by Buljan et al. [41], but the authors observed that the strongest OS expressed in 8-OHdG concentration was induced by polymer brackets, which most likely resulted from the presence of polyether polyol. Moreover, the researchers demonstrated that not only the mentioned polymers, but also zirconium dioxide and synthetic sapphire used in the production of elements of aesthetic braces were not indifferent to salivary redox balance, as expressed by increased 8-OHdG concentration in the L929 murine fibroblast cell line.

All orthodontic appliances induce OS. Its intensity depends on the time and the metal alloys used. Initial severity of OS is believed to be associated with intensified nickel release.

11. Fixations and Dental Implants

Titanium and its alloys are commonly applied for the production of medical implants. They are widely used in maxillofacial surgery and orthopedics as bone fixations, joint prostheses, dental implants, and other devices used in reconstructive surgery. Implants made of titanium and its alloys are very popular due to their good mechanical properties, corrosion resistance and biocompatibility. Their higher biocompatibility in human tissues, compared to other metallic materials, is related to the presence of an inactive layer of titanium dioxide (TiO_2) on the implant surface. However, clinical and experimental studies showed that ions and particles of titanium and its alloys are found in peri-implantation tissues, blood and distant organs after the placement of the implants. Gholinejad et al. [114] observed that titanium dioxide nanoparticles were internalized to HUVECs and induced intracellular ROS production as well as cell membrane oxidative modifications. Borys et al. [48,50] demonstrated that exposure to the titanium alloy Ti-6Al-4V stimulated antioxidative mechanisms in the periosteal cells covering titanium implants in the jaw and mandible. However, this defensive reaction was insufficient as it did not prevent oxidative damage to proteins (↑protein carbonyl) and lipids (↑MDA) in the periosteum-like tissue in the area adjacent to the implants [46]. The results obtained by the authors indicate the persistence of OS phenomena around the fixations of maxillary bones regardless of the time that passed from the surgery of facial bone defects, but these phenomena were not accompanied by any clinical symptoms [48]. Moreover, the authors indicate that the production of ROS results, among others, from mitochondrial dysfunction (decreased activity of complex I and citrate synthase) [46] as well as increased activity of NADPH oxidase and xanthine oxidase [49]. Mitochondrial function disorders in muscle cells and their morphological changes (swelling and vacuolization) were confirmed by the studies of Wang et al. and Pereira et al. [115,116]. Furthermore, Pereira et al. [115] showed that exposure of rat liver mitochondria to TiNPs (titanium nanoparticles) + AgNPs (silver nanoparticles) lowered the respiratory control ratio, which resulted in reduced oxidative phosphorylation efficiency. 21-day exposure of mitochondria to both types of nanoparticles maintained the increased ROS levels and depleted the endogenous antioxidant system. AgNPs and TiNPs acted synergistically: the intensity of the toxic effect on the mitochondrial redox balance was more significant in the presence of both types of nanoparticles. Borys et al. [49] also observed a positive relationship between the production of ROS/RNS and the concentration of titanium, aluminum and vanadium in tissues surrounding the titanium implants, which is explained by the observations of Shanbhag et al. [117] and Mouthuy et al. [118]. These authors demonstrated that the said ions released from the implants stimulate macrophages and osteoclasts to increase ROS and RNS production, and that ROS/RNS boost the release of metal ions from the implant surface through ROS/RNS-induced corrosion. According to these researchers, these observations highlight the need to improve the quality of the applied jawbone fixations by increasing the passive TiO_2 layer thickness in miniplates and screws in the process of hard anodizing, or search for other materials, preferably biodegradable in human tissues, for the production of dental fixations.

In recent years, we witnessed rapid development of implantology as a field of dentistry. Implantation is a more and more common method of filling in missing teeth [63]. The maintenance of an implant in the oral cavity depends on numerous factors. Peri-implantitis has an inflammatory etiology, therefore the effect of OS on the phenomenon of implant rejection is sought. However, the results of these studies are contradictory, depending on the type of the examined material or clinical situation. At the beginning, it is worth mentioning that ROS act as mediators of cytoskeletal remodeling and cell proliferation, while too low intracellular ROS concentration was found to slow down cell adhesion and proliferation. The results of Wei et al. [45] demonstrate that ROS content in DPSC and MC3T3-E1 cells that stuck to the surface of titanium and zirconium after 24 h of incubation is high enough to allow for the correct process of cell adhesion and spreading. These processes are more efficient for the zirconia surface [47]. Pietropaoli et al. [47] believe that both the excessive production of ROS and, consequently, AGEs in the tissues adjacent to the implant are factors that favor the implant rejection process. In the opinion of these authors, ROS-derived AGEs that irreversibly accumulate in the tissues surrounding the implant, disturb the collagen structure and induce inflammation. However, the redox imbalance in the course of peri-implantitis is less severe than in periodontal diseases. Similar results of redox equilibrium changes were obtained by Guo et al. [54]. but it should be emphasized that these observations were found in patients' saliva. Cabaña-Muñoz et al. observed that patients with long-term (10 years) dental titanium and amalgams have systemic oxidative stress expressed as a significant increase in MDA concentration and decrease in Mo/Co and Mo/Fe^{2+} ratios in hair samples than those with amalgam alone [119]. On the other hand, Sánchez-Siles et al. [120] found that salivary concentration of myeloperoxidase and MDA in patients with peri-implantitis and without periodontal diseases did not differ from the healthy control. According to the results of Mousavi et al. [55], there is a positive correlation between periodontal pocket depth (PPD) around the implant and MDA and TAC concentrations. However, the concentration of the tested OS markers (MDA, SOD, TAC) in an osmotically mediated transudate/inflammatory exudate around dental implants (PICF) in diseased implants (PPD $\geq$ 4 mm, gingival index GI $\geq$ 1, bleeding on probing BOP = 1) did not differ from "healthy implants" (PPD < 3 mm, GI = 0, BOP = 0). According to the authors, the study on the aforementioned OS markers does not allow for the differentiation between peri-implant health and disease conditions.

As a result of processes such as friction, titanium implants contribute to the increased production of ROS and increase the carbonyl, MDA, AGE proteins in the tissue around the implant. These observations call into question the safety of leaving titanium implants permanently.

12. Periodontology

Periodontal diseases are a very common problem in dental practice. Interestingly, a key role in periodontitis is played by oxidative stress [121,122]. In response to bacterial microflora and local inflammation, polymorphonuclear leukocytes (but also peripheral blood leukocytes) produce large amounts of ROS, which by oxidizing lipids, proteins, and nucleic acids, lead to the destruction of periodontal connective tissue. Thus, periodontitis may lead to increased tooth mobility and even tooth loss [52].

A question arises: can periodontal treatment influence the intensity of salivary oxidative stress? Tamaki et al. [53] demonstrated that scaling and root planning (SRP) significantly reduced the level of reactive oxygen metabolites (ROMs) in the plasma of patients with chronic periodontitis. Moreover, the rate of ROMs production correlated significantly with the severity of periodontal disease (a positive correlation with bleeding on probing [BOP] and clinical attachment loss [CAL]) both before and after the surgery [53]. SRP also considerably reduced the concentration of salivary malondialdehyde (MDA), which may—to some extent—explain the therapeutic success in patients with non-surgical periodontal treatment [53].

The salivary content of GSH is significantly lower in the saliva of patients with chronic periodontitis [52,123], which is not surprising as this compound is used intensively by periodontal tissues in response to increased ROS production. However, SRP together with 7-day antibiotic therapy (amoxicillin + metronidazole, 500 mg each, 3 times daily) does not change salivary levels of GSH or C-reactive protein (CRP) in patients with periodontitis [52]. Boia et al. [52] demonstrated that non-surgical periodontal therapy lowered ROMs levels in plasma. This parameter correlates positively with CAL, which confirms previous reports on the relationship between ROS production in blood and periodontal inflammation [52,53].

Recently, antimicrobial photodynamic therapy (aPDT) has become a popular method of treatment of periodontitis patients. The term aPDT means a laser therapy in which the photosensitizer produces oxygen free radicals that destroy microorganisms in the gingival pocket biofilm [51]. Indeed, it was demonstrated that laser light in the presence of methylene blue (MB) in 20% ethanol generates significant amounts of ROS, which determines its bactericidal effect. Pillusky et al. [51] also showed that aPDT increases the concentration of erythrocytic GSH, which is the systemic adaptive response to the applied treatment. Photodynamic therapy can be performed as an additional procedure to standard periodontal treatment to enhance the systemic protective response against oxidative stress, boosting and accelerating periodontium healing, particularly when the photosensitizer is dissolved in ethanol (which facilitates its penetration into periodontal tissues) [51].

Ozone (O_3) is also very popular in periodontology. It was demonstrated that O_3 increases ROS production in periodontal tissues, thus leading to the activation of numerous transcription factors such as mitogen-activated protein kinase (MAPK), cellular proto-oncogene encoding the transcription factor FOS (c-Fos), AP-1 (transcription factor activator protein 1) and the nuclear factor erythroid 2 (NF-E2)-related factor 2 (Nrf2). Importantly, Nrf2 is related to the promoter region of metallothionein that participates in the response to OS [56]. Leewananthawet et al. [56] proved that aqueous ozone ultrafine bubble water (OUFBW) increases the antioxidant defense of periodontal ligament fibroblasts, while the stimulation of c-Fos and c-Jun pathways further differentiates osteoblasts involved in periodontal tissue regeneration [56]. A study on an animal model showed that blue light increases the amount of ROS, which results in vasospasm in the aorta. Moreover, researchers suggest that the elevated ROS level under the influence of blue light also occurs in gingival fibroblasts. The alternating vasospasms and vasodilatations due to ROS lead to the subsequent generation of reactive oxygen species, which is called the vicious circle effect [124,125].

The ROS generated in the treatment of periodontal diseases seems to positively affect the healing process: they support the elimination of periopathogenic bacteria and accelerate periodontium healing.

13. Whitening

Tooth whitening is one of the most frequently chosen procedures to restore the esthetics of discolored teeth. Whitening can be performed both in the dental clinic and at home [126,127]. Hydrogen peroxide (H_2O_2) is the most commonly used substance for this purpose due to its low price and high effectiveness [83]. H_2O_2 is characterized by high reactivity, although it is not a free radical. It participates in oxidation reactions, the most biologically significant of which is the oxidation of sulfhydryl groups. [128]. It leads to the formation of disulfide bridges, which changes the conformations as well as biological functions of proteins. H_2O_2 also has the ability to oxidize unsaturated fatty acids during the process of lipid peroxidation. [129]. Moreover, hydrogen peroxide is capable of oxidizing ferrous or copper ions (the proper Fenton reaction: $Fe^{2+} + H_2O_2 \rightarrow Fe^{3+} + \cdot OH + OH^-$, the catalysts for this reaction are also Cu^{2+} ions). During these reactions, hydrogen peroxide is transformed into hydroxyl radical ·OH. The redox reaction under the influence of H_2O_2 results in the formation of: superoxide anion, hydroxyl radical and singlet oxygen, all of which have an oxidizing effect on the organic components of the enamel, leading to the whitening of tissues [67,72]. It is suggested that low concentrations of hydrogen peroxide do not exhibit a destructive effect on the oral cavity cells [125]. ROS generated during the whitening process induce a sequence of reactions that increase the expression of heme oxygenase 1 (HO-1) in fibroblasts and osteoblasts [83]. Considering the antioxidant and anti-inflammatory properties of this enzyme, it can be concluded that increased expression of HO-1 in cells exposed to H_2O_2 is a defensive mechanism against the adverse effects of whitening.

Del Real Garcia et al. [57] demonstrated that in patients exposed to 10% H_2O_2 contained in whitening strips (Crest® 3D Whitestrips® premium plus), the concentration of salivary 8-OHdG increased compared to non-exposed subjects. Moreover, the positive correlation between the genotoxicity test and 8-OHdG concentration indicates that hydrogen peroxide is the cause of DNA damage in patients using whitening strips. Indeed, in the study group the authors observed chromosome damage, impaired cytokinesis and increased apoptosis of the oral epithelial cells after 15 and 30 days of using whitening strips [57]. Interestingly, no DNA damage was demonstrated after professional whitening treatments with 35% hydrogen peroxide. Whitening procedures are only suggested when performed by qualified dentists [57].

Interestingly, hydrogen peroxide can diffuse through the enamel to a concentration of about 0.01% in the pulp. Recent studies suggested that the higher the content of whitening agents such as hydrogen peroxide, the greater the cytotoxic effect on the pulp [127]. Cytotoxicity increases significantly after using a LED lamp with a wavelength from 400 to 505 nm. In the study group using 0.01% hydrogen peroxide, a considerable increase in ROS production as well as boosted apoptosis on the mitochondrial pathway were demonstrated, which was associated with a decreased number of living cells in this group [127]. However, it was shown that the pulp after whitening undergoes regeneration within 24 to 72 h, which indicated a temporary cytotoxic effect [127]. Lima et al. [130] also demonstrated that the use of antioxidants such as sodium ascorbate (0.25 mM/0.5 mM) reduces ROS production, thus limiting the risk of OS development (85). Vargas et al. observed that the use of alpha-tocopherol (1, 3, 5 and 10 mM) reduced hydrogen peroxide-induced cytotoxicity (0.035%, 0.018%, 0.009% and 0.045%) in odontoblasts and pulp cells [131].

The use of appropriate concentrations of bleaching agents generates ROS while simultaneously induces antioxidant defense systems. Consequently, the whitening process takes place without adverse effects on the redox equilibrium of the oral cavity.

14. Summary

As a result of OS, cell components—mainly proteins, lipids and nucleic acids—are damaged, which leads not only to structural changes of the cell, but also to its death through apoptosis and necrosis. Moreover, oxidative stress is associated with the pathogenesis of numerous systemic diseases, including those related to the oral cavity. Interestingly, not only the diseases of the oral cavity, but also their treatment induce OS. The source of ROS in the oral cavity can be filling materials such as amalgam, composites, glass-ionomer materials, or bonding systems, but also agents used in endodontic treatment, periodontal and surgical procedures, or materials used in orthodontic treatment.

Although some of the listed ROS/RNS sources in the oral cavity are inevitable and, in some situations, beneficial (periodontal treatment), the search for therapeutic solutions to avoid materials and treatment procedures leading to ROS overproduction seems extremely important.

Author Contributions: Conceptualization, A.Z. and M.M.; Data curation, I.Z. and A.Z.; Formal analysis, I.Z. and M.M.; Funding acquisition, A.Z.; Investigation, I.Z., A.Z., and M.M.; Methodology, I.Z., A.Z., and M.M.; Writing—original draft, I.Z. and A.Z.; Writing—review and editing, A.Z. and M.M. All authors have read and agreed to the published version of the manuscript.

References

1. Maciejczyk, M.; Mikoluc, B.; Pietrucha, B.; Heropolitanska—Pliszka, E.; Pac, M.; Motkowski, R.; Car, H. Oxidative stress, mitochondrial abnormalities and antioxidant defense in Ataxia-telangiectasia, Bloom syndrome and Nijmegen breakage syndrome. *Redox Biol.* **2017**. [CrossRef] [PubMed]
2. Chatterjee, S. *Oxidative Stress, Inflammation, and Disease*; Elsevier Inc.: Amsterdam, The Netherlands, 2016; pp. 35–58.
3. Sardaro, N.; della Vella, F.; Incalza, M.A.; Stasio, D.D.I.; Lucchese, A.; Contaldo, M.; Laudadio, C.; Petruzzi, M. Oxidative stress and oral mucosal diseases: An overview. *In Vivo* **2019**, *33*, 289–296. [CrossRef] [PubMed]

4. Gallorini, M.; Cataldi, A.; di Giacomo, V. HEMA-induced cytotoxicity: Oxidative stress, genotoxicity and apoptosis. *Int. Endod. J.* **2014**, *47*, 813–818. [CrossRef] [PubMed]
5. Zalewska, A.; Maciejczyk, M.; Szulimowska, J.; Imierska, M.; Błachnio-Zabielska, A. High-fat diet affects ceramide content, disturbs mitochondrial redox balance, and induces apoptosis in the submandibular glands of mice. *Biomolecules* **2019**, *9*, 877. [CrossRef] [PubMed]
6. Pawlukianiec, C.; Gryciuk, M.E.; Mil, K.M.; Żendzian-Piotrowska, M.; Zalewska, A.; Maciejczyk, M. A New Insight into Meloxicam: Assessment of Antioxidant and Anti-Glycating Activity in In Vitro Studies. *Pharmaceuticals* **2020**, *13*, 240. [CrossRef] [PubMed]
7. Davies, M.J. Protein oxidation and peroxidation. *Biochem. J.* **2016**, *473*, 805–825. [CrossRef] [PubMed]
8. Reeg, S.; Grune, T. Protein Oxidation in Aging: Does It Play a Role in Aging Progression? *Antioxid. Redox Signal.* **2015**, *23*, 239–255. [CrossRef] [PubMed]
9. Maciejczyk, M.; Szulimowska, J.; Taranta-Janusz, K.; Wasilewska, A.; Zalewska, A. Salivary Gland Dysfunction, Protein Glycooxidation and Nitrosative Stress in Children with Chronic Kidney Disease. *J. Clin. Med.* **2020**, 1285. [CrossRef] [PubMed]
10. Branco, V.; Canário, J.; Holmgren, A.; Carvalho, C. Inhibition of the thioredoxin system in the brain and liver of zebra-seabreams exposed to waterborne methylmercury. *Toxicol. Appl. Pharmacol.* **2011**, *251*, 95–103. [CrossRef] [PubMed]
11. Morita, M.; Naito, Y.; Yoshikawa, T.; Niki, E. Redox Biology Plasma lipid oxidation induced by peroxynitrite, hypochlorite, lipoxygenase and peroxyl radicals and its inhibition by antioxidants as assessed by diphenyl-1-pyrenylphosphine. *Redox Biol.* **2016**, *8*, 127–135. [CrossRef] [PubMed]
12. Skutnik-Radziszewska, A.; Maciejczyk, M.; Fejfer, K.; Krahel, J.; Flisiak, I.; Kołodziej, U.; Zalewska, A. Salivary Antioxidants and Oxidative Stress in Psoriatic Patients: Can Salivary Total Oxidant Status and Oxidative Status Index Be a Plaque Psoriasis Biomarker? *Oxid. Med. Cell. Longev.* **2020**. [CrossRef] [PubMed]
13. Gerreth, P.; Maciejczyk, M.; Zalewska, A.; Gerreth, K.; Hojan, K. Comprehensive Evaluation of the Oral Health Status, Salivary Gland Function, and Oxidative Stress in the Saliva of Patients with Subacute Phase of Stroke: A Case-Control Study. *J. Clin. Med.* **2020**, 2252. [CrossRef] [PubMed]
14. Sawczuk, B.; Maciejczyk, M.; Sawczuk-Siemieniuk, M.; Posmyk, R.; Zalewska, A.; Car, H. Salivary gland function, antioxidant defence and oxidative damage in the saliva of patients with breast cancer: Does the BRCA1 mutation disturb the salivary redox profile? *Cancers* **2019**, *11*, 1501. [CrossRef] [PubMed]
15. Waddington, R.J.; Moseley, R.; Embery, G. Reactive oxygen species: A potential role in the pathogenesis of periodontal diseases. *Oral. Dis.* **2000**, *6*, 138–151. [CrossRef] [PubMed]
16. Zińczuk, J.; Maciejczyk, M.; Zaręba, K.; Romaniuk, W.; Markowski, A.; Kędra, B.; Zalewska, A.; Pryczynicz, A.; Matowicka-Karna, J.; Guzińska-Ustymowicz, K. Antioxidant Barrier, Redox Status, and Oxidative Damage to Biomolecules in Patients with Colorectal Cancer. Can Malondialdehyde and Catalase Be Markers of Colorectal Cancer Advancement? *Biomolecules* **2019**, *9*, 637. [CrossRef] [PubMed]
17. Maciejczyk, M.; Szulimowska, J.; Skutnik, A.; Taranta-Janusz, K.; Wasilewska, A.; Wiśniewska, N.; Zalewska, A. Salivary Biomarkers of Oxidative Stress in Children with Chronic Kidney Disease. *J. Clin. Med.* **2018**, *7*, 209. [CrossRef]
18. Żukowski, P.; Maciejczyk, M.; Waszkiel, D. Sources of free radicals and oxidative stress in the oral cavity. *Arch. Oral Biol.* **2018**, *92*, 8–17. [CrossRef]
19. Celik, N.; Binnetoglu, D.; Ozakar Ilday, N.; Hacimuftuoglu, A.; Seven, N. The cytotoxic and oxidative effects of restorative materials in cultured human gingival fibroblasts. *Drug Chem. Toxicol.* **2019**, *31*, 1–6. [CrossRef]
20. Ramezani, G.H.; Moghadam, M.M.; Saghiri, M.A.; Garcia-Godoy, F.; Asatourian, A.; Aminsobhani, M.; Scarbecz, M.; Sheibani, N. Effect of dental restorative materials on total antioxidant capacity and calcium concentration of unstimulated saliva. *J. Clin. Exp. Dent.* **2017**, *9*, e71–e77. [CrossRef]
21. Daokar, S.G.; Shahu, C.; Shikshan, M.; Mustafa, M. Assessment of Oxidative Stress Induced by Various Restorative Materials: An In Vivo Biochemical Study. *J. Int. Oral Health* **2016**, *8*, 1–6.
22. Al-Saleh, I.; Al-Sedairi, A.; Elkhatib, R. Effect of mercury (Hg) dental amalgam fillings on renal and oxidative stress biomarkers in children. *Sci. Total Environ.* **2012**, *431*, 188–196. [CrossRef] [PubMed]
23. Cabaña-Muñoz, M.E.; Parmigiani-Izquierdo, J.M.; Bravo-González, L.A.; Kyung, H.M.; Merino, J.J. Increased Zn/glutathione levels and higher superoxide dismutase-1 activity as biomarkers of oxidative stress in women with long-term dental amalgam fillings: Correlation between mercury/aluminium levels (in hair) and antioxidant systems in plasma. *PLoS ONE* **2015**, *10*, 1–11. [CrossRef] [PubMed]

24. Yıldız, M.; Alp, H.H.; Gül, P.; Bakan, N.; Özcan, M. Lipid peroxidation and DNA oxidation caused by dental filling materials. *J. Dent. Sci.* **2017**, *12*, 233–240. [CrossRef] [PubMed]
25. Jiao, Y.; Ma, S.; Wang, Y.; Li, J.; Shan, L.; Liu, Q.; Liu, Y.; Song, Q.; Yu, F.; Yu, H.; et al. N-Acetyl cysteine depletes reactive oxygen species and prevents dental monomer-induced intrinsic mitochondrial apoptosis in vitro in human dental pulp cells. *PLoS ONE* **2016**, *11*, 1–20. [CrossRef] [PubMed]
26. Schneider, T.R.; Hakami-Tafreshi, R.; Tomasino-Perez, A.; Tayebi, L.; Lobner, D. Effects of dental composite resin monomers on dental pulp cells. *Dent. Mater. J.* **2019**, *38*, 579–583. [CrossRef] [PubMed]
27. Chang, H.H.; Guo, M.K.; Kasten, F.H.; Chang, M.C.; Huang, G.F.; Wang, Y.L.; Wang, R.S.; Jeng, J.H. Stimulation of glutathione depletion, ROS production and cell cycle arrest of dental pulp cells and gingival epithelial cells by HEMA. *Biomaterials* **2005**, *26*, 745–753. [CrossRef]
28. Lefeuvre, M.; Amjaad, W.; Goldberg, M.; Stanislawski, L. TEGDMA induces mitochondrial damage and oxidative stress in human gingival fibroblasts. *Biomaterials* **2005**, *26*, 5130–5137. [CrossRef]
29. Diomede, F.; Marconi, G.D.; Guarnieri, S.; D'Attilio, M.; Cavalcanti, M.F.X.B.; Mariggiò, M.A.; Pizzicannella, J.; Trubiami, O. A Novel Role of Ascorbic Acid in Anti-Inflammatory Pathway and ROS Generation in HEMA Treated Dental Pulp Stem Cells. *Materials* **2020**, 130. [CrossRef]
30. Di Nisio, C.; Zara, S.; Cataldi, A.; di Giacomo, V. 2-Hydroxyethyl methacrylate inflammatory effects in human gingival fibroblasts. *Int. Endod. J.* **2013**, *46*, 466–476. [CrossRef]
31. Perduns, R.; Volk, J.; Schertl, P.; Leyhausen, G.; Geurtsen, W. HEMA modulates the transcription of genes relatedto oxidative defense, inflammatory response andorganization of the ECM in human oral cells. *Dent. Mater.* **2019**, *35*, 501–510. [CrossRef]
32. Jiao, Y.; Niu, T.; Liu, H.; Tay, F.R.; Chen, J. Protection against HEMA-Induced Mitochondrial Injury In Vitro by Nrf2 Activation. *Oxid. Med. Cell. Longev.* **2019**, *2019*. [CrossRef] [PubMed]
33. Teti, G.; Orsini, G.; Salvatore, V.; Focaroli, S.; Mazzotti, M.C.; Ruggeri, A.; Mattioli-belmonte, M.; Falconi, M. HEMA but not TEGDMA induces autophagy in human gingival fibroblasts. *Front. Physiol.* **2015**, *6*, 1–8. [CrossRef] [PubMed]
34. Krifka, S.; Seidenader, C.; Hiller, K.A.; Schmalz, G.; Schweikl, H. Oxidative stress and cytotoxicity generated by dental composites in human pulp cells. *Clin. Oral Investig.* **2012**, *16*, 215–224. [CrossRef] [PubMed]
35. Pauly, K.; Fritz, K.; Furey, A.; Lobner, D. Insulin-like Growth Factor 1 and Transforming Growth Factor-β Stimulate Cystine/Glutamate Exchange Activity in Dental Pulp Cells. *J. Endod.* **2011**, *37*, 943–947. [CrossRef]
36. Huang, F.; Li, Y.; Lee, S.; Chang, Y. Cytotoxicity of dentine bonding agents on human pulp cells is related to intracellular glutathione levels. *Int. Endod. J.* **2010**, *43*, 1091–1097. [CrossRef]
37. Gul, P.; Akgul, N.; Hakan, H. Effects of composite restorations on oxidative stress in saliva: An in vivo study. *J. Dent. Sci.* **2015**, *10*, 394–400. [CrossRef]
38. Blasiak, J.; Synowiec, E. Dental methacrylates may exert genotoxic effects via the oxidative induction of DNA double strand breaks and the inhibition of their repair. *Mol. Biol. Rep.* **2012**, *39*, 7487–7496. [CrossRef] [PubMed]
39. Ferrúa, C.P.; Leal, F.B.; de Oliveira Gazal, M.; Ghisleni, G.C.; de Carvalho, R.V.; Demarco, F.F.; Ogliari, F.A.; Nedel, F. Iodonium salt incorporation in dental adhesives and its relation with degree of conversion, ultimate tensile strength, cell viability, and oxidative stress. *Clin. Oral Investig.* **2019**, *23*, 1143–1151. [CrossRef] [PubMed]
40. Spalj, S.; Mlacovic Zrinski, M.; Tudor Spalj, V.; Ivankovic Buljan, Z. In-vitro assessment of oxidative stress generated by orthodontic archwires. *Am. J. Orthod. Dentofac. Orthop.* **2012**, *141*, 583–589. [CrossRef] [PubMed]
41. Buljan, Z.I.; Ribaric, S.P.; Abram, M.; Ivankovic, A.; Spalj, S. In vitro oxidative stress induced by conventional and self-ligating brackets. *Angle Orthod.* **2012**, *82*, 340–345. [CrossRef]
42. Portelli, M.; Militi, A.; Cervino, G.; Lauritano, F.; Sambataro, S.; Mainardi, A.; Nucera, R. Oxidative Stress Evaluation in Patients Treated with Orthodontic Self-ligating Multibracket Appliances: An in Vivo Case-Control Study. *Open Dent. J.* **2017**, *11*, 257–265. [CrossRef] [PubMed]
43. Atuğ Özcan, S.S.; Ceylan, I.; Özcan, E.; Kurt, N.; Dağsuyu, I.M.; Çanakçi, C.F. Evaluation of oxidative stress biomarkers in patients with fixed orthodontic appliances. *Dis. Mark.* **2014**, *2014*. [CrossRef] [PubMed]
44. Buczko, P.; Knaś, M.; Grycz, M.; Szarmach, I.; Zalewska, A. Orthodontic treatment modifies the oxidant–antioxidant balance in saliva of clinically healthy subjects. *Adv. Med. Sci.* **2017**, *62*, 129–135. [CrossRef] [PubMed]
45. Wei, C.; Gong, T.; Pow, E.H.N.; Botelho, M.G. Adhesive and oxidative response of stem cell and pre-osteoblasts on titanium and zirconia surfaces in vitro. *J. Investig. Clin. Dent.* **2019**, *10*, e12407. [CrossRef] [PubMed]

46. Borys, J.; Maciejczyk, M.; Antonowicz, B.; Krętowski, A.; Sidun, J.; Domel, E.; Dąbrowski, J.; Ładny, J.; Morawska, K.; Zalewska, A. Glutathione Metabolism, Mitochondria Activity, and Nitrosative Stress in Patients Treated for Mandible Fractures. *J. Clin. Med.* **2019**, *8*, 127. [CrossRef] [PubMed]
47. Pietropaoli, D.; Ortu, E.; Severino, M.; Ciarrocchi, I.; Gatto, R.; Monaco, A. Glycation and oxidative stress in the failure of dental implants: A case series. *BMC Res. Notes* **2013**, *6*, 1. [CrossRef]
48. Borys, J.; Maciejczyk, M.; Krętowski, A.J.; Antonowicz, B.; Ratajczak-Wrona, W.; Jablonska, E.; Zaleski, P.; Waszkiel, D.; Ladny, J.R.; Zukowski, P.; et al. The redox balance in erythrocytes, plasma, and periosteum of patients with titanium fixation of the jaw. *Front. Physiol.* **2017**, *8*, 386. [CrossRef]
49. Borys, J.; Maciejczyk, M.; Antonowicz, B.; Sidun, J.; Świderska, M.Z.A. Free Radical Production, Inflammation and Apoptosis in Patients Treated With Titanium Mandibular Fixations—An Observational Study. *Front. Immunol.* **2019**, *10*, 1–12. [CrossRef]
50. Borys, J.; Maciejczyk, M.; Antonowicz, B.; Krętowski, A.; Waszkiel, D.; Bortnik, P.; Czarniecka-Bargłowska, K.; Kocisz, M.; Szulimowska, J.; Czajkowski, M.; et al. Exposure to Ti4Al4V titanium alloy leads to redox abnormalities, oxidative stress, and oxidative damage in patients treated for mandible fractures. *Oxid. Med. Cell. Longev.* **2018**, *2018*. [CrossRef]
51. Pillusky, F.M.; Barcelos, R.C.S.; Vey, L.T.; Barin, L.M.; de Mello Palma, V.; Maciel, R.M.; Kantorski, K.Z.; Bürger, M.E.; Danesi, C.C. Antimicrobial photodynamic therapy with photosensitizer in ethanol improves oxidative status and gingival collagen in a short-term in periodontitis. *Photodiagnosis Photodyn. Ther.* **2017**, *19*, 119–127. [CrossRef]
52. Boia, S.; Stratul, Ş.I.; Boariu, M.; Ursoniu, S.; Goţia, S.L.; Boia, E.R.; Borza, C. Evaluation of antioxidant capacity and clinical assessment of patients with chronic periodontitis treated with non-surgical periodontal therapy and adjunctive systemic antibiotherapy. *Rom. J. Morphol. Embryol.* **2018**, *59*, 1107–1113. [PubMed]
53. Tamaki, N.; Tomofuji, T.; Ekuni, D.; Yamanaka, R.; Yamamoto, T. Short—Term Effects of Non-Surgical Periodontal Treatment on Plasma Level of Reactive Oxygen Metabolites in Patients With Chronic Periodontitis. *J. Periodontol.* **2009**, *80*, 901–906. [CrossRef]
54. Guo, M.; Liu, L.; Zhang, J.; Liu, M. Role of Reactive Oxygen Species and Advanced Glycation End Products in the Malfunctioning of Dental Implants. *West. Indian Med. J.* **2015**, *64*, 419–423. [PubMed]
55. Mousavi Jazi, M.; Sadeghi Pour Rodsari, H.R.; Mirmiran, F. Level of Oxidative Stress Markers in Peri-Implant Crevicular Fluid and Their Correlation with Clinical Parameters. *J. Dent.* **2015**, *12*, 340–346.
56. Leewananthawet, A.; Arakawa, S.; Okano, T.; Daitoku Kinoshita, R.; Ashida, H.; Izumi, Y.; Suzuki, T. Ozone ultrafine bubble water induces the cellular signaling involved in oxidative stress responses in human periodontal ligament fibroblasts. *Sci. Technol. Adv. Mater.* **2019**, *20*, 589–598. [CrossRef] [PubMed]
57. Del Real García, J.F.; Saldaña-Velasco, F.R.; Sánchez-de la Rosa, S.V.; Ortiz-García, Y.M.; Morales-Velazquez, G.; Gómez-Meda, B.C.; Zúñiga-González, G.M.; Sánchez-Parada, M.G.; Zamora-Perez, A.L. In vivo evaluation of the genotoxicity and oxidative damage in individuals exposed to 10% hydrogen peroxide whitening strips. *Clin. Oral Investig.* **2019**, *23*, 3033–3046. [CrossRef] [PubMed]
58. Farina, M.; Aschner, M.; Rocha, J.B.T. Oxidative stress in MeHg-induced neurotoxicity. *Toxicol. Appl. Pharmacol.* **2011**, *256*, 405–417. [CrossRef] [PubMed]
59. Franco, J.L.; Posser, T.; Dunkley, P.R.; Dickson, P.W.; Mattos, J.J.; Martins, R.; Bainy, A.C.D.; Marques, M.R.; Dafre, A.L.; Farina, M. Methylmercury neurotoxicity is associated with inhibition of the antioxidant enzyme glutathione peroxidase Jeferson. *Free Radic. Biol. Med.* **2009**, *47*, 449–457. [CrossRef]
60. Glaser, V.; Leipnitz, G.; Raniel, M.; Oliveira, J.; Wannmacher, D.; Fabro, A.; Bem, D.; Valgas, V. Oxidative stress-mediated inhibition of brain creatine kinase activity by methylmercury. *NeuroToxicology* **2010**, *31*, 454–460. [CrossRef]
61. Glaser, V.; Maria, E.; Maria, Y.; Müller, R.; Feksa, L.; Milton, C.; Wannmacher, D.; Batista, J.; Rocha, T.; Fabro, A.; et al. Effects of inorganic selenium administration in methylmercury-induced neurotoxicity in mouse cerebral cortex. *Int. J. Dev. Neurosci.* **2010**, *28*, 631–637. [CrossRef]
62. Rocha, J.B.; Freitas, A.J.; Marques, M.B.; Pereira, M.E.; Emanuelli, T.; Souza, D. Effects of methylmercury exposure during the second stage of rapid postnatal brain growth on negative geotaxis and on delta-aminolevulinate dehydratase of suckling rats. *Braz J. Med. Biol Res.* **1993**, *10*, 1077–1083.
63. Barbosa, A.C.; Jardim, W.; Dórea, J.G.; Fosberg, B.; Souza, J. Hair Mercury Speciation as a Function of Gender, Age, and Body Mass Index in Inhabitants of the Negro River Basin, Amazon, Brazil. *Arch. Environ. Contam. Toxicol.* **2001**, *40*, 439–444. [PubMed]

64. Dorea, J. Environmental contaminants as biomarkers of fish intake: A case for hair mercury concentrations. *Eur. J. Clin. Nutr.* **2011**, *65*, 419–420. [CrossRef] [PubMed]
65. Nogueira, C.W.; Rocha, J.B. Diphenyl Diselenide a Janus-Faced Molecule. *J. Braz. Chem. Soc.* **2010**, *21*, 2055–2071. [CrossRef]
66. Araie, H.; Shiraiwa, Y. Selenium Utilization Strategy by Microalgae. *Molecules* **2009**, *14*, 4880–4891. [CrossRef]
67. Hollenberg, S.M.; Cinel, I. Bench-to-bedside review: Nitric oxide in critical illness—Update 2008. *Crit. Care* **2009**, *9*. [CrossRef]
68. Lobanov, A.V.; Hatfield, D.L.; Gladyshev, V.N. Eukaryotic selenoproteins and selenoproteomes. *Biochim. Biophys. Acta Gen. Subj.* **2012**, *1790*, 1424–1428. [CrossRef]
69. Tsuzuki, Y.Y.T. Inhibitory actions of mercury compounds against glucose-6-phosphate dehydrogenase from yeast. *J. Toxicol. Sci.* **1979**, *4*, 105–113. [CrossRef]
70. Stringari, J.; Nunes, A.K.C.; Franco, J.L.; Bohrer, D.; Solange, C.; Dafre, A.L.; Milatovic, D.; Souza, D.O.; Rocha, J.B.T.; Farina, M. Prenatal methylmercury exposure hampers glutathione antioxidant system ontogenesis and causes long-lasting oxidative stress in the mouse brain. *Toxicol. Appl. Pharmacol.* **2010**, *227*, 147–154. [CrossRef]
71. Farina, M.; Campos, F.; Vendrell, I.; Berenguer, J.; Barzi, M. Probucol Increases Glutathione Peroxidase-1 Activity and Displays Long-Lasting Protection against Methylmercury Toxicity in Cerebellar Granule Cells. *Toxicol. Sci.* **2009**, *112*, 416–426. [CrossRef]
72. Wagner, C.; Sudati, H.; Nogueira, W.; Rocha, J. In vivo and in vitro inhibition of mice thioredoxin reductase by methylmercury. *Biometals* **2010**, *23*, 1171–1177. [CrossRef] [PubMed]
73. Hirayama, N.M.A.Y.K. Comparative study of activities in reactive oxygen species production/defense system in mitochondria of rat brain and liver, and their susceptibility to methylmercury toxicity. *Arch. Toxicol* **2007**, 769–776.
74. Wu, L.L.; Chiou, C.; Chang, P.; Wu, J.T. Urinary 8-OHdG: A marker of oxidative stress to DNA and a risk factor for cancer, atherosclerosis and diabetics. *Clin. Chim. Acta* **2004**, *339*, 1–9. [CrossRef] [PubMed]
75. Kim, J.Y.; Mukherjee, S.; Ngo, L.; Christiani, D.C. Urinary 8-hydroxy-2′-deoxyguanosine as a biomarker of oxidative DNA damage in workers exposed to fine particulates. *Environ. Health Perspect.* **2004**, *112*, 666–671. [CrossRef] [PubMed]
76. Chen, C.; Qu, L.; Li, B.; Xing, L.; Jia, G.; Wang, T.; Gao, Y.; Zhang, P.; Li, M.; Chen, W.; et al. Increased Oxidative DNA Damage, as Assessed by Urinary 8-Hydroxy-2′-Deoxyguanosine Concentrations, and Serum Redox Status in Persons Exposed to Mercury. *Clin. Chem.* **2005**, *767*, 759–767. [CrossRef]
77. Ohno, T.; Sakamoto, M.; Kurosawa, T.; Dakeishi, M. Total mercury levels in hair, toenail, and urine among women free from occupational exposure and their relations to renal tubular function. *Environ. Res.* **2007**, *103*, 191–197. [CrossRef] [PubMed]
78. Selimović-Dragaš, M.; Huseinbegović, A.; Kobašlija, S.; Hatibović-Kofman, Š. A comparison of the in vitro cytotoxicity of conventional and resin modifi ed glass ionomer cements. *Assoc. Basic Med. Sci. FBIH* **2012**, *12*, 273–278. [CrossRef]
79. Van Landuyt, K.L.; Nawrot, T.; Geebelen, B.; De Munck, J.; Snauwaert, J.; Yoshihara, K.; Scheers, H.; Godderis, L.; Hoet, P.; Van Meerbeek, B. How much do resin-based dental materials release? A meta-analytical approach. *Dent. Mater.* **2011**, *27*, 723–747. [CrossRef] [PubMed]
80. Schweikl, H.; Spagnuolo, G.; Schmalz, G. Genetic and cellular toxicology of dental resin monomers. *J. Dent. Res.* **2006**, *85*, 870–877. [CrossRef] [PubMed]
81. Maciejczyk, M.; Heropolitanska-Pliszka, E.; Pietrucha, B.; Sawicka-Powierza, J.; Bernatowska, E.; Wolska-Kusnierz, B.; Pac, M.; Car, H.; Zalewska, A.; Mikoluc, B. Antioxidant defense, redox homeostasis, and oxidative damage in children with ataxia telangiectasia and nijmegen breakage syndrome. *Front. Immunol.* **2019**, *10*, 1–11. [CrossRef]
82. Coelho, A.S.; Laranjo, M.; Gonçalves, A.C.; Paula, A.; Paulo, S.; Abrantes, A.M.; Caramelo, F.; Ferreira, M.M.; Silva, M.J.; Carrilho, E.; et al. Cytotoxic effects of a chlorhexidine mouthwash and of an enzymatic mouthwash on human gingival fibroblasts. *Odontology* **2020**, *108*, 260–270. [CrossRef] [PubMed]
83. Samuelsen, J.T.; Kopperud, H.M.; Holme, J.A.; Dragland, I.S.; Christensen, T.; Dahl, J.E. Role of thiol-complex formation in 2-hydroxyethyl- methacrylate-induced toxicity in vitro. *J. Biomed. Mater. Res.* **2010**, *96*, 395–401. [CrossRef] [PubMed]

84. Nocca, G.; De Palma, F.; Minucci, A.; De Sole, P.; Martorana, G.E.; Callà, C.; Morlacchi, C.; Gozzo, M.L.; Gambarini, G.; Chimenti, C.; et al. Alterations of energy metabolism and glutathione levels of HL-60 cells induced by methacrylates present in composite resins. *J. Dent.* **2007**, *35*, 187–194. [CrossRef] [PubMed]
85. Krifka, S.; Hiller, K.; Spagnuolo, G.; Jewett, A.; Schmalz, G.; Schweikl, H. The influence of glutathione on redox regulation by antioxidant proteins and apoptosis in macrophages exposed to 2-hydroxyethyl methacrylate (HEMA). *Biomaterials* **2012**, *33*, 5177–5186. [CrossRef] [PubMed]
86. Schweikl, H.; Petzel, C.; Bolay, C.; Hiller, K.; Buchalla, W.; Krifka, S. 2-Hydroxyethyl methacrylate-induced apoptosis through the ATM- and p53-dependent intrinsic mitochondrial pathway. *Biomaterials* **2014**, *35*, 2890–2904. [CrossRef] [PubMed]
87. Zalewska, A.; Szarmach, I.; Żendzian-Piotrowska, M.; Maciejczyk, M. The effect of N-acetylcysteine on respiratory enzymes, ADP/ATP ratio, glutathione metabolism, and nitrosative stress in the salivary gland mitochondria of insulin resistant rats. *Nutrients* **2020**, 458. [CrossRef]
88. Mikulás, K.; Hermann, P.; Gera, I.; Komlódi, T. Triethylene glycol dimethacrylate impairs bioenergetic functions and induces oxidative stress in mitochondria via inhibiting respiratory Complex. *Dent. Mater.* **2018**, 1–16. [CrossRef]
89. Gomes, A.P.; Price, N.L.; Ling, A.J.Y.; Moslehi, J.J.; Montgomery, M.K.; Rajman, L.; Teodoro, S.; Wrann, C.D.; Hubbard, B.P.; Mercken, E.M.; et al. Declining NAD+ Induces a Pseudohypoxic State Disrupting Nuclear-Mitochondrial Communication during Aging. *Cell* **2013**, *155*. [CrossRef]
90. Styllou, P.; Styllou, M.; Hickel, R.; Högg, C.; Reichl, F.X.; Scherthan, H. NAC ameliorates dental composite-induced DNA double-strand breaks and chromatin condensation. *Dent. Mater. J.* **2017**, *36*, 638–646. [CrossRef]
91. Ma, Q. Role of Nrf2 in Oxidative Stress and Toxicity. *Annu. Rev. Pharmacol. Toxicol.* **2013**, *53*, 401–426. [CrossRef]
92. Durante, W. Protective Role of Heme Oxygenase-1 against Inflammation in Atherosclerosis. *Front. Biosci* **2018**, *16*, 2372–2388. [CrossRef] [PubMed]
93. Gozzelino, R.; Jeney, V.; Soares, M.P. Mechanisms of Cell Protection by Heme Oxygenase-1. *Annu. Rev. Pharmacol. Toxicol.* **2010**, *50*, 323–354. [CrossRef] [PubMed]
94. Gallorini, M.; Petzel, C.; Bolay, C.; Hiller, K.; Cataldi, A.; Buchalla, W.; Krifka, S.; Schweikl, H. Biomaterials Activation of the Nrf2-regulated antioxidant cell response inhibits HEMA-induced oxidative stress and supports cell viability. *Biomaterials* **2015**, *56*, 114–128. [CrossRef] [PubMed]
95. Lee, D.H.; Lim, B.S.; Lee, Y.K.; Ahn, S.J.; Yang, H.C. Involvement of oxidative stress in mutagenicity and apoptosis caused by dental resin monomers in cell cultures. *Dent. Mater.* **2006**, *22*, 1086–1092. [CrossRef] [PubMed]
96. Krifka, S.; Spagnuolo, G.; Schmalz, G.; Schweikl, H. A review of adaptive mechanisms in cell responses towards oxidative stress caused by dental resin monomers. *Biomaterials* **2013**, *34*, 4555–4563. [CrossRef] [PubMed]
97. Jones, R.M.; Petermann, E. Replication fork dynamics and the DNA damage response. *Biochem. J.* **2012**, *26*, 13–26. [CrossRef]
98. Ansteinsson, V.; Solhaug, A.; Samuelsen, J.T.; Holme, J.A.; Dahl, J.E. DNA-damage, cell-cycle arrest and apoptosis induced in BEAS-2B cells by 2-hydroxyethyl methacrylate (HEMA). *Mutat. Res. Genet. Toxicol. Environ. Mutagen.* **2011**, *723*, 158–164. [CrossRef] [PubMed]
99. Ansteinsson, V. In Vitro Toxicity of Filler Particles and Methacrylates Used in Dental Composite Materials Cytokine Release and Cell Death. Ph.D. Thesis, The University of Bergen, Bergen, Norway, 2013.
100. Popal, M.; Volk, J.; Leyhausen, G.; Geurtsen, W. Cytotoxic and genotoxic potential of the type I photoinitiators BAPO and TPO on human oral keratinocytes and V79 fibroblasts. *Dent. Mater.* **2018**, *34*, 1783–1796. [CrossRef] [PubMed]
101. Yoshino, F.; Yoshida, A.; Okada, E.; Okada, Y.; Maehata, Y.; Miyamoto, C.; Kishimoto, S.; Otsuka, T.; Nishimura, T.; Lee, M.C. Il Dental resin curing blue light induced oxidative stress with reactive oxygen species production. *J. Photochem. Photobiol. B Biol.* **2012**, *114*, 73–78. [CrossRef] [PubMed]
102. Oktay, E.A.; Tort, H.; Yıldız, O.; Ulusoy, K.G.; Topcu, F.T.; Ozer, C. Dental resin curing blue light induces vasoconstriction through release of hydrogen peroxide. *J. Photochem. Photobiol. B Biol.* **2018**, *185*, 41–45. [CrossRef]
103. Botton, G.; Pires, C.W.; Cadoná, F.C.; Machado, A.K.; Azzolin, V.F.; Cruz, I.B.M.; Sagrillo, M.R.; Praetzel, J.R. Toxicity of irrigating solutions and pharmacological associations used in pulpectomy of primary teeth. *Int. Endod. J.* **2016**, *49*, 746–754. [CrossRef] [PubMed]

104. Saghiri, M.A.; Delvarani, A.; Mehrvarzfar, P.; Nikoo, M.; Lotfi, M.; Karamifar, K.; Asgar, K.; Dadvand, S. The impact of pH on cytotoxic effects of three root canal irrigants. *Saudi Dent. J.* **2011**, *23*, 149–152. [CrossRef] [PubMed]
105. Soares, J.; Marins, R.; Sassone, L.M.; Fidel, S.R.; Ribeiro, D.A. In Vitro Genotoxicity and Cytotoxicity in Murine Fibroblasts Exposed to EDTA, NaOCl, MTAD and Citric Acid. *Braz. Dent. J.* **2012**, *23*, 527–533.
106. Singh, H.; Khurana, H.; Singh, H.; Singh, M. Photodynamic therapy: Truly a marriage between a drug and a light. *Muller J. Med. Sci. Res.* **2014**, *5*, 48–55. [CrossRef]
107. Pires, C.W.; Botton, G.; Cadoná, F.C.; Machado, A.K.; Azzolin, V.F.; da Cruz, I.B.M.; Sagrillo, M.R.; Praetzel, J.R. Induction of cytotoxicity, oxidative stress and genotoxicity by root filling pastes used in primary teeth. *Int. Endod. J.* **2016**, *49*, 737–745. [CrossRef] [PubMed]
108. Barbin, L.E.; Estrela, C.; Guedes, D.F.C.; Spanó, J.C.E.; Sousa-Neto, M.D.; Pécora, J.D. Detection of para-chloroaniline, reactive oxygen species, and 1-chloro-4-nitrobenzene in high concentrations of chlorhexidine and in a mixture of chlorhexidine and calcium hydroxide. *J. Endod.* **2013**, *5*, 664–668. [CrossRef]
109. Victoria-Escandell, A.; Ibañez-Cabellos, J.S.; De Cutanda, S.B.; Berenguer-Pascual, E.; Beltrán-García, J.; García-López, E.; Pallardó, F.V.; García-Giménez, J.L.; Pallarés-Sabater, A.; Zarzosa-López, I.; et al. Cellular Responses in Human Dental Pulp Stem Cells Treated with Three Endodontic Materials. *Stem. Cells Int.* **2017**, *2017*. [CrossRef] [PubMed]
110. Kim, T.G.; Lee, Y.H.; Lee, N.H.; Bhattarai, G.; Lee, I.K.; Yun, B.S.; Yi, H.K. The Antioxidant Property of Pachymic Acid Improves Bone Disturbance against AH Plus–induced Inflammation in MC-3T3 E1 Cells. *J. Endod.* **2013**, *39*, 461–466. [CrossRef]
111. Chang, S.-W.; Lee, S.-Y.; Ann, H.-J.; Kum, K.-Y.; Kim, E.-C. Effects of Calcium Silicate Endodontic Cements on Biocompatibility and Mineralization-inducing Potentials in Human Dental Pulp Cells. *J. Endod.* **2014**, *40*, 1194–1200. [CrossRef]
112. Loison-robert, L.S.; Tassin, M.; Bonte, E. In vitro effects of two silicate-based materials, Biodentine and BioRoot RCS, on dental pulp stem cells in models of reactionary and reparative dentinogenesis. *PLoS ONE* **2018**, *13*, 1–19. [CrossRef]
113. Trombetta, D.; Mondello, M.R.; Cimino, F.; Cristani, M.; Pergolizzi, S.; Saija, A. Toxic effect of nickel in an in vitro model of human oral epithelium. *Toxicol. Lett.* **2005**, *159*, 219–225. [CrossRef] [PubMed]
114. Gholinejad, Z.; Ansari, M.H.K.; Rasmi, Y. Titanium dioxide nanoparticles induce endothelial cell apoptosis via cell membrane oxidative damage and p38, PI3K/Akt, NF-κB signaling pathways modulation. *J. Trace Elem. Med. Biol.* **2019**, *54*, 27–35. [CrossRef] [PubMed]
115. Pereira, L.C.; Pazin, M.; Franco-Bernardes, M.F.; Martins, C.; Barcelos, R.M.; Pereira, C.M.; Rodrigues, J.L.; Barbosa, F., Jr.; Dorta, D.J. A Perspective of Mitochondrial Dysfunction in Rats Treated with Silver and Titanium Nanoparticles (AgNPs and TiNPs). *J. Trace Elem. Med. Biol.* **2018**. [CrossRef] [PubMed]
116. Wang, G.; Xu, Y.; Zhang, L.; Ye, D.; Feng, X.; Fu, T. Enhancement of Apoptosis by Titanium Alloy Internal Fixations during Microwave Treatments for Fractures: An Animal Study. *PLoS ONE* **2015**. [CrossRef] [PubMed]
117. Shanbhag, A.S.; Macaulay, W.; Stefanovic-racic, M.; Rubash, H.E. Nitric oxide release by macrophages in response to particulate wear debris. *J. Biomed. Maters Res.* **1998**, *3*, 497–503. [CrossRef]
118. Mouthuy, P.; Snelling, S.J.B.; Dakin, S.G.; Milković, L.; Gašparović, Č.; Carr, A.J.; Žarković, N. Biocompatibility of implantable materials: An oxidative stress viewpoint. *Biomaterials* **2016**. [CrossRef]
119. Cabaña-Muñoz, M.E.; Parmigiani-Izquierdo, J.M.; Alonso, F.C.; Merino, J. Increased Systemic Malondialdehyde Levels and Decreased Mo/Co, Mo/Hg^{2+}, Co/Fe^{2+} Ratios in Patients with Long-Term Dental Titanium Implants and Amalgams. *J. Clin. Med.* **2019**, *8*, 86. [CrossRef]
120. Sánchez-Siles, M.; Lucas-Azorin, J.; Salazar-Sánchez, N.; Carbonell-Meseguer, L.; Camacho-Alonso, F. Salivary Concentration of Oxidative Stress Biomarkers in a Group of Patients with Peri-Implantitis: A Transversal Study. *Clin. Implant. Dent.* **2015**, *18*, 1015–1022. [CrossRef] [PubMed]
121. Toczewska, J.; Maciejczyk, M.; Konopka, T.; Zalewska, A. Total Oxidant and Antioxidant Capacity of Gingival Crevicular Fluid and Saliva in Patients with Periodontitis: Review and Clinical Study. *Antioxidants* **2020**, *9*, 450. [CrossRef] [PubMed]
122. Toczewska, J.; Konopka, T.; Zalewska, A. Nitrosative Stress Biomarkers in the Non-Stimulated and Stimulated Saliva, as well as Gingival Crevicular Fluid of Patients with Periodontitis: Review and Clinical Study. *Antioxidants* **2020**, *9*, 259. [CrossRef]

123. Yeung, S.Y.; Huang, C.S.; Chan, C.P.; Lin, C.P.; Lin, H.N.; Lee, P.H.; Jia, H.W.; Huang, S.K.; Jeng, J.H.; Chang, M.C. Antioxidant and pro-oxidant properties of chlorhexidine and its interaction with calcium hydroxide solutions. *Int. Endod. J.* **2007**, *40*, 837–844. [CrossRef] [PubMed]
124. Yoshida, A.; Iwata, S.; Iizuka, J.; Takahashi, S.; Wada-takahashi, S.; Miyamoto, C.; Maehata, Y.; Ogura, Y.; Lee, M.; Yo, F. Blue Light from Dental Resin Curing Unit Causes Light-Induced Vasocon- striction in Isolated Rat Aorta. *OHDM* **2014**, *13*, 1147–1151.
125. Jha, N.; Ryu, J.J.; Choi, E.H.; Kaushik, N.K. Generation and Role of Reactive Oxygen and Nitrogen Species Induced by Plasma, Lasers, Chemical Agents, and Other Systems in Dentistry. *Oxid. Med. Cell. Longev.* **2017**, *2017*. [CrossRef] [PubMed]
126. Wu, T.T.; Li, L.F.; Du, R.; Jiang, L.; Zhu, Y.Q. Hydrogen peroxide induces apoptosis in human dental pulp cells via caspase-9 dependent pathway. *J. Endod.* **2013**, *39*, 1151–1155. [CrossRef]
127. Marto, C.M.; Laranjo, M.; Paula, A.; Coelho, A.S.; Abrantes, A.M.; Casalta-Lopes, J.; Gonçalves, A.C.; Sarmento-Ribeiro, A.B.; Ferreira, M.M.; Cabrita, A.; et al. Cytotoxic effects of zoom® whitening product in human fibroblasts. *Materials* **2020**, *13*, 1491. [CrossRef]
128. Zalewska, A.; Ziembicka, D.; Zendzian-Piotrowska, M.; MacIejczyk, M. The impact of high-fat diet on mitochondrial function, free radical production, and nitrosative stress in the salivary glands of wistar rats. *Oxid. Med. Cell. Longev.* **2019**. [CrossRef]
129. Matczuk, J.; Zendzian-Piotrowska, M.; Maciejczyk, M.; Kurek, K. Salivary lipids: A review. *Adv. Clin. Exp. Med.* **2017**. [CrossRef]
130. Lima, A.F.; Lessa, F.C.; Hebling, J.; de Souza Costa, C.A.; Marchie, G.M. Protective Effect of Sodium Ascorbate on MDPC-23 Odontoblast-Like Cells Exposed to a Bleaching Agent. *Eur. J. Dent.* **2010**, *4*, 238–244.
131. Vargas, S.; Soares, D.G.; Paula, A.; Ribeiro, D.; Hebling, J.; Alberto, C.; Costa, D.S. Protective Effect of Alpha-Tocopherol Isomer from Vitamin E against the H_2O_2 Induced Toxicity on Dental Pulp Cells. *Biomed. Res. Int.* **2014**, *2014*, 1–5. [CrossRef]

2

Influence of Dental Prosthesis and Restorative Materials Interface on Oral Biofilms

Yu Hao [1,2,3,†], Xiaoyu Huang [1,2,3,†], Xuedong Zhou [1,2,3], Mingyun Li [1,3], Biao Ren [1,3], Xian Peng [1,3,*] and Lei Cheng [1,2,3,*]

1 State Key Laboratory of Oral Diseases, Sichuan University, Chengdu 610041, China; haoyu_dentist@sina.com (Y.H.); 2013181641007@stu.scu.edu.cn (X.H.); zhouxd@scu.edu.cn (X.Z.); limingyun@scu.edu.cn (M.L.); renbiao@scu.edu.cn (B.R.)

2 Department of Cariology and Endodontics, West China School of Stomatology, Sichuan University, Chengdu 610041, China

3 National Clinical Research Center for Oral Diseases, Sichuan University, Chengdu 610041, China

* Correspondence: pengx07@hotmail.com (X.P.); chenglei@scu.edu.cn (L.C.)

† These authors contributed equally to this work.

Abstract: Oral biofilms attach onto both teeth surfaces and dental material surfaces in oral cavities. In the meantime, oral biofilms are not only the pathogenesis of dental caries and periodontitis, but also secondary caries and peri-implantitis, which would lead to the failure of clinical treatments. The material surfaces exposed to oral conditions can influence pellicle coating, initial bacterial adhesion, and biofilm formation, due to their specific physical and chemical characteristics. To define the effect of physical and chemical characteristics of dental prosthesis and restorative material on oral biofilms, we discuss resin-based composites, glass ionomer cements, amalgams, dental alloys, ceramic, and dental implant material surface properties. In conclusion, each particular chemical composition (organic matrix, inorganic filler, fluoride, and various metallic ions) can enhance or inhibit biofilm formation. Irregular topography and rough surfaces provide favorable interface for bacterial colonization, protecting bacteria against shear forces during their initial reversible binding and biofilm formation. Moreover, the surface free energy, hydrophobicity, and surface-coating techniques, also have a significant influence on oral biofilms. However, controversies still exist in the current research for the different methods and models applied. In addition, more in situ studies are needed to clarify the role and mechanism of each surface parameter on oral biofilm development.

Keywords: biofilm; dental restorative material; surface characteristics; surface roughness; resin-based composite

1. Introduction

From the widely applied dental amalgams [1] to esthetic resin-based composites [2,3] and ion-release glass ionomer cements [4], direct restorative materials are generally used to reconstruct the tooth when its structure is compromised by trauma or dental caries. Besides, indirect crown restorations and dental implants have been applied to tooth and dentition defect restorations for decades [5,6]. Although these restorative materials had significant evolvement in the past few decades, the failure rates of restorations are still problems to the dentists and investigators.

As it stands, direct restorations showed an annual failure rate up to 7.9% with the main reasons of secondary caries and bulk fracture [3,7,8]. It was reported that the 5-year failure rate of fixed dental prostheses was more than 10%, due to the common complications of caries and endodontic diseases [9–11]. Although the implant survival reached 92.8–97.1% over a follow-up period of

10 years, we cannot ignore peri-implantitis, which is mainly caused by biofilm accumulation [12,13]. The prevalence of peri-implantitis varies from 11% to 47%, because of the different threshold of bone loss [14]. However, Schwendicke's study showed that an implant might cost more than 300 Euro when it comes to peri-implantitis, by comparison with a healthy implant [15]. Dental restorative materials placed in oral cavity are subjected to aggressive attack by bacteria. Components in materials will be biodegraded by the dental plaque, which will probably compromise the marginal integrity and induce the development and progression of secondary caries and peri-implantitis [12,16–18].

The oral cavity is a complex environment, where high humidity, moderate temperature, and abundance of nutrients promote the formation of differentiated microorganisms and microbial biofilms [19–21]. Biofilm formation in the oral cavity is a gradated process consisting of four stages (Figure 1) [22]:

1 acquired pellicle formation;
2 primary colonization;
3 coaggregation;
4 mature biofilm establishment.

To generate a biofilm, all surfaces exposed to the oral environment are steadily covered by a pellicle derived from the adsorption of organic and inorganic molecules in saliva. The receptors of salivary pellicle offer binding sites for floating initial bacteria cells to attach to these surfaces and form microcolonies. As time goes by, the bacteria cells aggregate, proliferate, and grow into a mushroom-shaped mature biofilm, firmly attaching to these surfaces [23,24]. Therefore, bacterial cells within the biofilm do not exist as independent entities but, rather, as a coordinated, metabolically integrated microbial community [22].

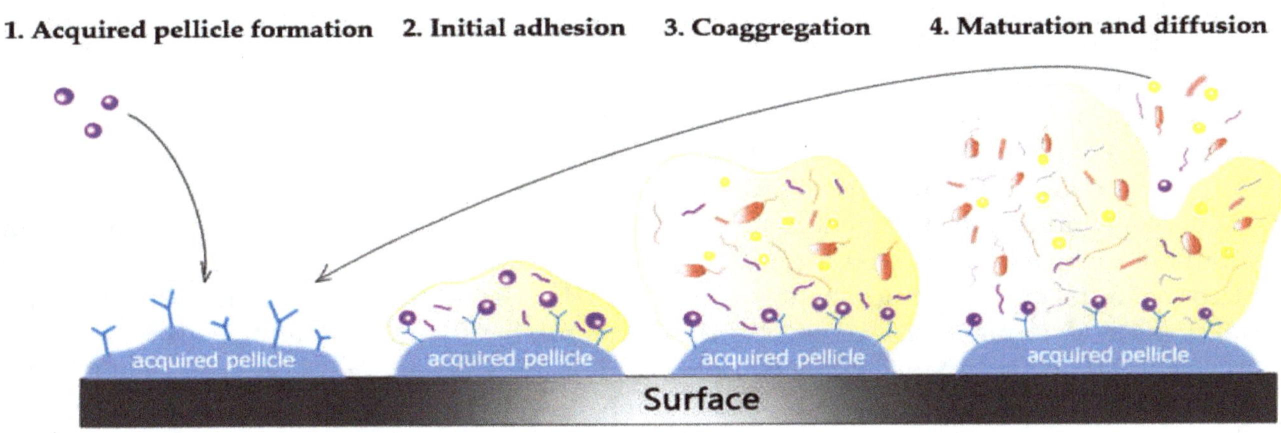

Figure 1. The process of biofilm formation in the oral cavity is divided into four stages: 1. acquired pellicle formation; 2. initial adhesion; 3. coaggregation; 4. maturation and diffusion.

Since adhesion is the crucial step of biofilm formation, understanding bacteria–surface interaction is essential for biofilm control and survival rate of restorations. The physical and chemical characteristics of dental prosthesis and restorative materials can influence pellicle coating, initial bacterial adhesion, and biofilm formation. The growing application of dental materials has presented an ever-increasing need to better understand the interactions between biofilm and material surfaces in the oral cavity. Thus, in this review, we discuss the effects of physical and chemical characteristics of different dental prosthesis and restorative material surfaces on oral biofilms.

2. Physical Characteristics of Dental Materials

2.1. *Surface Roughness*

Nowadays, some clinical procedures, polishing and finishing, are usually applied for smoother surfaces. Among these polishing and finishing techniques, the lowest surface roughness (SR) values could be achieved by Mylar, and followed by Al_2O_3 discs, one-step rubber points, diamond bur, and multi-blade carbide bur [25].

Many researches have demonstrated that unpolished materials surfaces could accumulate more dental biofilm than polished ones, including resin-based composites, ceramics, implant abutments, and denture bases [22,26,27]. Kim [28] investigated the surface ultrastructure, roughness of four ceramic materials (Vita Enamic, Lava Ultimate, Vitablocs Mark II, and Wieland Reflex), and assessed their promotion of biofilm development following adjustments and simulated intraoral polishing methods. It was proved that surface roughness values (Ra) were greater in all materials following these methods, resulting in more biofilm accumulation, which implied the main cause of biofilm accumulation was surface roughness. A previous study evaluated the surface roughness of 20 commercial dental composite resins after abrasive wear, with the average roughness ranging from 0.49 to 0.79 μm [29]. According to Bollen's study, the surface roughness above the threshold roughness (Ra = 0.2 μm) results in a simultaneous increase in biofilm accumulation, and no further reduction in bacterial adhesion could be observed under the threshold value [30]. In the same way, Yuan et al. demonstrated that the area of adherent bacteria was a highly linear correlation coefficient ($r = 0.893$, $P < 0.01$) when Ra < 0.80 μm, and weakly correlated with SR when Ra $\leq$ 0.20 μm ($r = 0.643$, $P < 0.01$) [31]. It indicated that factors other than SR influence biofilm formation when Ra $\leq$ 0.20 μm.

According to Ionescu et al., surface topography, the 3D characteristics of a surface with peaks and valleys distribution, could explain the crucial role of SR in biofilm formation [26]. The deeper and larger depressions may increase the contact area and provide more favorable interfaces for bacterial colonization and biofilm formation, protecting bacteria against shear forces (rinsing and brushing) during their initial reversible binding, leading to irreversible and stronger attachment [17,32]. Hence, it is difficult to eliminate microcolonies on the rough surfaces, resulting in the formation of mature biofilm [33].

The studies mentioned above were mostly done in vitro. All surfaces in the oral cavity are covered by the salivary pellicle, and the SR, one of the physical characteristics of material surfaces, is, in part, counterbalanced by the presence of the salivary pellicle [33]. Besides, as the biofilm maturing, the effect of SR on biofilm development is reduced, with the new bacteria adhering to the initial formed biofilm but not to the tested material surface [34–36]. Hence, the roughness of material surface mainly influences the initial bacterial colonization. Lorenzo [37] revealed that biofilms developed by single bacterial species or simple microbial associations are more readily influenced by surface roughness and topography than biofilm formed by complex communities. The different outcomes of the above research could be related to different methods and the development of the genetic technology.

Although improving implant osseointegration, the surface roughness has been proposed as the main feature inducing biofilm development [38]. Many studies showed that the increase of the SR could cause an exponential growth in bacterial cells [39] and facilitate biofilm formation [22]. However, compared to the resin-based composites (RBCs) and ceramic, SR is not always detrimental to the treatment because it is benefit for the attachment of osteoblast. Thus, the role of SR seems a little contradictory in this field.

With respect to the biofilm composition, Marcos [40] affirmed that there seems to be no reason to believe that implants with rough surfaces are more susceptive to fail, and his results are in accordance with the study [41] that showed a similar microbiota composition on titanium of different SR. The controversial views, above, may result from different kinds of biofilms, different incubation times and, most importantly, the different kind of titanium discs used. Some of these studies employed the commercially available ones provided by companies, and some of them employed titanium discs only for labs, which differed in more than just roughness. Marcos [40] also found no significant difference of succession kinetics of 23 microorganism species on titanium, with different Ra values, in 1, 3, 7, 14, and 21 days. Regardless, in manufacturing advanced implants, new surface treatment technology should be applied to establish a balance between osteoblast and oral bacterial attachment.

2.2. *Other Physical Characteristics*

The surface free energy (SFE) is related to the wettability of the material surface as an equivalent to the surface of a fluid. To determine the SFE, the contact angles (θ) are measured by three liquids differing in hydrophobicity on a specific surface [26]. A smaller contact angle implies higher SFE and higher surface hydrophilia of the material [33]. It has been reported that less biofilm formation occurred on RBC surfaces with low SFE, probably because of the similar hydrophilic properties between salivary pellicle and substratum surfaces [26,30]. The effects of SFE on biofilm formation may be inaccurate when Ra > 0.1 μm, and SR plays the primary role in biofilm accumulation, indeed. In other words, SFE influenced early adhesion of *Streptococcus mutans* (*S. mutans*) on super smooth surfaces (Ra $\leq$ 0.06 μm) [31].

The parameters of clinical dental materials influence on oral biofilms are intricate and co-occurring. Higher surface hydrophilia implies higher SFE, which induces more microorganism accumulation [33]. Also, the SR partially depends on inorganic filler size. Nanofilled RBCs wear by breaking out of individual primary particles. However, for microhybrid RBCs, the relatively soft matrix is worn before the fillers plucked out [29]. It is essential to control variables to study single parameters of clinical dental materials influencing oral biofilms.

3. Chemical Characteristics of Dental Materials

3.1. *Resin-Based Composite*

Resin-based dental materials have substantially evolved since they have been brought into the market, more than 60 years ago [2,42]. Resin-based composites, as a kind of versatile direct restorative materials, are widely used due to their excellent esthetic properties, improved mechanical characteristics, and ease of clinical handling [2,3]. Conventional RBCs are composed of four major components: a polymeric matrix, inorganic fillers, a silane coupling agent to produce a strong interface between the two phases mentioned, and initiators that induce or modulate the polymerization reaction [2]. Although the composite resin has been widely used in recent years, it has more biofilm accumulation, more frequent replacement, and shorter longevity, when compared with amalgam [43,44]. The failure of RBCs, mainly on account of secondary caries along the tooth–composite interfaces, is frequently related to biofilm formation on dental restorations [3,8].

Different kinds of components imply that the surface of a RBC is not a homogeneous interface, because of the distribution of physical-chemical phases with different chemical properties. The main base monomers of polymeric matrix used in commercial dental composites are Bis-GMA (bis-phenyl glycidyl dimethacrylate), Bis-EMA (bisphenol A ethoxylated dimethacrylate), PEGDMA (polyethylene glycol dimethacrylate), and UDMA (urethane dimethacrylate) with high viscosity, mixed with TEGDMA (triethylene glycol dimethacrylate) for dilution [2,31]. By tailoring RBC surfaces with either high carbon (matrix-rich) or high silicon (filler-rich) content from several commercially available RBCs without any antimicrobial agent, Ionescu et al. suggested that minimization of resin-matrix exposure might reduce biofilm formation on RBC surfaces because of the correlation between RBC surface carbon content and viable *S. mutans* biomass [26]. Recently, it was discovered that RBCs with a UDMA/aliphatic dimethacrylate matrix blend showed significantly higher biofilm formation on the surfaces than specimens with a Bis-GMA/TEGDMA matrix blend and analogous filler fraction, except for nanosized filler particles [45]. Another matrix, the silorane-based composite, was demonstrated to be less prone to *S. mutans* biofilm development compared with a generally used methacrylate-based composite, due to the increased hydrophobicity by silorane [46]. It was investigated that a reduced light-curing time can significantly increase the amount of unpolymerized monomers on the material surface, which might be responsible for increasing in vitro colonization on resin composite surfaces by *S. mutans* [47]. Kawai et al. reported that the specific resin components, a diglycidyl methacrylate and TEGDMA, significantly promoted glucosyltransferase (GTF) enzymes activity [48]. The GTF enzymes involved in the synthesis of water-insoluble glucan in situ entail an extracellular slime layer that promotes adhesion and the formation of dental plaque biofilms [49,50]. Consistently, the biodegradation byproduct (BBP) triethylene glycol (TEG), derived from methacrylate monomers, promotes the growth of *S. mutans* via upregulating the expression of glucosyltransferase B (*gtfB*) (involved in biofilm formation) and *yfiV* (a putative transcription regulator) in *S. mutans* [49]. Meanwhile, another BBP bishydroxypropoxyphenyl propane (BisHPPP) of Bis-GMA can also enhance the GTF enzyme activity of *S. mutans* biofilms, and modulate genes and proteins involved in biofilm formation, carbohydrate transport, and acid tolerance [51]. In conclusion, further studies are needed to explore the appropriate proportions of resin matrix and filler particles on the surface of RBCs, as well as to explore better ways to prevent resin biodegradation.

There are different sized inorganic fillers of the resin composites, including macrofill, microfill, nanofill, and hybrids. The RBC's strength and polishing ability mostly depend on the size and proportion of inorganic fillers [2]. Pereira et al. demonstrated the least biofilm formation on a nanofilled RBC (Filtek Z350™) compared with nanohybrid, microhybrid, and bulk-filled RBCs. The nanosized inorganic fillers could obtain the extensive distribution of the fillers and smoother composite surfaces after the same finishing and polishing procedures, consequently decreasing *S. mutans* adhesion [25,29,52]. Resin composites containing surface pre-reacted glass ionomer (S-PRG) filler have been reported to show less biofilm accumulation and reduced bacterial attachment. The pre-reacted glass-ionomer bioactive fillers have been fabricated by the acid–base reaction between a fluoroaluminosilicate glass and polyalkenoic acid in the presence of water. The antibacterial effects of S-PRG filler-containing resin composite is mainly attributed to release of BO_3^{3-} and F^-, and fluoride-recharging abilities [53,54]. Yoshihara et al. investigated that bioactive glass filler may promote bacterial adhesion because of the unstable surface integrity, releasing ions and dissolving, which results in rougher restoration surfaces [55].

Up to now, there is still a high secondary caries rate, probably because of relatively few commercially antibacterial resins materials applied in clinic. However, more and more experimental antibacterial components and materials have been produced in the lab [44,56–58], among which, 12-methacryloyloxydodecylpyridinium bromide (MDPB), fluoride, and nanoparticles, have been translated into clinical materials. Both experimental antibacterial materials and new commercial antibacterial materials will soon pioneer a new materials field [54,59,60].

These experimental findings (Table 1) suggest that biofilm formation is influenced by the surface chemical composition of the material, including filler size, shape, and distribution, as well as matrix composition.

Table 1. The effect of the resin-based composites on biofilm formation.

Author, Year	Resin-Based Composite	Brief	Ref.
Ionescu et al., 2012	Filtek Supreme XT; Filtek Silorane™; Grandio	The proportions of resin matrix and filler particles on the surface of resin-based composite strongly influence biofilm formation in vitro.	[26]
Brambilla et al., 2016	Filtek Silorane™; Filtek Z250™	Silorane-based composite is less prone to *S. mutans* biofilm development.	[46]
Brambilla et al., 2009	Filtek Z250™	Unpolymerized monomers on the material surface are responsible for increasing in vitro colonization by *S. mutans*.	[47]

Table 1. *Cont.*

Author, Year	Resin-Based Composite	Brief	Ref.
Kawai et al., 2000	Clearfil F II; Silux	The diglycidyl methacrylate and TEGDMA significantly promoted GTF enzymes activity	[48]
Pereira et al., 2011	Filtek Z 350™; Esthet X™; Vit-l-escence™	The least biofilm forms on a nanofilled RBC compared with nanohybrid, microhybrid, and bulk-filled RBCs.	[52]
Hahnel et al., 2014	Beautifil II	The inclusion of S-PRG fillers may reduce biofilm formation on resin composite.	[53]
Yoshihara et al., 2017	Beautifil ll; Herculite XRV Ultra	Bioactive glass filler may promote bacterial adhesion because of unstable surface integrity, releasing ions and dissolving.	[53]

3.2. Glass Ionomer Cements

Glass ionomer cements (GICs), applied as direct restorative materials and cements, feature some desirable characters, such as a chemical adhesion to enamel and dentin, and the ability to release fluoride over time [4]. It is well known that conventional GICs have biological effects and caries-inhibiting properties because of the release of surface fluoride ions [61].

Recently, many studies have reported that the fluoride of GICs can affect the acid production, acid tolerance, and extracellular polymetric substance (EPS) formation of dental plaques, especially cariogenic biofilms, such as *S. mutans* biofilms. The fluoride can reduce the proportion of *S. mutans* but increase *S. oralis* (*Streptococcus oralis*) in the dual-species biofilm, subsequently inhibiting the formation of cariogenic bacteria-dominant biofilms [62]. This phenomenon lasts during both the initial rapid and second slow release phases, which is called the biphasic pattern of fluoride release of GICs [63–66]. The release of fluoride showed a significant dependence on the experimental conditions applied, such as sterile broth, bacteria, and acid. The bacterial condition leads to the highest decrease in the release of fluoride, which can be explained by the extracellular matrix of biofilm serving as a layer that modulates the release of fluoride from the substratum materials. Furthermore, the acidic conditions can enhance the constant release of fluoride, due to its high bioavailability at low pH [67]. The result agreed with Jennifer's study, that more fluoride is released at pH 4, the acidic and cariogenic pH, than at pH 5.5 or pH 7, when these ions are most needed to inhibit caries [68]. It can be concluded that the efficiency of fluoride ions depends not only on their amount, but also on the pH value of the material during setting.

Acidic conditions promote the free fluoride ions to be released and form a weak electrolyte, hydrogen fluoride (HF, unionized fluoride) [66], and the combination of F-/HF and enzymes can modulate bacterium metabolism [69]. Adjacent to GIC restorations, an anti-caries environment is established by the fluoride, which may inhibit acidic pH efficiently due to the relatively high pKa value, 3.15, of hydrogen fluoride (HF) in vivo [70], by affecting bacterial metabolism (Figure 2), both directly (e.g., inhibition of enolase and ATPase) and indirectly (e.g., intracellular acidification) [71]. In addition, the aluminum released from Vitremer plays a vital role in inhibiting bacterial metabolism and has a synergistic effect with fluoride [71,72].

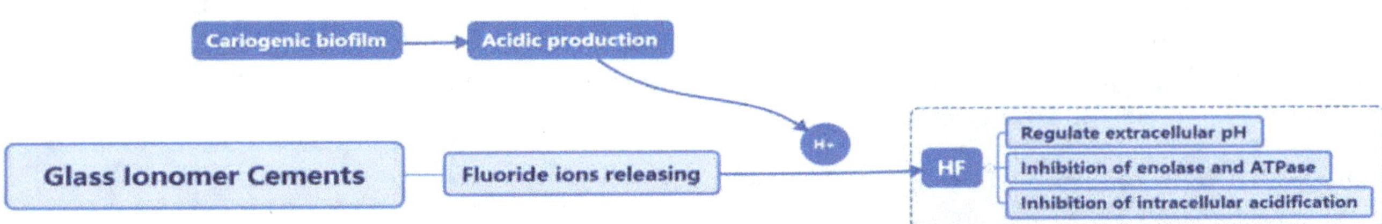

Figure 2. The relationship between fluoride of glass ionomer cements and bacterial metabolism.

Although the acid conditions of biofilms can promote fluoride release to inhibit biofilm formation, the microbial environment changes the morphology of GICs, and accelerates material aging (Figure 3). Meanwhile, the changed morphology and increased roughness can enhance the initial bacterial attachment and oral biofilm formation [17]. To demonstrate the actual effects on biofilm formation of dental material in a pragmatic way, the study models evolved consistently, from the previous water aging model to a biological aging model, from a primary caries animal model to a secondary caries animal model, and from in vitro to the in situ model used nowadays [73–75].

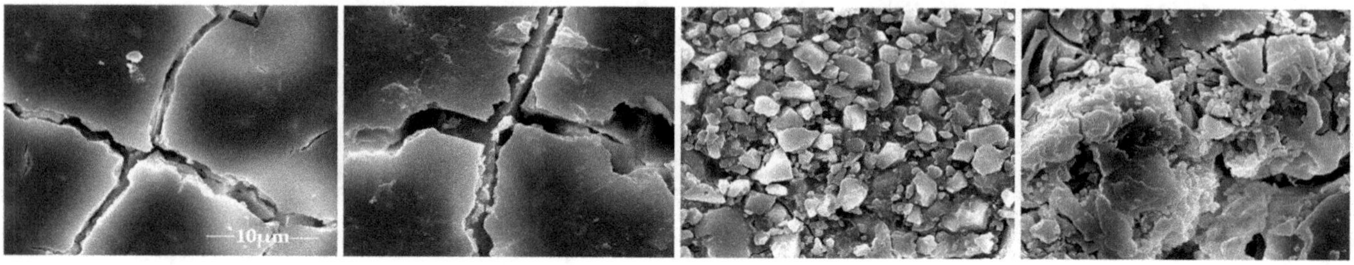

A B C D

Figure 3. Representative SEM images of glass ionomer cement (GIC) surfaces before and after aging treatments. **A**: without any aging treatments; **B**: the GICs were immersed in water; **C**: *S. mutans* suspensions; **D**: salivary microbes' suspensions.

3.3. *Amalgams*

Over its long clinical history, dental amalgams have evolved and served the profession successfully and at low cost. Amalgam restorations are being phased out because of the environmental pollution and inferior esthetic appearance [1]. However, they cannot be replaced by other restoratives because of their perfect mechanical properties, longevity, and low cost [15]. The longevity of amalgam is inseparable from the lower incidence of secondary caries caused by oral biofilms.

After clinical placement, amalgam restorations undergo a series of corrosion to release a variety of metallic ions in oral cavities. It was discovered that the mercury of amalgams could deposit in the dental plaque for up to 2 μg in 24 h, whereas the aged amalgams released little mercury because of the presence of the formed passive tarnish layer on the surface of amalgams [76]. In the 1980s, the amalgam was proved to have bacteriostatic and bactericidal properties due to the metallic ions being released from the surface of the materials, such as Ag, Cu, Sn, and Hg [77]. The low biomass of oral biofilms on amalgam surfaces is probably a result of the release of toxic ions from amalgam, which mainly consists of Hg and Ag [69]. Specifically, amalgam showed lasting inhibition of both *S. mutans* and *Actinomyces viscosus* (*A. viscosus*) which played crucial roles in biofilm formation [78]. Morrier et al. investigated that the order of antimicrobial potential of elements in amalgams would be Hg > Cu > Zn, by testing a suspension of *S. mutans* and *A. viscosus* [79]. Among those metallic ions, Cu^{2+} and Zn^{2+} showed synergistic effects on the reduction in acid production in dental biofilm [80]. Amalgam also showed a robust acid-buffering ability, which can neutralize bacteria-produced acids of oral biofilm by increasing the start pH of all solutions to around 7 to 8. This should be attributed to the release of corrosion products on the amalgams surface. The tin and copper oxides are amphoteric compounds that react as a base in acidic conditions [81]. This can be related to the fact that biofilms accumulated more on composites than amalgams in the clinic. Even in the in situ study, the amalgam showed, visually, a prevalence of non-viable cells forming small clusters distributed by the biofilm compared to other materials [69]. However, no research has yet explored the mechanisms of bacteriostatic and bactericidal properties of amalgam clearly.

3.4. *Dental Alloys of Indirect Restoration*

After 1975, the alloys for full-cast restorations, porcelain-fused-to-metal restorations, and removable partial denture frameworks, can be divided into three kinds, high-noble alloys (Au–Pt,

Au–Pd, Au–Cu–Ag–Pd), noble alloys (Au–Cu–Ag–Pd, Pd–Cu, Pd–Ag), and base-metal alloys (Ni–Cr, Co–Cr, Ti) [5]. Oral microbial metabolites, such as acids, sulfide, and ammonia, can induce the microbial corrosion of metallic materials [82]. Dental alloys corrode and release metal irons in the oral environment which may compromise material biocompatibility and mechanical properties, and lead to the esthetic loss of dental restorations, and influence health [83].

Among the noble alloys, a high gold content alloy (88% by weight), Captek™, showed a 71% reduction in total bacterial numbers when compared to natural tooth surfaces [84]. This could be attributed to the low porosity of high nobility gold inherent in the manufacturing process and the unique electrochemical corrosion resistance [85]. Besides, metallic copper and copper-containing alloys possess a strong and rapid bactericidal effect, named "contact killing". This was induced by successive membrane damage, oxidative damage, cell death, and DNA degradation [20,86]. The surface-released free copper ions are toxic to bacteria because of their soft ionic character and their thiophilicity [86,87]. As for the base-metal alloys, a higher amount of viable microbial cells and biofilm density on prosthetic structures based on cobalt–chromium (Co–Cr) alloys was demonstrated, when compared to those based on titanium [21,88]. Mystkowska found that there were more corrosion pits on cobalt alloys than on titanium alloys [88], and that these corrosion pits increase the surfaces roughness of dental alloys, which may facilitate the subsequent accumulation of biofilm [82]. However, there was a significant increase in biofilm density and number of microbial cells of biofilm growing on both titanium and Co–Cr alloy, from 24 up to 48 h [21]. The acid produced by microorganisms induces the corrosion of Cr_2O_3 and TiO_2, the passive films, which are responsible for corrosion resistance and biocompatibility of the alloys [82,89–91] (Table 2).

Table 2. The influence of different dental alloys on the biofilm formation.

Author, Year	Resin-Based Composite	Brief	Ref.
Zappala et al., 1996	Gold alloy	High-noble alloys showed a significant reduction in biofilm because of the low porosity and unique electrochemical corrosion resistance.	[85]
Grass et al., 2011	Metallic copper	Metallic copper processes strong and rapid bactericidal effect, named "contact killing".	[20]
Mystkowska et al., 2016	Co–Cr-based alloy	Co–Cr alloys developed more pits and viable microbial cells than titanium alloys after degradation.	[88]
McGinley et al., 2013	Ni-based alloy	Ni-based dental casting alloys induced elevated levels of cellular toxicity compared with *S. mutans*-treated Co–Cr-based dental casting alloys.	[91]
Souza et al., 2013	Titanium	The presence of *S. mutans* colonies on the titanium negatively affected its corrosion resistance due to the titanium-passive film.	[21]

Zhang et al. discovered that corroded alloy surfaces could upregulate gene expression of the glucosyltransferase BCD, glucan-binding proteins B, fructosyltransferase, and lactate dehydrogenase in *S. mutans*, which play critical roles in bacteria adherence and biofilm accumulation [82]. Microorganisms of biofilm decrease the pH by producing acidic substances and dissolve the surface oxides of the dental alloys to reduce the corrosion resistance of the metal [92]. In turn, the changed surfaces of the dental alloys can accelerate the virulence gene expression and biofilm formation [82]. Therefore, this bacteria-adhesion and corrosion cycle can accelerate the corrosion process and, finally, induce failure of the dental alloys' restoration.

3.5. Ceramic

In recent years, adhesively cemented ceramic restorations, such as inlays/onlays, veneers, and crowns, have been used as the main approach for minimally invasive esthetic restorations in anterior and posterior teeth [93]. However, its clinical failure is related to a lot of factors, such as marginal misfit, surface irregularities, and cement excess, which may favor the accumulation of microorganisms, compromising clinical restoration longevity [94].

Both surface roughness and surface free energy have been found to influence initial microbial adherence decisively [40], due to compositional and microstructural differences, and bacterial colonization was thought to differ from one ceramic material to another. Sebastian [95] employed different kind of ceramics, glass/lithium disilicate glass/glass-infiltrated zirconia/partially sintered zirconia/hipped zirconia ceramic as the specimens, and the glass plates were used as a control. He found that the lithium disilicate glass ceramic had the highest values for Ra, whereas the lowest values were found for the glass ceramic, the partially sintered zirconia, and the hipped zirconia ceramic. Furthermore, salivary protein coating caused a significant increase in surface free energy and the polarity of these ceramics, except for the control material. However, after salivary protein coating, only the control material showed higher values for streptococcal adhesion than all ceramic materials. The same study [96], which was performed in vivo, demonstrated significant differences in biofilm formation with various types of dental ceramics. In particular, zirconia exhibited low biofilm accumulation. Thus, except for its high intensity, low biofilm accumulation makes zirconia a promising material for various indications. The different results of the two studies [95,96] may be related to the different models (in vitro, in vivo) they applied (Table 3).

Table 3. The influence of different ceramic on the biofilm formation.

Author, Year	Ceramic	Brief	Ref.
Hahnel et al., 2009	Glass, lithium disilicate glass, glass-infiltrated zirconia, partially sintered zirconia, hipped zirconia ceramic	Only slight and random differences in streptococcal adhesion were found between the various ceramic materials, and control material showed higher values for streptococcal adhesion than all ceramic materials.	[95]
Bremer et al., 2011	Veneering glass-ceramic, lithium disilicate glass-ceramic, yttrium-stabilized zirconia (Y-TZP), hot isostatically pressed (HIP) Y-TZP ceramic, and HIP Y-TZP ceramic with 25% alumina	The study in vivo showed significant difference in biofilm formation with various types of dental ceramics; especially zirconia exhibited low biofilm accumulation.	[96]
Kim et al., 2017	Commercially available ceramic materials: Vita Enamic, Lava Ultimate, Vitablocs Mark II, and Wieland Reflex	All materials, except for Vitablocs Mark II, promoted significantly greater biofilm growth.	[28]

3.6. Dental Implant

Over the last decades, the use of dental implants has become a common way of restoring dentition defect [6]. The implant survival rate reaches to 92.8–97.1% over a follow-up period of 10 years, but dental implants easily become infectious, due to oral pathogenic bacteria [12,13,97]. Two main etiologies of peri-implantitis are oral biofilms and occlusal overload [98], among which, oral biofilms developed on dental implants play a significant role in peri-implantitis' pathogenesis. The peri-implantitis can cause implant loss in the absence of prevention and therapy [99,100]. The implant may be attached by saliva, blood, and oral bacterial cells during and after the implant surgery, and bacterial cells attached to the abutment harm the surrounding gingiva. All the above-mentioned points would affect the healing and restoration following surgery [101].

We begin with the abutment, since pathogenic bacteria usually attach on it first, causing peri-implant mucositis [102]. Hence, peri-implant tissue inflammation, as a consequence of biofilms on abutments in the subgingival region, is currently considered as a major contributor to implant loss [103]. Avila [103] found that, in the case of saliva-derived biofilm, the number of cells and the density of the biofilm on ZrO_2 were lower than on titanium materials. Zirconia abutments have a lower possibility for bacterial attachment, which is similar to the study above [104,105], and some researchers thought that the surface free energy is more critical on zirconia abutment surfaces [106]. Cássio's [107] 16S rDNA sequencing results agreed with previous studies [108,109] that the titanium accumulated more biofilm and more species of microorganisms. Two studies [110,111] found that the early bacterial communities were low in genome counts at the very beginning of implant surgery for both the zirconia and titanium abutment materials. As time goes by, both materials showed similar microbial counts and diversity, the same as on teeth. The different results may be related to no criterion for these products and testing methods. Zirconia is used widely for its esthetic property nowadays, and maybe the zirconia abutment will replace the titanium abutment for the lower bacteria attachment. However, substantial evidence is needed to prove its excellent properties in microbiological field.

When the peri-implant mucositis progress to peri-implantitis, more attention should be paid to the implant surface (Figure 4). About implant surface treatment techniques, there are mainly four kinds of coating techniques: alumina coating, titanium plasma spraying (TPS), biomimetic calcium phosphate (CaP) coating and plasma sprayed hydroxyapatite (HA) coating [112]. The coating techniques contribute to critical positive effects of dental implant application. Most authors [113,114] agreed that a suitable coating technique may enhance the mechanical properties of the dental implants. However, these techniques have several limitations including poor long-term adherence of the coating to the substrate material [115], nonuniformity in thickness of the deposited layer, variations in crystallinity [116], and composition of the coating, which influence the biofilm formation on the surface [112] (Table 4). However, none of studies shows the single factor of different coating techniques so far, because different coating techniques are related to different surface characteristics, which we have discussed in other sections of this review, further studies about the coating techniques should be performed.

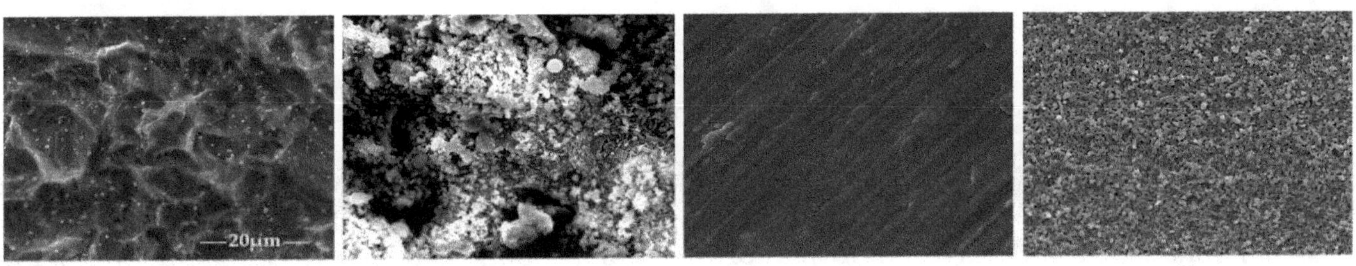

A B C D

Figure 4. Four kinds of titanium implant surface treatment show different SEM imagines. **A**: Sandblasting and acid etching technique (SLA); **B**: plasma sprayed hydroxyapatite coating (HA); **C**: machined treatment (machined); **D**: microarc oxidation (MAO).

It has been found out that, except for surface roughness and surface free energy [119], the type of the biomaterial itself can also influence biofilm formation and subsequent plaque accumulation on implant surfaces [21]. Two investigations have shown less inflammatory cells in the peri-implant soft tissue of zirconia in comparison with titanium or other metals [104,105]. Additionally, Zhao's [106] study showed that neither roughness nor hydrophobicity had a decisive influence on the biofilm formation that occurred on three different implant materials, comprising titanium (Ti, cold-worked, grade 4), titanium–zirconium alloy (TiZr, 15% (wt) Zr) and zirconium oxide (ZrO_2, Y-TZP). Same as Zhao's result, in the 3-species biofilm (*Streptococcus sanguinis*, *Fusobacterium nucleatum*, and *Porphyromonas gingivalis*), the analysis showed that there were no significant differences between titanium and zirconia in terms of total biofilm mass and metabolism. However, zirconia revealed significantly reduced plaque thickness. Regarding human plaque biofilms, microbiological techniques showed statistically significant reduction in biofilm formation for zirconia compared to titanium. The result suggested that not only surface roughness or surface hydrophilicity might be important factors for biofilm formation, but also material composition—metals compared to ceramics—suggesting a reduced disposition for peri-implant plaque and subsequent potential peri-implant infections on zirconia compared to titanium implant surfaces [32,120]. Nowadays, topography, surface charge, roughness, hydrophobicity, and chemistry have been investigated for many years. Besides, some new techniques have been studied, like nanoscale surface roughness, negatively charged surfaces, super hydrophilic surfaces and super hydrophobic surfaces, and they have all been demonstrated to reduce bacterial adhesion [32].

Table 4. The influence of different titanium surface treatments on the biofilm formation.

Author, Year	Different Titanium Surfaces	Brief	Ref.
Patrick et al., 2013	Machined, stained, acid-etched, or sandblasted/ acid-etched (SLA)	After the colonization for 2, 4, and 8 h, there seems no difference between these titanium discs. Up to 16.5 h, the SLA surface showed the highest trend for the bacterial colonization	[117]
Matos et al., 2011	Micro-arc oxidation (MAO), glow discharge plasma (GDP), machined, and sandblasted surfaces	The counts of *F. nucleatum* were lower for MAO treatment at early biofilm phase (16.5 h), while the plasma treatment did not affect the viable microorganism counts. Biofilm extracellular matrix was similar among these groups, except for GDP, with the lowest protein content.	[118]
Al-Ahmad et al., 2010	Machined titanium (Tim), modified titanium (TiUnite)	No significant differences in biofilm composition on the implant surfaces. Besides, the influence of roughness and material on biofilm formation was compensated by biofilm maturation	[35]
de Freitas et al., 2011	Machined, blasted, HA-coated	The titanium discs were put into volunteers' oral cavity and were tested after 1, 3, 7, 14, and 21 days. There was no statistically significant difference between the kinetics of bacterial species succession and the different surfaces.	[40]
Bevilacqua et al., 2018	Machined surface(M), laser-treated surface (LT), sandblasted surface (SB)	The biofilm developed in vivo for 1 day and 4 days showed no statistical difference between 3 kinds of discs. In vitro, when the biofilm was formed by *P. aeruginosa*, M showed less biomass and biofilm average thickness. As for the biofilm developed by mixed salivary bacteria, SB showed less biomass and average biofilm thickness.	[37]

4. Conclusions

As discussed in this review, bacterial adhesion and biofilm formation can be strongly influenced by surface characteristics of dental materials, which include chemical compositions, surface roughness, surface free energy, surface topography, ions release, and others. In conclusion, every possible particular chemical composition (organic matrix, inorganic filler, fluoride, and various metallic ions) can enhance or inhibit biofilm formation. Irregular topography and rough surfaces provide favorable interfaces for bacterial colonization, protecting bacteria against shear forces during their initial reversible binding and biofilm formation. Besides, the surface free energy, hydrophobicity, surfaces coating techniques also have a significant influence on oral biofilm.

However, the "ideal" surface characteristics have not been identified yet, and results have varied from different methods and models. One of the major drawbacks of current research is the limitation of the in vitro study. In vitro studies are not always able to completely simulate the complicated conditions presented in the oral environment. Thus, further in situ studies are much needed to clarify the role and mechanism of each surface parameter on oral biofilm formation. Finally, the goal is to produce robust, long-lasting dental materials which will reduce costly replacements and significantly ameliorate oral health.

Author Contributions: Y.H. and X.H. drafted the manuscript. X.Z., M.L., B.R., X.P., L.C. edited and added valuable insights into the manuscript. All authors read and approved the final manuscript.

Acknowledgments: This research was supported by The National Key Research Program of China 2017YFC0840100 and 2017YFC0840107 (L.C.), National Natural Science Foundation of China (81870759), the Youth Grant of the Science and Technology Department of Sichuan Province, China 2017JQ0028 (L.C.), Innovative Research Team Program of Sichuan Province (L.C.)

References

1. Shenoy, A. Is it the end of the road for dental amalgam? A critical review. *J. Conserv. Dent.* **2008**, *11*, 99–107. [CrossRef] [PubMed]
2. Ferracane, J.L. Resin composite—State of the art. *Dent. Mater.* **2011**, *27*, 29–38. [CrossRef] [PubMed]
3. Demarco, F.F.; Correa, M.B.; Cenci, M.S. Longevity of posterior composite restorations: Not only a matter of materials. *Dent. Mater.* **2012**, *28*, 87–101. [CrossRef] [PubMed]

4. Joel, H. Berg, Glass ionomer cements. *Pediatr. Dent.* **2002**, *24*, 430–438.
5. Wataha, J.C. Alloys for prosthodontic restorations. *J. Prosthet. Dent.* **2002**, *87*, 351–363. [CrossRef] [PubMed]
6. Renvert, S.; Quirynen, M. Risk indicators for peri-implantitis. A narrative review. *Clin. Oral Implants Res.* **2015**, *26*, 15–44. [CrossRef] [PubMed]
7. Laske, M.; Opdam, N.J.; Bronkhorst, E.M. Longevity of direct restorations in Dutch dental practices. Descriptive study out of a practice based research network. *J. Dent.* **2016**, *46*, 12–17. [CrossRef] [PubMed]
8. Delaviz, Y.; Finer, Y.; Santerre, J.P. Biodegradation of resin composites and adhesives by oral bacteria and saliva: A rationale for new material designs that consider the clinical environment and treatment challenges. *Dent. Mater.* **2014**, *30*, 16–32. [CrossRef] [PubMed]
9. Goodacre, C.J. Bernal, Guillermo, Rungcharassaeng, Kitichai,, Clinical complications in fixed prosthodontics. *J. Prosthet. Dent.* **2003**, *90*, 31–41. [CrossRef]
10. Toman, M.; Toksavul, S. Clinical evaluation of 121 lithium disilicate all-ceramic crowns up to 9 years. *Quintessence Int.* **2015**, *46*, 189–197. [CrossRef] [PubMed]
11. Layton, D. A critical appraisal of the survival and complication rates of tooth-supported all-ceramic and metal-ceramic fixed dental prostheses the application of evidence-based dentistry. *Int. J. Prosthodont.* **2011**, *24*, 417–427. [PubMed]
12. Albrektsson, T.; Donos, N. Implant survival and complications. In Proceedings of the Third EAO Consensus Conference, Pfäffikon, Schwyz, Switzerland, 15–18 February 2012; pp. 63–65.
13. Srinivasan, M.; Vazquez, L.; Rieder, P.; Moraguez, O. Survival rates of short (6 mm) micro-rough surface implants: A review of literature and meta-analysis. *Clin. Oral Implants Res.* **2014**, *25*, 539–545. [CrossRef] [PubMed]
14. Robertson, K.; Shahbazian, T.; MacLeod, S. Treatment of peri-implantitis and the failing implant. *Dent. Clin. N. Am.* **2015**, *59*, 329–343. [CrossRef] [PubMed]
15. Schwendicke, F.; Tu, Y.K.; Stolpe, M. Preventing and Treating Peri-Implantitis: A Cost-Effectiveness Analysis. *J. Periodontol.* **2015**, *86*, 1020–1029. [CrossRef] [PubMed]
16. Li, Y.; Carrera, C.; Chen, R.; Li, J. Degradation in the dentin-composite interface subjected to multi-species biofilm challenges. *Acta Biomater.* **2014**, *10*, 375–383. [CrossRef] [PubMed]
17. Park, J.W.; Song, C.W.; Jung, J.H. The effects of surface roughness of composite resin on biofilm formation of Streptococcus mutans in the presence of saliva. *Oper. Dent.* **2012**, *37*, 532–539. [CrossRef] [PubMed]
18. Cheng, L.; Zhang, K.; Zhang, N.; Melo, M.A.S.; Weir, M.D.; Zhou, X.D.; Bai, Y.X.; Reynolds, M.A.; Xu, H.H.K. Developing a New Generation of Antimicrobial and Bioactive Dental Resins. *J. Dent. Res.* **2017**, *96*, 855–863. [CrossRef] [PubMed]
19. Dewhirst, F.E.; Chen, T.; Izard, J. The human oral microbiome. *J. Bacteriol.* **2010**, *192*, 5002–5017. [CrossRef] [PubMed]
20. Grass, G.; Rensing, C.; Solioz, M. Metallic copper as an antimicrobial surface. *Appl. Environ. Microbiol.* **2011**, *77*, 1541–1547. [CrossRef] [PubMed]
21. Souza, J.; Mota, R.R.; Sordi, M.B.; Passoni, B.B. Biofilm Formation on Different Materials Used in Oral Rehabilitation. *Braz. Dent. J.* **2016**, *27*, 141–147. [CrossRef] [PubMed]
22. Teughels, W.; Van Assche, N.; Sliepen, I.; Quirynen, M. Effect of material characteristics and/or surface topography on biofilm development. *Clin. Oral Implants Res.* **2006**, *17*, 68–81. [CrossRef] [PubMed]
23. Wang, Z.; Shen, Y.; Haapasalo, M. Dental materials with antibiofilm properties. *Dent. Mater.* **2014**, *30*, e1–e16. [CrossRef] [PubMed]
24. Teranaka, A.; Tomiyama, K.; Ohashi, K. Relevance of surface characteristics in the adhesiveness of polymicrobial biofilms to crown restoration materials. *J. Oral Sci.* **2017**, *60*, 129–136. [CrossRef] [PubMed]
25. Cazzaniga, G.; Ottobelli, M.; Ionescu, A.C. In vitro biofilm formation on resin-based composites after different finishing and polishing procedures. *J. Dent.* **2017**, *67*, 43–52. [CrossRef] [PubMed]
26. Ionescu, A.; Wutscher, E.; Brambilla, E. Influence of surface properties of resin-based composites on in vitro Streptococcus mutans biofilm development. *Eur. J. Oral Sci.* **2012**, *120*, 458–465. [CrossRef] [PubMed]
27. Haralur, S.B. Evaluation of efficiency of manual polishing over autoglazed and overglazed porcelain and its effect on plaque accumulation. *J. Adv. Prosthodont.* **2012**, *4*, 179–186. [CrossRef] [PubMed]
28. Kim, K.H.; Loch, C.; Waddell, J.N.; Tompkins, G. Surface Characteristics and Biofilm Development on Selected Dental Ceramic Materials. *Int. J. Dent.* **2017**, *2017*, 7627945. [CrossRef] [PubMed]

29. Han, J.M.; Zhang, H.; Choe, H.S.; Lin, H.; Zheng, G.; Hong, G. Abrasive wear and surface roughness of contemporary dental composite resin. *Dent. Mater. J.* **2014**, *33*, 725–732. [CrossRef] [PubMed]
30. Curd, M.L.; Bollen, P.L. Marc Quirynen Comparison of surface roughness of oral hard materials to the threshold surface roughness for bacterial plaque retention: A review of the literature. *Dent. Mater.* **1997**, *13*, 258. [CrossRef]
31. Yuan, C.; Wang, X.; Gao, X. Effects of surface properties of polymer-based restorative materials on early adhesion of Streptococcus mutans in vitro. *J. Dent.* **2016**, *54*, 33–40. [CrossRef] [PubMed]
32. Song, F.; Koo, H.; Ren, D. Effects of Material Properties on Bacterial Adhesion and Biofilm Formation. *J. Dent. Res.* **2015**, *94*, 1027–1034. [CrossRef] [PubMed]
33. Cazzaniga, G.; Ottobelli, M.; Ionescu, A. Surface properties of resin-based composite materials and biofilm formation A review of the current literature. *Am. J. Dent.* **2015**, *28*, 311–320. [PubMed]
34. Frojd, V.; Chavez de Paz, L. In situ analysis of multispecies biofilm formation on customized titanium surfaces. *Mol. Oral Microbiol.* **2011**, *26*, 241–252. [CrossRef] [PubMed]
35. Al-Ahmad, A.; Wiedmann-Al-Ahmad, M.; Faust, J.; Bachle, M.; Follo, M.; Wolkewitz, M.; Hannig, C.; Hellwig, E.; Carvalho, C.; Kohal, R. Biofilm formation and composition on different implant materials in vivo. *J. Biomed. Mater. Res. B Appl. Biomater.* **2010**, *95*, 101–109. [CrossRef] [PubMed]
36. Dezelic, T.G.B.; Schmidlin, P.R. Multi-species Biofilm Formation on Dental Materials and an Adhesive Patch. *Oral Health Prev. Dent.* **2009**, *7*, 47–53. [CrossRef] [PubMed]
37. Bevilacqua, L.; Milan, A.; Del Lupo, V.; Maglione, M.; Dolzani, L. Biofilms Developed on Dental Implant Titanium Surfaces with Different Roughness: Comparison Between In Vitro and In Vivo Studies. *Curr. Microbiol.* **2018**, *75*, 766–772. [CrossRef] [PubMed]
38. Wennerberg, A.; Albrektsson, T. Effects of titanium surface topography on bone integration: A systematic review. *Clin. Oral Implants Res.* **2009**, *20* (Suppl. S4), 172–184. [CrossRef] [PubMed]
39. Da Silva, C.H.F.P.; Vidigal, G.M., Jr.; de Uzeda, M.; de Almeida Soares, G. Influence of Titanium Surface Roughness on Attachment of Streptococcus Sanguis: An in vitro study. *Implant Dent.* **2005**, *14*, 88–93. [CrossRef]
40. De Freitas, M.M.; da Silva, C.H.; Groisman, M.; Vidigal, G.M., Jr. Comparative analysis of microorganism species succession on three implant surfaces with different roughness: An in vivo study. *Implant Dent.* **2011**, *20*, e14–e23. [CrossRef] [PubMed]
41. Größner-Schreiber, B.; Teichmann, J.; Hannig, M.; Dörfer, C.; Wenderoth, D.F.; Ott, S.J. Modified implant surfaces show different biofilm compositions under in vivo conditions. *Clin. Oral Implants Res.* **2009**, *20*, 817–826. [CrossRef] [PubMed]
42. Pfeifer, C.S. Polymer-Based Direct Filling Materials. *Dent. Clin. N. Am.* **2017**, *61*, 733–750. [CrossRef] [PubMed]
43. Spencer, P.; Ye, Q.; Misra, A. Proteins, pathogens, and failure at the composite-tooth interface. *J. Dent. Res.* **2014**, *93*, 1243–1249. [CrossRef] [PubMed]
44. Zhang, N.; Melo, M.A.S.; Weir, M.D. Do Dental Resin Composites Accumulate More Oral Biofilms and Plaque than Amalgam and Glass Ionomer Materials? *Materials* **2016**, *9*, 888. [CrossRef] [PubMed]
45. Ionescu, A.; Brambilla, E.; Wastl, D.S. Influence of matrix and filler fraction on biofilm formation on the surface of experimental resin-based composites. *J. Mater. Sci. Mater. Med.* **2015**, *26*, 1–7. [CrossRef] [PubMed]
46. Brambilla, E.; Ionescu, A.; Cazzaniga, G.; Ottobelli, M. Influence of Light-curing Parameters on Biofilm Development and Flexural Strength of a Silorane-based Composite. *Oper. Dent.* **2016**, *41*, 219–227. [CrossRef] [PubMed]
47. Brambilla, E.; Gagliani, M.; Ionescu, A. The influence of light-curing time on the bacterial colonization of resin composite surfaces. *Dent. Mater.* **2009**, *25*, 1067–1072. [CrossRef] [PubMed]
48. Kawai, K.; Tsuchitani, Y. Effects of resin composite components on glucosyltransferase of cariogenic bacterium. *J. Biomed. Mater. Res.* **2000**, *51*, 123–127. [CrossRef]
49. Khalichi, P.; Singh, J.; Cvitkovitch, D.G. The influence of triethylene glycol derived from dental composite resins on the regulation of Streptococcus mutans gene expression. *Biomaterials* **2009**, *30*, 452–459. [CrossRef] [PubMed]
50. Bowen, W.H.; Koo, H. Biology of Streptococcus mutans-derived glucosyltransferases: Role in extracellular matrix formation of cariogenic biofilms. *Caries Res.* **2011**, *45*, 69–86. [CrossRef] [PubMed]

51. Sadeghinejad, L.; Cvitkovitch, D.G.; Siqueira, W.L. Mechanistic, genomic and proteomic study on the effects of BisGMA-derived biodegradation product on cariogenic bacteria. *Dent. Mater.* **2017**, *33*, 175–190. [CrossRef] [PubMed]
52. Pereira, C.A.; Eskelson, E.; Cavalli, V. Streptococcus mutansBiofilm Adhesion on Composite Resin Surfaces After Different Finishing and Polishing Techniques. *Oper. Dent.* **2011**, *36*, 311–317. [CrossRef] [PubMed]
53. Hahnel, S.; Wastl, D.S. Streptococcus mutans biofilm formation and release of fluoride from experimental resin-based composites depending on surface treatment and S-PRG filler particle fraction. *J. Adhes. Dent.* **2014**, *16*, 313–321. [CrossRef] [PubMed]
54. Miki, S.; Kitagawa, H.; Kitagawa, R. Antibacterial activity of resin composites containing surface pre-reacted glass-ionomer (S-PRG) filler. *Dent. Mater.* **2016**, *32*, 1095–1102. [CrossRef] [PubMed]
55. Yoshihara, K.; Nagaoka, N.; Maruo, Y. Bacterial adhesion not inhibited by ion-releasing bioactive glass filler. *Dent. Mater.* **2017**, *33*, 723–734. [CrossRef] [PubMed]
56. Liang, J.; Li, M.; Ren, B.; Wu, T. The anti-caries effects of dental adhesive resin influenced by the position of functional groups in quaternary ammonium monomers. *Dent. Mater.* **2018**, *34*, 400–411. [CrossRef] [PubMed]
57. Khurshid, Z.; Naseem, M.; Sheikh, Z.; Najeeb, S. Oral antimicrobial peptides: Types and role in the oral cavity. *Saudi Pharm. J.* **2016**, *24*, 515–524. [CrossRef] [PubMed]
58. Ge, Y.; Wang, S.; Zhou, X.; Wang, H.; Xu, H.H.; Cheng, L. The Use of Quaternary Ammonium to Combat Dental Caries. *Materials* **2015**, *8*, 3532–3549. [CrossRef] [PubMed]
59. Carlo, H.L.; Bonan, P.R.F.; Franklin, G.G. In vitro effect of S. mutans biofilm on fluoride/MDPB-containing adhesive system bonded to caries-affected primary dentin. *Am. J. Dent.* **2014**, *37*, 227–232.
60. Khurshid, Z.; Zafar, M.; Qasim, S.; Shahab, S. Advances in Nanotechnology for Restorative Dentistry. *Materials* **2015**, *8*, 717–731. [CrossRef] [PubMed]
61. Kramer, N.; Schmidt, M.; Lücker, S. Glass ionomer cement inhibits secondary caries in an in vitro biofilm model. *Clin. Oral Investig.* **2018**, *22*, 1019–1031. [CrossRef] [PubMed]
62. Jung, J.E.; Cai, J.N.; Cho, S.D. Influence of fluoride on the bacterial composition of a dual-species biofilm composed of Streptococcus mutans and Streptococcus oralis. *Biofouling* **2016**, *32*, 1079–1087. [CrossRef] [PubMed]
63. Neilands, J.; Troedsson, U.; Sjodin, T.; Davies, J.R. The effect of delmopinol and fluoride on acid adaptation and acid production in dental plaque biofilms. *Arch. Oral Biol.* **2014**, *59*, 318–323. [CrossRef] [PubMed]
64. Pandit, S.; Kim, H.J.; Song, K.Y.; Jeon, J.G. Relationship between fluoride concentration and activity against virulence factors and viability of a cariogenic biofilm: In vitro study. *Caries Res.* **2013**, *47*, 539–547. [CrossRef] [PubMed]
65. Chau, N.P.; Pandit, S.; Jung, J.-E. Long-term anti-cariogenic biofilm activity of glass ionomers related to fluoride release. *J. Dent.* **2016**, *47*, 34–40. [CrossRef] [PubMed]
66. Mayanagi, G.; Igarashi, K.; Washio, J.; Domon-Tawaraya, H.; Takahashi, N. Effect of fluoride-releasing restorative materials on bacteria-induced pH fall at the bacteria–material interface: An in vitro model study. *J. Dent.* **2014**, *42*, 15–20. [CrossRef] [PubMed]
67. Hahnel, S.; Ionescu, A.C.; Cazzaniga, G.; Ottobelli, M.; Brambilla, E. Biofilm formation and release of fluoride from dental restorative materials in relation to their surface properties. *J. Dent.* **2017**, *60*, 14–24. [CrossRef] [PubMed]
68. Moreau, J.L.; Xu, H.H. Fluoride releasing restorative materials: Effects of pH on mechanical properties and ion release. *Dent. Mater.* **2010**, *26*, e227–e235. [CrossRef] [PubMed]
69. Padovani, G.C.; Fucio, S.B.; Ambrosano, G.M.; Correr-Sobrinho, L.; Puppin-Rontani, R.M. In situ bacterial accumulation on dental restorative materials. CLSMCOMSTAT analysis. *Am. J. Dent.* **2016**, *28*, 3–8.
70. Nakajo, K.; Takahashi, Y.; Kiba, W.; Imazato, S.; Takahashi, N. Fluoride ion released from glass-ionomer cement is responsible to inhibit the acid production of caries-related oral streptococci. *Interface Oral Health Sci.* **2007**, *25*, 263–264. [CrossRef]
71. Hayacibara, M.F.; Rosa, O.P.; Koo, H. Effects of fluoride and aluminum from ionomeric materials on S. mutans biofilm. *J. Dent. Res.* **2003**, *82*, 267–271. [CrossRef] [PubMed]
72. Fucio, S.B.; Paula, A.B.; Sardi, J.C.O. Streptococcus Mutans Biofilm Influences on the Antimicrobial Properties of Glass Ionomer Cements. *Braz. Dent. J.* **2016**, *27*, 681–687. [CrossRef] [PubMed]

73. Zhou, X.; Wang, S.; Peng, X.; Hu, Y.; Ren, B. Effects of water and microbial-based aging on the performance of three dental restorative materials. *J. Mech. Behav. Biomed. Mater.* **2018**, *80*, 42–50. [CrossRef] [PubMed]
74. Wu, T.; Li, B.; Zhou, X.; Hu, Y.; Zhang, H. Evaluation of Novel Anticaries Adhesive in a Secondary Caries Animal Model. *Caries Res.* **2018**, *52*, 14–21. [CrossRef] [PubMed]
75. Xue, Y.; Lu, Q.; Tian, Y.; Zhou, X. Effect of toothpaste containing arginine on dental plaque-A randomized controlled in situ study. *J. Dent.* **2017**, *67*, 88–93. [CrossRef] [PubMed]
76. Lyttle, H.A.; Bowden, G.H. The level of mercury in human dental plaque and interaction in vitro between biofilms of Streptococcus mutans and dental amalgam. *J. Dent. Res.* **1993**, *72*, 1320–1324. [CrossRef] [PubMed]
77. Morrier, J.J.; Barsotti, O.; Blanc-Benon, J.; Rocca, J.P.; Dumont, J. Antibacterial properties of five dental amalgams an in vitro study. *Dent. Mater.* **1989**, *5*, 310–313. [CrossRef]
78. Beyth, N.; Domb, A.J.; Weiss, E.I. An in vitro quantitative antibacterial analysis of amalgam and composite resins. *J. Dent.* **2007**, *35*, 201–206. [CrossRef] [PubMed]
79. Morrier, J.J.; Suchett-Kaye, G.; Nguyen, D.; Rocca, J.P.; Blanc-Benon, J.; Barsotti, O. Antimicrobial activity of amalgams, alloys and their elements and phases. *Dent. Mater.* **1998**, *5*, 310–313. [CrossRef]
80. Afseth, J.; Oppermann, R.V.; Rolla, G. Thein vivoeffect of glucose solutions containing Cu^{++} and Zn^{++} on the acidogenicity of dental plaque. *Acta Odontol. Scand.* **2009**, *38*, 229–233. [CrossRef]
81. Nedeljkovic, I.; De Munck, J.; Slomka, V. Lack of Buffering by Composites Promotes Shift to More Cariogenic Bacteria. *J. Dent. Res.* **2016**, *95*, 875–881. [CrossRef] [PubMed]
82. Zhang, S.; Qiu, J.; Ren, Y. Reciprocal interaction between dental alloy biocorrosion and Streptococcus mutans virulent gene expression. *J. Mater. Sci. Mater. Med.* **2016**, *27*, 78. [CrossRef] [PubMed]
83. Lu, C.; Zheng, Y.; Zhong, Q. Corrosion of dental alloys in artificial saliva with Streptococcus mutans. *PLoS ONE* **2017**, *12*, e0174440. [CrossRef] [PubMed]
84. Goodson, J.M.; Shoher, I.; Imber, S.; Som, S.; Nathanson, D. Reduced dental plaque accumulation on composite gold alloy margins. *J. Periodontal Res.* **2001**, *36*, 252–259. [CrossRef] [PubMed]
85. Zappala, C.; Shoher, I.; Battaini, P. Microstructural Aspects of the Captek™ Alloy for PorcelainFused-to-Metal Restorations. *J. Esthet. Dent.* **1996**, *8*, 151. [CrossRef] [PubMed]
86. HansSalima, M. Physicochemical properties of copper important for its antibacterial activity and development of a unified model. *Biointerphases* **2016**, *11*, 018902. [CrossRef]
87. Molteni, C.; Abicht, H.K.; Solioz, M. Killing of bacteria by copper surfaces involves dissolved copper. *Appl. Environ. Microbiol.* **2010**, *76*, 4099–4101. [CrossRef] [PubMed]
88. Mystkowska, J. Biocorrosion of dental alloys due to Desulfotomaculum nigrificans bacteria. *Acta Bioeng. Biomech.* **2016**, *18*, 87–96. [CrossRef] [PubMed]
89. Ward, B.C.; Webster, T.J. The effect of nanotopography on calcium and phosphorus deposition on metallic materials in vitro. *Clin. Oral Implants Res.* **2006**, *27*, 3064–3074. [CrossRef] [PubMed]
90. Souza, J.C.; Ponthiaux, P. Corrosion behaviour of titanium in the presence of Streptococcus mutans. *J. Dent.* **2013**, *41*, 528–534. [CrossRef] [PubMed]
91. McGinley, E.L.; Dowling, A.H.; Moran, G.P. Influence of S. mutans on base-metal dental casting alloy toxicity. *J. Dent. Res.* **2013**, *92*, 92–97. [CrossRef] [PubMed]
92. Lucchetti, M.C.; Fratto, G.; Valeriani, F. Cobalt-chromium alloys in dentistry: An evaluation of metal ion release. *J. Prosthet. Dent.* **2015**, *114*, 602–608. [CrossRef] [PubMed]
93. Pereira, S.; Anami, L.C.; Pereira, C.A. Bacterial Colonization in the Marginal Region of Ceramic Restorations: Effects of Different Cement Removal Methods and Polishing. *Oper. Dent.* **2016**, *41*, 642–654. [CrossRef] [PubMed]
94. Anami, L.C.; Pereira, C.A.; Guerra, E. Morphology and bacterial colonisation of tooth/ceramic restoration interface after different cement excess removal techniques. *J. Dent.* **2012**, *40*, 742–749. [CrossRef] [PubMed]
95. Hahnel, S.; Rosentritt, M.; Handel, G. Surface characterization of dental ceramics and initial streptococcal adhesion in vitro. *Dent. Mater.* **2009**, *25*, 969–975. [CrossRef] [PubMed]
96. Bremer, F.; Grade, S.; Kohorst, P.; Stiesch, M. In vivo biofilm formation on different dental ceramics. *Quintessence Int.* **2011**, *42*, 565. [PubMed]
97. Klinge, B.; Meyle, J. Peri-implant tissue destruction. The Third EAO Consensus Conference 2012. *Clin. Oral Implants Res.* **2012**, *23* (Suppl. S6), 108–110. [CrossRef] [PubMed]

98. Serino, G.; Strom, C. Peri-implantitis in partially edentulous patients: Association with inadequate plaque control. *Clin. Oral Implants Res.* **2009**, *20*, 169–174. [CrossRef] [PubMed]
99. Lindhe, J.; Meyle, J.; Group, D. Peri-implant diseases: Consensus Report of the Sixth European Workshop on Periodontology. *J. Clin. Periodontol.* **2008**, *35*, 282–285. [CrossRef] [PubMed]
100. Zitzmann, N.U.; Berglundh, T. Definition and prevalence of peri-implant diseases. *J. Clin. Periodontol.* **2008**, *35*, 286–291. [CrossRef] [PubMed]
101. Subramani, K.; Jung, R.E.; Molenberg, A.; Hämmerle, C.H. Biofilm on dental implants: A review of the literature. *Int. J. Oral Maxillofac. Implants* **2009**. [CrossRef]
102. De Avila, E.D.; Avila-Campos, M.J.; Vergani, C.E.; Spolidorio, D.M.; Mollo Fde, A., Jr. Structural and quantitative analysis of a mature anaerobic biofilm on different implant abutment surfaces. *J. Prosthet. Dent.* **2016**, *115*, 428–436. [CrossRef] [PubMed]
103. Elter, C.; Heuer, W.; Demling, A.; Hannig, M.; Heidenblut, T.; Bach, F.W.; Stiesch-Scholz, M. Supra- and subgingival biofilm formation on implant abutments with different surface characteristics. *Int. J. Oral Maxillofac. Implants* **2008**, *23*, 327–334. [PubMed]
104. Degidi, M.; Artese, L.; Scarano, A.; Perrotti, V.; Gehrke, P.; Piattelli, A. Inflammatory Infiltrate, Microvessel Density, Nitric Oxide Synthase Expression, Vascular Endothelial Growth Factor Expression, and Proliferative Activity in Peri-Implant Soft Tissues Around Titanium and Zirconium Oxide Healing Caps. *J. Periodontol.* **2006**, *77*, 73–80. [CrossRef] [PubMed]
105. Welander, M.; Abrahamsson, I.; Berglundh, T. The mucosal barrier at implant abutments of different materials. *Clin. Oral Implants Res.* **2008**, *19*, 635–641. [CrossRef] [PubMed]
106. Zhao, B.; van der Mei, H.C.; Subbiahdoss, G.; de Vries, J.; Rustema-Abbing, M.; Kuijer, R.; Busscher, H.J.; Ren, Y. Soft tissue integration versus early biofilm formation on different dental implant materials. *Dent. Mater.* **2014**, *30*, 716–727. [CrossRef] [PubMed]
107. Nascimento, C.; Pita, M.S.; Santos Ede, S.; Monesi, N.; Pedrazzi, V.; Albuquerque Junior, R.F.; Ribeiro, R.F. Microbiome of titanium and zirconia dental implants abutments. *Dent. Mater.* **2016**, *32*, 93–101. [CrossRef] [PubMed]
108. Do Nascimento, C.; Pita, M.S.; Pedrazzi, V. In vivo evaluation of Candida spp. adhesion on titanium or zirconia abutment surfaces. *Arch. Oral Biol.* **2013**, *58*, 853–861. [CrossRef] [PubMed]
109. Nascimento, C.D.; Pita, M.S.; Fernandes, F.H.N.C.; Pedrazzi, V.; de Albuquerque Junior, R.F.; Ribeiro, R.F. Bacterial adhesion on the titanium and zirconia abutment surfaces. *Clin. Oral Implants Res.* **2014**, *25*, 337–343. [CrossRef] [PubMed]
110. De Freitas, A.R.; Silva, T.S.O.; Ribeiro, R.F.; de Albuquerque Junior, R.F.; Pedrazzi, V.; do Nascimento, C. Oral bacterial colonization on dental implants restored with titanium or zirconia abutments: 6-month follow-up. *Clin. Oral Investig.* **2018**. [CrossRef] [PubMed]
111. Raffaini, F.C.; Freitas, A.R.; Silva, T.S.O.; Cavagioni, T.; Oliveira, J.F.; Albuquerque Junior, R.F.; Pedrazzi, V.; Ribeiro, R.F.; do Nascimento, C. Genome analysis and clinical implications of the bacterial communities in early biofilm formation on dental implants restored with titanium or zirconia abutments. *Biofouling* **2018**, *34*, 173–182. [CrossRef] [PubMed]
112. Jemat, A.; Ghazali, M.J.; Razali, M.; Otsuka, Y. Surface Modifications and Their Effects on Titanium Dental Implants. *Biomed. Res. Int.* **2015**, *2015*, 791725. [CrossRef] [PubMed]
113. Aparicio, C.; Rodriguez, D.; Gil, F.J. Variation of roughness and adhesion strength of deposited apatite layers on titanium dental implants. *Mater. Sci. Eng. C Mater. Biol. Appl.* **2011**, *31*, 320–324. [CrossRef]
114. San Thian, E.; Huang, J.; Barber, Z.H.; Best, S.M.; Bonfield, W. Surface modification of magnetron-sputtered hydroxyapatite thin films via silicon substitution for orthopaedic and dental applications. *Surf. Coat. Technol.* **2011**, *205*, 3472–3477. [CrossRef]
115. He, F.M.; Yang, G.L.; Li, Y.N. Early bone response to sandblasted, dual acid-etched and H2O2/HCl treated titanium implants: An experimental study in the rabbit. *Int. J. Oral Maxillofac. Surg.* **2009**, *38*, 677–681. [CrossRef] [PubMed]
116. Yang, C.Y.; Lee, T.M.; Lu, Y.Z.; Yang, C.W.; Lui, T.S.; Kuo, A.; Huang, B.W. The influence of plasma spraying parameters on the characteristics of fluorapatite coatings. *J. Med. Biol. Eng.* **2010**, *30*, 91–98.
117. Schmidlin, P.R.; Mueller, P.; Attin, T.; Wieland, M.; Hofer, D.; Guggenheim, B. Polyspecies biofilm formation on implant surfaces with different surface characteristics. *J. Appl. Oral Sci.* **2013**, *21*, 48–55. [CrossRef] [PubMed]

118. Matos, A.O.; Ricomini-Filho, A.P.; Beline, T.; Ogawa, E.S.; Costa-Oliveira, B.E.; de Almeida, A.B.; Nociti Junior, F.H.; Rangel, E.C.; da Cruz, N.C.; Sukotjo, C.; et al. Three-species biofilm model onto plasma-treated titanium implant surface. *Colloids Surf. B Biointerfaces* **2017**, *152*, 354–366. [CrossRef] [PubMed]
119. Al-Ahmad, A.; Wiedmann-Al-Ahmad, M.; Fackler, A.; Follo, M.; Hellwig, E.; Bachle, M.; Hannig, C.; Han, J.S.; Wolkewitz, M.; Kohal, R. In vivo study of the initial bacterial adhesion on different implant materials. *Arch. Oral Biol.* **2013**, *58*, 1139–1147. [CrossRef] [PubMed]
120. Roehling, S.; Astasov-Frauenhoffer, M.; Hauser-Gerspach, I.; Braissant, O.; Woelfler, H.; Waltimo, T.; Kniha, H.; Gahlert, M. In Vitro Biofilm Formation on Titanium and Zirconia Implant Surfaces. *J. Periodontol.* **2017**, *88*, 298–307. [CrossRef] [PubMed]

3

Antibacterial, Hydrophilic Effect and Mechanical Properties of Orthodontic Resin Coated with UV-Responsive Photocatalyst

Akira Kuroiwa [1], Yoshiaki Nomura [2,*], Tsuyoshi Ochiai [3,4,5], Tomomi Sudo [1], Rie Nomoto [6], Tohru Hayakawa [6], Hiroyuki Kanzaki [1], Yoshiki Nakamura [1] and Nobuhiro Hanada [2]

1 Department of Orthodontics, Tsurumi University School of Dental Medicine, Yokohama 230-8501, Japan; 2711005@stu.tsurumi-u.ac.jp (A.K.); sudo-tomomi@tsurumi-u.ac.jp (T.S.); kanzaki-h@tsurumi-u.ac.jp (H.K.); nakamura-ys@tsurumi-u.ac.jp (Y.N.)

2 Department of Translational Research, Tsurumi University School of Dental Medicine, Yokohama 230-8501, Japan; hanada-n@tsurumi-u.ac.jp

3 Photocatalyst Group, Research and Development Department, Local Independent Administrative Agency Kanagawa Institute of industrial Science and TEChnology (KISTEC), 407 East Wing, Innovation Center Building, KSP, 3-2-1 Sakado, Takatsu-ku, Kawasaki, Kanagawa 213-0012, Japan; pg-ochiai@newkast.or.jp

4 Materials Analysis Group, Kawasaki Technical Support Department, KISTEC, Ground Floor East Wing, Innovation Center Building, KSP, 3-2-1 Sakado, Takatsu-ku, Kawasaki, Kanagawa 213-0012, Japan

5 Photocatalysis International Research Center, Tokyo University of Science, 2641 Yamazaki, Noda, Chiba 278-8510, Japan

6 Department of Dental Engineering, Tsurumi University School of Dental Medicine, Yokohama 230-8501, Japan; nomoto-r@tsurumi-u.ac.jp (R.N.); hayakawa-t@tsurumi-u.ac.jp (T.H.)

* Correspondence: nomura-y@tsurumi-u.ac.jp

Abstract: Photocatalysts have multiple applications in air purifiers, paints, and self-cleaning coatings for medical devices such as catheters, as well as in the elimination of xenobiotics. In this study, a coating of a UV-responsive photocatalyst, titanium dioxide (TiO_2), was applied to an orthodontic resin. The antibacterial activity on oral bacteria as well as hydrophilic properties and mechanical properties of the TiO_2-coated resin were investigated. ultraviolet A (UVA) (352 nm) light was used as the light source. Antibacterial activity was examined with or without irradiation. Measurements of early colonizers and cariogenic bacterial count, i.e., colony forming units (CFU), were performed after irradiation for different time durations. Hydrophilic properties were evaluated by water contact angle measurements. While, for the assessment of mechanical properties, flexural strength was measured by the three-point bending test. In the coat(+)light(+) samples the CFU were markedly decreased compared to the control samples. Water contact angle of the coat(+)light(+) samples was decreased after irradiation. The flexural strength of the specimen irradiated for long time showed a higher value than the required standard value, indicating that the effect of irradiation was weak. We suggest that coating with the ultraviolet responsive photocatalyst TiO_2 is useful for the development of orthodontic resin with antimicrobial properties.

Keywords: orthodontic resin; photocatalyst TiO_2; antibacterial; cariogenic; early colonizer; hydrophilic properties; irradiation

1. Introduction

Maintenance of good oral hygiene after an active orthodontic treatment is one of the most important procedures. In general, after an active orthodontic treatment, moved teeth and jawbone are retained by acrylic resin based retainer [1]. The retainer is typically used for at least two years.

The longer the retainer is used, the more unhygienic it becomes. Gradually, micro-organisms colonize on the surfaces of retainers, just as on dentures, and they often cause stomatitis, dental caries, periodontal disease, chronic atrophic or candidiasis [2–11]. Porosities on the outer and inner surfaces of retainer also provide favorable conditions for microbial colonization [12]. Therefore, prevention of micro-organism colonization is essential for the maintenance of good oral hygiene and prevention of oral diseases.

Management of oral biofilm is important to maintain a good oral status. Common oral diseases, dental caries and periodontitis, are caused by an imbalance between biofilms and host defenses [13]. The initial process in the oral biofilm formation starts with pellicle, covering the tooth surface within a few minutes after mechanical cleaning. The pellicle plays a major role in the development and maintenance of bacterial communities. Then, the complex bacterial communities develop on the pellicle within a few days, and their components can be divided into two categories—early colonizers, and late colonizers [14]. Early colonizers that directly adhere to the pellicles are predominantly streptococci [15]. Streptococci constitute 60% to 90% of the bacteria that colonize on the teeth in the first 4 h after professional cleaning [16]. These species are mainly Gram-positive and have minor pathogenic effects on periodontal tissue. Late colonizers, such as *Fusobacterium nucleatum*, *Porphyromonas gingivalis*, *Tannerella forsythia*, *Treponema denticola*, and *Aggregatibacter actinomycetemcomitans* tend to be more pathogenic than the early colonizers. The late colonizers alone cannot form a biofilm on the tooth surface, but they form a biofilm by their parasitical adherence to the early colonizers [14].

In the formation of a biofilm it is inevitable that colonizing bacteria primarily adhere to the surface of the retainer [17]. Therefore, it is critical to prevent the bacteria from adhering to the retainers. As the orthodontic acrylic resin and denture base acrylic resin have similar requirements for clinical use (ISO 20795), the results for the denture base resin are also applicable for orthodontic acrylic resin. Various approaches have been employed for the prevention of microbial biofilms. These include dental disinfection, denture cleaner, mixing resin with antibacterial agents, and coating resin with antiseptic [6,18–32]. However, the biofilms are resistant to antibacterial and antifungals agents [33,34]. Moreover, a long-term use of denture cleanser corrodes metals such as clasps [35,36]. Denture cleanser affects the color stability of the denture base acrylic resin [37]. Mechanical cleaning with the adjunctive use of antimicrobial solutions is helpful in reducing biofilm growth or preventing its formation. However, such approaches rely primarily on a patient's compliance, and may be compromised in pediatric, geriatric, and handicapped individuals. Silver nanoparticles impregnated in acrylic resin make the appliance antibacterial, but releasing silver nanoparticles from the resin is a limiting factor [24,25,27,31]. Incorporating fluorine and silver ions into resin elutes antimicrobials but it is available only for the first few weeks [27]. Moreover, elution of antimicrobial agents may result in deterioration of the mechanical properties of the retainer over time. This reduction renders the appliance more susceptible to fracture, due to its low resistance to impact, low flexural strength, or low fatigue strength [38]. Hence, novel and alternative methods to prevent the micro-organism colonization are required.

Application of a photocatalyst is one of the effective and safe approaches to remove biofilm from the dentures or retainer [39,40]. Photocatalyst reaction is defined as a photocatalyst promoted reaction on a solid surface, usually a semiconductor [41]. Titanium dioxide (TiO_2) is the most studied photocatalyst [39,41–50]. TiO_2 is biocompatible, nontoxic, and inexpensive. TiO_2 generates reactive oxygen species (ROSs) upon ultraviolet A (UVA) irradiation, and its strong oxidative power decomposes micro-organisms and organic materials [33,42–44,46,50]. Further, the photocatalyst reaction can obtain superhydrophilic properties by UV irradiation, and superhydrophilicity prevents dirt accumulation on the device.

The purpose of the present study was to test the clinical applications TiO_2 coated orthodontic resin based retainer. To this end, we investigated the antibacterial effects as well as mechanical, and hydrophilic properties of acrylic based orthodontic resin coated with the photocatalyst TiO_2 after irradiation with UVA. Thus, we determined its clinical suitability for use as an orthodontic retainer material. First, we examined the effect of the orthodontic resin coated with TiO_2 on bacteria for various irradiation durations. Further, we investigated the antimicrobial effect against early colonizers, the bacteria which are first attached to the appliances. The effects on *S. mutans* and *S. sobrinus*, which are the most well-known cariogenic bacteria, were investigated. Second, mechanical properties of the orthodontic resin are evaluated by irradiating for about 2 years, which is the recommended usage period of the orthodontic retainer. Third, the hydrophilic properties were investigated as one of the photocatalytic effects. Acquiring hydrophilic properties by decreasing the contact angle could lead to the prevention of bacterial adhesion and a self-cleaning function.

2. Materials and Methods

Autopolymerizable orthodontic acrylic resin (Ortho Crystal, Nissin Co., Tokyo, Japan), which consisted of a liquid component and a powder component, was used for this study. In the following sections, autopolymerizable orthodontic acrylic resin are referred to as 'resin'.

2.1. Sample Preparation

According to the manufacturer's instructions, a powder-to-liquid ratio of 10 g:4.5 mL was used. Powder and liquid components were mixed under vibration for homogenization and removal of the trapped air. The slurry was poured into an aluminum open mold and pressed using a pair of glass plates to fabricate the specimens of different dimensions: 50 mm × 50 mm × 3.0 mm (n = 60), 50 mm × 50 mm × 3.0 mm (n = 20), and 64 mm × 10 mm × 3.5 mm (n = 35) for the antibacterial properties tests, photoinduced hydrophilic tests, and mechanical properties tests, respectively. The slurry resin was immediately transferred in the polymerization equipment for a dental technique at 40 °C (manufacturer's recommendation: 30–40 °C), and 0.25 MPa for 30 min to enhance curing (Fit Resin Multicure, Shofu Inc., Kyoto, Japan). Following preparation, each specimen was kept at room temperature in water for 12 h to eliminate the residual monomer. All test specimens were gradually grinded with waterproof polishing paper, having a grain size of approximately 30 μm (P500), 18 μm (P1000), and 15 μm (P1200). The specimens were then divided into four test groups for the assessment of the antibacterial properties and water contact angle measurement of base resin coated with thin film of photocatalytic TiO_2. Uncoated resin and non-lighted resin were used as control groups for their respective experimental group.

A spin-coating methods was used to apply ultraviolet-light-responsive photocatalytic titanium dioxide (UV-TiO_2) to the surface of the materials. The surface modification of the specimen with commercialized photocatalytic TiO_2 (NRC 350A and 360C, Nippon Soda Co., Ltd., Tokyo, Japan) was carried out by a sol-gel thin film spin-coating method according to the manufacturer's instructions. NRC 350A was coated to the surface of the materials. After coating, they were dried in a desiccator under 30 °C for 48 h. Then NRC 360Cwas coated, and dried in a desiccator in the same way. After the coating, the surface conditions of the materials were observed by a scanning electron microscope (SEM; JSM-5600LV, JEOL, Tokyo, Japan) at an accelerating voltage of 15 kV. Specimens were sputter-coated with Au prior to the SEM observations.

We covered samples with a glass to prevent drying, and irradiation was carried out from above. UVA from a black light source (wavelength: 352 nm, FL15BLB, Toshiba Co., Tokyo, Japan) was selected as the light source for catalytic excitation. The irradiation was performed at a distance of 10 cm (1.0 mW/cm^2 under the glass).

2.2. Bacterial Strains

Streptococcus mutans ATCC 25175 (*S. mutans*), *Streptococcus sobrinus* ATCC33478 (*S. sobrinus*), *Streptococcus gordonii* ATCC 10558 (*S. gordonii*), *Streptococcus oralis* ATCC 35037 (*S. oralis* ATCC), *Streptococcus oralis* GTC 276 (*S. oralis* GTC), *Streptococcus sanguinis* ATCC 10556 (*S. sanguinis*), and *Streptococcus mitis* MRS 08-31 (*S. mitis*) were used in this study. *S. mutans* and *S. sobrinus* are cariogenic bacteria. *S. gordonii*, *S. oralis* ATCC, *S. oralis* GTC, *S. sanguinis*, and *S. mitis* are the early colonizers. These bacterial species were inoculated into 4 mL of Tryptic Soy (TS) broth (Becton, Dickinson and Company, Sparks, MD, USA) and were cultured aerobically at 37 °C for 16 h. They were harvested by centrifugation at 3000× rpm for 15 min and then suspended with phosphate buffered saline (PBS) resulting in an optical density at 540 nm (OD_{540} equal to 1.0).

2.3. Antibacterial Test

A micro-organism suspension (500 μL) adjusted to $OD_{540} = 1.0$ was dropped directly on the surface of the coated and non-coated specimen on ice, and UV irradiation was performed for 0, 15, 30, 60, 90, 120, 150, and 180 min. After irradiation, each bacterial cell pellet was suspended in 1 mL PBS and subjected to serial 10-fold dilutions in PBS. The dilutions of each bacteria were inoculated on MS agar (Difico Mitis Salivarius Agar (semi-selective medium for streptococci); BD Biosciences, Flanklin Lakes, NJ, USA) in petri dishes with spiral plating equipment (Eddy Jet, IUL SA, Barcelona, Spain), and petri dishes were incubated under anaerobic conditions in an AnaeroPack-Anaero box (AnaeroPack System, Mitsubishi Gas Chemical Co., Inc., Tokyo, Japan) at 37 °C for 48 h. The number of colonies was counted in accordance with the spiral plater instruction manual. Each measurement was repeated three times.

2.4. Bending Test

The rectangular plates (64 mm × 10 mm × 3.5 mm) were immersed in distilled water at 37 °C for 0, 200, 400, 600, 800, 1000, 1200 h under UVA irradiation from a distance of 10 cm. The three-point bending test was conducted using a universal testing machine (EZ Test 500 N, Shimadzu Co., Kyoto, Japan) at a crosshead speed of 5 mm/min and a span length of 50.0 mm ($n = 5$). Then, load-displacement curves were plotted to measure bending strength, elastic modulus, and toughness. The test was conducted according to ISO20795-2 standard.

2.5. Water Contact Angle Measurement

The rectangular plates (50 mm × 50 mm × 3.0 mm) were prepared as indicated above and spin-coated with 125 μL of the experimental coating materials on each sample. The water contact angles were measured using a contact angle device (FTA125, First Ten Ångstroms, Portsmouth, VA, USA) at 25 °C. For surface analysis of the hydrophilic characteristics, 3.5 μL of deionized water (Milli-Q Plus system, Japan Millipore, Tokyo, Japan) was dropped on the surface, and video images were taken. Video images were automatically inputted to an attached computer in which the contact angles were measured using an image analysis program (FTA32 video, First Ten Ångstroms). Water contact angles were measured every 30 min for a period of 20 s at 25 °C.

2.6. Statistical Analysis

Antibacterial effects were analyzed by three factors: TiO_2 coating, presence of UVA, and irradiated time ($n = 3$). The significance of differences in the antibacterial effects was examined using three-way ANOVA or two-way ANOVA. Mechanical properties were examined using one-way ANOVA, with irradiated time included as a factor ($n = 5$). Tukey's HSD test was then used to determine the positions of significance. All statistical analyses were performed using IBM SPSS Statistics version 22.0 (IBM, Tokyo, Japan). A significance level of $p < 0.05$ was used.

3. Results

Antibacterial Test

The antimicrobial activity of the resin coated with TiO_2 was examined by bacterial count of the early colonizers and cariogenic bacteria under UV irradiation. Figure 1 shows the antibacterial activity of the TiO_2-coated resin surfaces against *S. gordonii* ATCC 10558, and *S. oralis* ATCC 35037 after irradiation. The coat(−)light(−) group was used as control group. The coat(+)light(−) group showed no significant differences compared with the control group. Hence, there was no effect with the coat alone. We also examined the activity with UV alone. Coat(−)light(+) induced a significant reduction in the number of colony. The number of *S. gordonii* was reduced from 1.6×10^7 colony-forming units/mL (CFU/mL) to 1.6×10^6 CFU/mL (after 120 min of UV irradiation), and that of *S. oralis* ATCC was reduced from 6.5×10^5 CFU/mL to 3.1×10^4 CFU/mL (after 90 min of UV irradiation). Consequently, about 90%, 95% colonies of *S. gordonii* and *S. oralis* ATCC were not formed on the coated plates upon irradiation (Figure 1A,B). On the other hand, coat(+)light(+) group showed a significant reduction in the CFU. The number of *S. gordonii* was reduced from 1.6×10^7 CFU/mL to 2.7×10^4 CFU/mL (after 120 min of UV irradiation) and that of *S. oralis* ATCC from 6.5×10^5 CFU/mL to 5.2×10^3 CFU/mL (after 90 min of UV irradiation). Thus, about 99.9% or more colonies of both *S. gordonii* and *S. oralis* ATCC were not formed on the coated plates upon irradiation (Figure 1A,B). Hence, coat(+)light(+) group showed a hundred times higher antibacterial effect, when compared with coat(−)light(+).

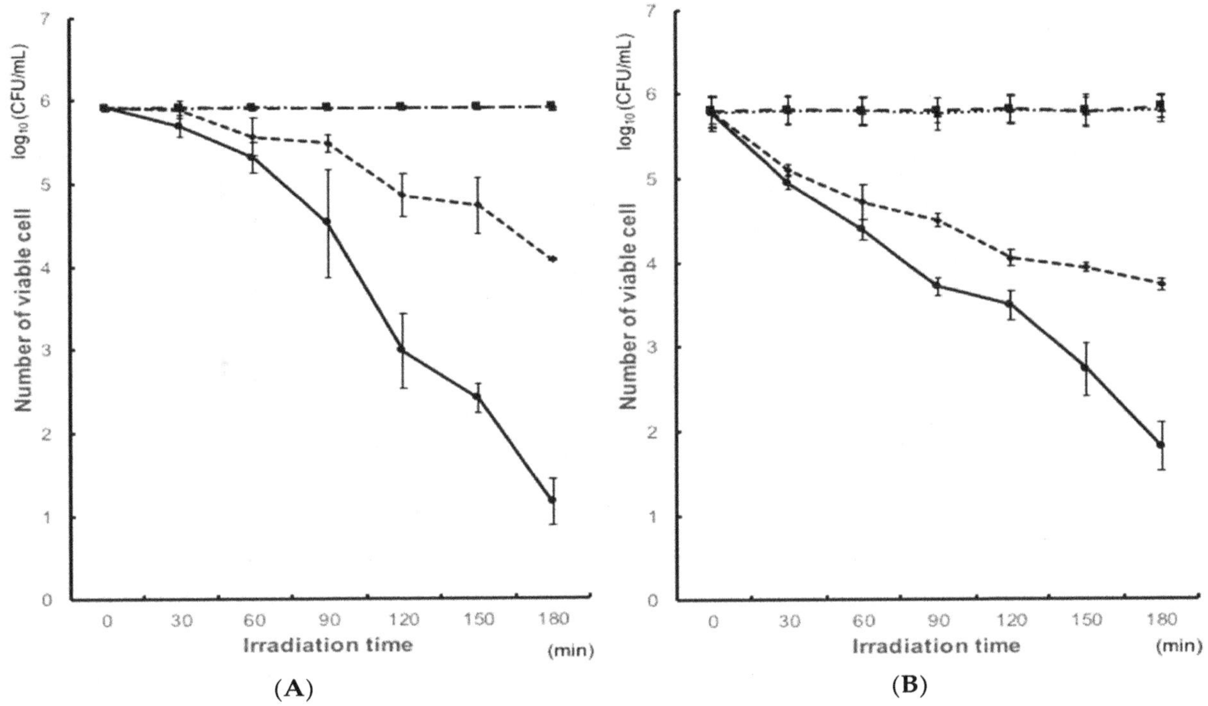

Figure 1. Antibacterial effects of TiO_2 photocatalysis against (**A**) *Streptococcus gordonii*; (**B**) *Streptococcus oralis* ATCC. coat(+)light(+): experiment group containing powdered TiO_2 with irradiation. coat(−)light(−): control group without both TiO_2 and irradiation. coat(+)light(−): experiment group in the presence of powdered TiO_2 without irradiation. coat(−)light(−): experiment group without TiO_2, but with irradiation.

Compared with the TiO_2-noncoated samples, TiO_2-coated samples showed a rapid decrease in the level of CFU of *Streptococcus gordonii*, particularly in the early stages (90 min and 120 min) of irradiation. Therefore, other strains were also examined at 90 and 120 min (Figure 2A,B). The cell viability on each sample before UV irradiation was set as 100%. The coat(+)light(+) clearly showed a great reduction in the cell viability. Cell viability was reduced to 0.2% for *S. sobrinus*, 0.9% for *S. oralis* GTC, 5.4% for *S. mutans*, and 9.9% for *S. sanguinis*. Clearly, the coat(+)light(+) samples exhibited the best antimicrobial performance in all microbes after 90 min UV irradiation. Similar results were observed even after 120 min of irradiation.

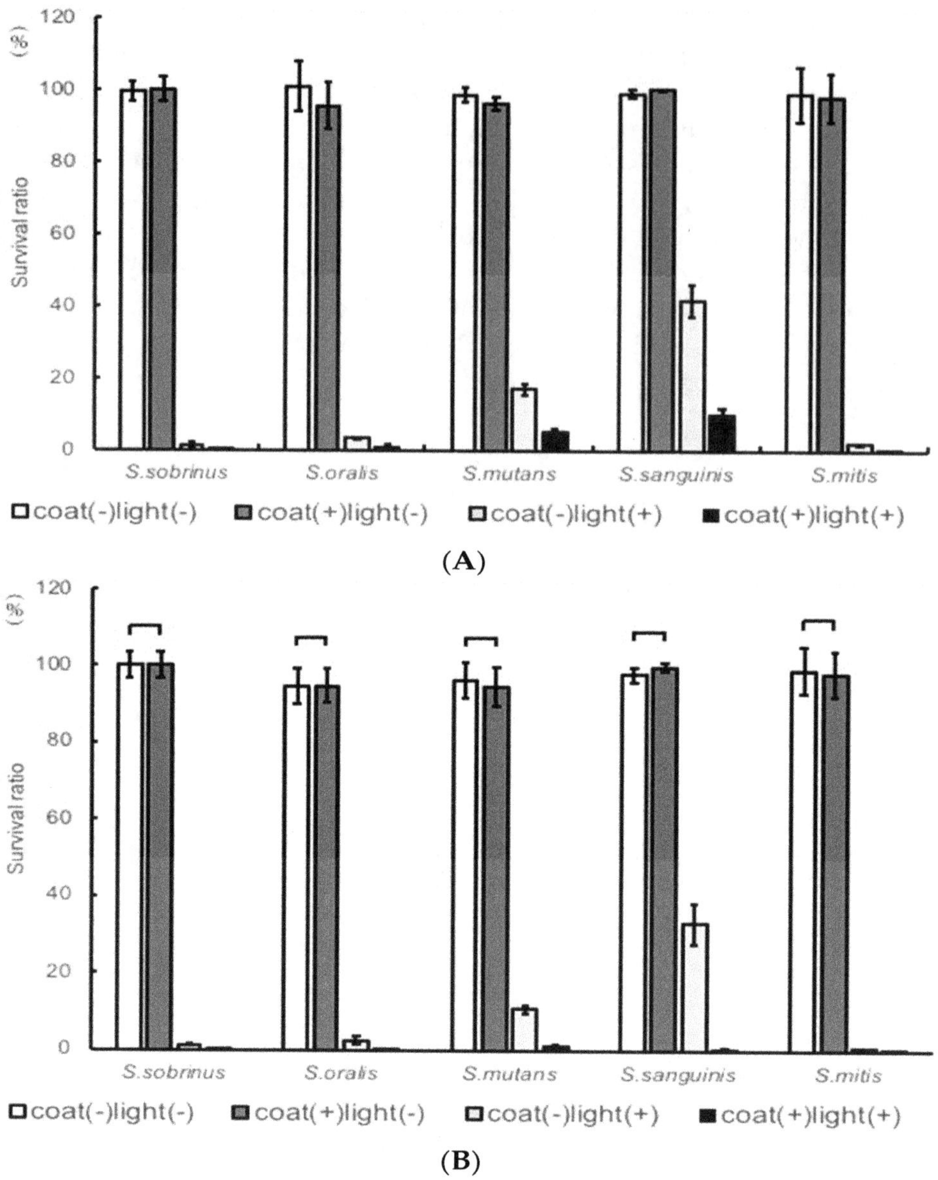

Figure 2. Antibacterial effects on various specimens of *Streptococcus sobrinus*, *Streptococcus oralis* GTC, *Streptococcus mutans*, and *Streptococcus sanguinis* at (**A**) 90 min, and (**B**) 120 min of ultraviolet A (UVA) irradiation.

Table 1 shows explanatory variables related to bacterial counts by three way ANOVA. The coefficients of bacterial counts in light(+) and interaction of light(+) and coat(+) were all negative. The coefficients of light(+) for *S. oralis* and *S. sobrinus* were higher than those by interaction of light(+) and coat(+). In contrast, the coefficients of light(+) of *S. gordonii*, *S. mutans*, and *S. sanguinis* were higher than those by interaction of light(+) and coat(+). The coefficient of both light(+) and interaction of light(+) and coat(+) of *S. mutans* was the highest in all the bacteria. The coefficient for irradiation time of 120 min were significantly different in all bacterial species. In all the bacteria, the coefficient of coat(+) was almost 0. On the other hand, the coefficient of light(+) and interaction of light(+) and coat(+) were statistically significant. These results indicated that the antibacterial effect of the photocatalyst was exerted by UVA irradiation. It also showed differences in susceptibility of oral bacteria to UVA.

Table 1. Models of three way ANOVA for changes in bacterial counts. *p*-values less than 0.05 were considered statistically significant.

		S. gordonii ATCC10558			*S. mitis*			*S. oralis* ATCC35037			*S. oralis GTC276*		
		Coefficient	95% CI	*p*-Value	Coefficient	95% CI	*p*-Value	Coefficient	95% CI	*p*-Value	Coefficient	95% CI	*p*-Value
Intercept		6.563	6.04–7.08	0.999<	8.267	7.57–8.96	0.999<	6.584	6.18–6.98	0.999<	8.840	8.30–9.37	0.999<
time	30 min	−0.061	−0.67–0.55	0.845	−0.306	−1.13–0.52	0.462	−0.372	−0.84–0.10	0.123	−0.498	−1.13–0.13	0.122
	60 min	−0.238	−0.85–0.37	0.444	−0.753	−1.57–0.07	0.073	−0.616	−1.09–−0.14	0.012	−0.700	−1.33–−0.06	0.031
	90 min	−0.458	−1.07–0.15	0.143	−1.246	−2.07–−0.42	<0.001	−0.846	−1.32–−0.37	<0.001	−0.877	−1.51–−0.24	<0.001
	120 min	−1.001	−1.61–−0.38	<0.001	−1.671	−2.49–−0.84	<0.001	−1.003	−1.47–−0.52	<0.001	−1.260	−1.89–−0.62	<0.001
	150 min	−1.175	−1.79–−0.55	<0.001	−1.935	−2.75–−1.10	<0.001	−1.231	−1.70–−0.75	<0.001	−1.576	−2.21–−0.94	<0.001
	180 min	−1.654	−2.27–−1.03	<0.001	−2.432	−3.25–−1.60	<0.001	−1.491	−1.96–−1.01	<0.001	−1.820	−2.45–−1,18	<0.001
coat(+)		−0.001	−0.46–0.46	0.996	−0.015	−0.63–0.60	0.963	0.017	−0.34–0.37	0.925	−0.008	−0.48–0.47	0.975
light(+)		−0.695	−1.16–−0.22	<0.001	−1.457	−2.08–−0.83	<0.001	−1.247	−1.60–−0.88	<0.001	−1.338	−1.81–−0.85	<0.001
interaction of light and coat		−1.216	−1.87–−0.55	<0.001	−1.845	−2.72–−0.96	<0.001	−0.727	−1.23–−0.21	0.006	−1.206	−1.88–−0.52	<0.001

		S. mutans			*S. sobrinus*			*S. sanguinis*		
		Coefficient	95% CI	*p*-Value	Coefficient	95% CI	*p*-Value	Coefficient	95% CI	*p*-Value
Intercept		5.609	5.38–5.83	0.999<	11.066	10.68–11.44	0.999<	9.280	8.90–9.65	0.999<
time	30 min	−0.119	−0.38–0.14	0.376	−0.585	−1.03–−0.13	0.011	−0.105	−0.54–0.33	0.638
	60 min	−0.272	−0.53–−0.01	0.044	−0.938	−1.38–−0.49	<0.001	−0.231	−0.67–0.20	0.299
	90 min	−0.347	−0.61–−0.82	0.011	−1.121	−1.56–−0.67	<0.001	−0.348	−0.78–0.09	0.120
	120 min	−0.512	−0.77–−0.24	<0.001	−1.146	−1.59–−0.70	<0.001	−0.718	−1.15–−0.27	0.002
	150 min	−0.512	−0.77–−0.24	<0.001	−1.404	−1.85–−0.95	<0.001	−0.848	−1.28–−0.40	<0.001
	180 min	−0.908	−1.17–−0.64	<0.001	−1.555	−2.00–−1.10	<0.001	−1.239	−1.67–−0.79	<0.001
coat(+)		<0.001	−0.20–0.20	0.998	0.001	−0.33–0.33	0.995	<0.001	−0.33–0.33	0.999<
light(+)		−0.480	−0.67–−0.27	<0.001	−1.587	−1.92–−1.25	<0.001	−0.514	−0.84–−0.18	0.003
interaction of light and coat		−0.557	−0.84–−0.27	<0.001	−0.680	−1.15–−0.20	0.006	−0.948	−1.41–−0.47	<0.001

SEM was used to observe the cross section of coating; cross sectional photographs are shown in Figure 3.

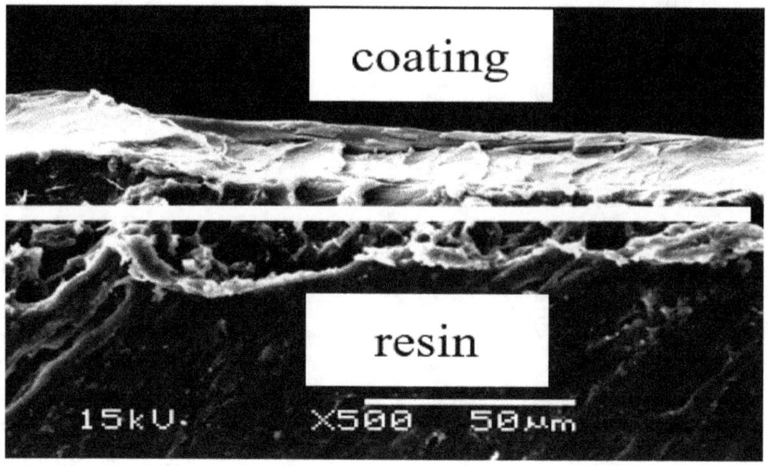

Figure 3. Scanning electron microscopy of cross sectional photographs of the TiO_2 coating.

The Flexural strength (Fs) and flexural modulus (Fm) of resin plates after UV irradiation are shown in Figure 4A,B, respectively. There was no difference between the irradiated test pieces, and all irradiated specimens fulfilled the requirements of the ISO 20795-2:2010 standard for Fs testing after 1200 h of UV irradiation (>65 MPa) (Figure 4A).

In the same way, all irradiated TiO_2-coated specimens fulfilled the requirements of the ISO 20795-2:2010 standard for Fm testing after 1200 h of UV irradiation (>2000 MPa) (Figure 4B).

(A) (b)

Figure 4. Flexural strength (**A**) and Flexural modulus (**B**) of the TiO_2-coated resin plates upon UV irradiation.

Figure 5A shows the water contact angle for TiO_2-noncoated groups and TiO_2-coated groups. Figure 5B shows the images illustrating the wettability of water on TiO_2-coated specimens or TiO_2-noncoated specimens after 120 min of UV irradiation.

The water contact angle of TiO_2-coated specimen was very small from the start of experiment, compared to that of TiO_2-noncoated and it gradually decreased with time.

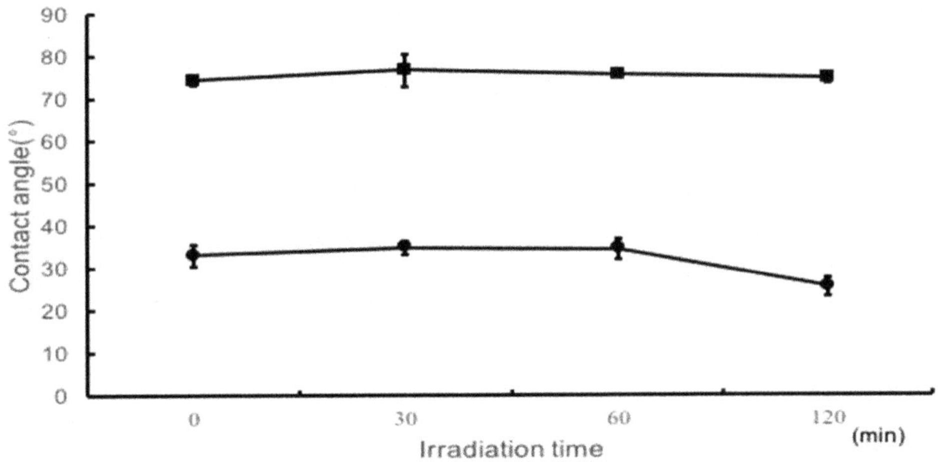

(A)

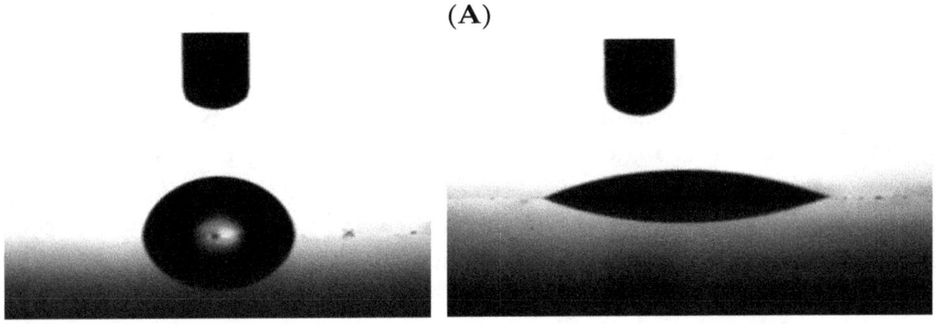

(B)

Figure 5. (**A**) Water contact angle of the resin plates with TiO_2-coating upon UV irradiation for 0, 30, 60, and 120 min. (**B**) Image shows contact angle of a water droplet on non-coated (**left**) and TiO_2-coated resin plate (**right**) after 120 min of UV irradiation.

4. Discussion

This study demonstrates the antibacterial effects of TiO_2-coating on *S. mutans*, *S. sobrinus*, and early colonizers upon UVA irradiation. When TiO_2-coating and UVA were used together, a significant reduction in the microbial count was observed. In a previous study, TiO_2 coated orthodontic arch wires showed the photocatalytic antibacterial effects on *S. mutans*, and its reduction rate was more than 99.99% by bacterial count after 1 h irradiation [51]. Also, a tissue conditioner containing a TiO_2 photocatalyst decreased bacterial counts for *Escherichia coli* (about 90%), *Staphylococcus aureus* (>99.99%), and *S. mutans* (about 90%) after 2 h of irradiation [52]. Moreover, the photocatalytic antibacterial effects of metal specimens coated with two crystalline forms of TiO_2 by thermal and anodic oxidation decreased bacterial counts for *S. mutans* (about 90%) after 60 min irradiation [43]. Furthermore, titanium disks coated with anatase-rich titanium dioxide (TiO_2) reduced amount of viable cells of *S. oralis* by 40% after 24 h UVA exposure [53]. Interestingly, anodized titanium (AO) decreased survival ratio of *S. sanguinis* (70%) upon 2 h of UV irradiation [50]. Also, after 20 min of UV exposure to TiO_2 surfaces, viabilities of *S. mutans* were reduced by 65% [54]. There were a few reports on *S. gordonii* and *S. sobrinus*. Finally, our results showed the bacterial count reduction rate of *S. gordonii* (>90%) (Figure 1), *S. mutans* (87%), *S. sobrinus* (>99%), *S. oralis* (98%), *S. sanguinis* (90%), and *S. mitis* (>99%) (Figure 2) after 90 min irradiation. The reduction rates of *S. oralis*, and *S. sanguinis* were better than those of past study [50,53]. The reduction rate of *S. mutans* was similar as previous studies [43,52–54]. However, a greater reduction rates of bacteria than those in our study were reported [51]. Although factors that contribute to the difference in the reduction rate are unknown, this may be due to the difference in the components of the photocatalyst used. This may also be due to the difference in the surface properties of the coating. Similar to the previous reports, the photocatalytic reaction induced a relatively mild decrease in the bacterial counts after the first 20 min of irradiation and showed a rapid decrease upon subsequent irradiation (Figure 1A) [55]. There is a difference in reaction by bacteria, but only upon irradiation for at least 90 min. Also, compared to conventional cleaning methods, cleaning is facilitated by coating TiO_2. This may lead to improvement in patient's compliance, reduced cost for equipment cleaning, and prevention of unpleasant odors.

UVA irradiation alone showed a decrease in bacterial counts. Furthermore, the photocatalytic activities of TiO_2 coating decreased significantly in bacterial counts of *S. gordonii*, *S. oralis* ATCC 35037 (Figure 1), *S. sobrinus*, *S. mutans*, *S. oralis* GTC, *S. sanguinis*, and *S. mitis* (Figure 2). When uncoated resins were irradiated with UVA light, all the bacteria reduced in counts. These reductions in the light(+)coat(−) groups were expected outcomes and followed a similar trend as a previous study, which reported that the viability of *S. mutans* decreased significantly after 60 min of UVA irradiation as compared to the control which was not irradiated [43]. The decrease may be associated with the cell-damaging effect of UVA. Coat(+)light(+) group showed a higher antibacterial effect, as compared to the coat(−)light(+) group. The difference of antibacterial effect between these group was explained in the Table 1.

The primary step in photocatalytic decomposition consists of hydroxyl radical attack on the bacterial cell wall [48]. This leads to increased permeability which allows radicals to reach and damage the cytoplasmic membrane causing lipid peroxidation and thereby causing membrane disorder [48]. The antibacterial effect of TiO_2 is associated to this disorder of cytoplasmic membrane [48,56]. We propose that the observed bacterial type-dependent variation in the antimicrobial effects may be due to differential effects of hydroxyl radicals on distinct bacterium species [57,58]. The antibacterial effect of the TiO_2 coating for various organisms is determined primarily by the complexity and density of the cell walls, as well as by the types of micro-organisms [59].

In this study, we observed that UVA irradiation has antibacterial effect. In cariogenic bacteria, *S. mutans* was more resistant to UVA than *S. sobrinus*. This may be because of the higher GC content of *S. sobrinus* than *S. mutans*. It has been proposed that species with genomes exhibiting a high GC content are more susceptible to UV-induced mutagenesis [60]. Also, our results showed that the coefficients for *S. sanguinis* and *S. gordonii* in light(+) treatment were low. Consistently, it has been demonstrated that *S. sanguinis* and *S. gordonii* have higher resistance to H_2O_2 [61].

In all bacteria, *S. mutans* was the most resistant to UVA. Conversely, *S. sobrinus* and *S. oralis* were highly susceptible to UVA. Several factors may contribute to the cause of these variable responses to UVA among species. For instance, the production of various ROSs involved in inducing UV damage may vary among species. In addition, the method of defending and repairing DNA damage differs among bacteria [61–63]. Also, the oxidative damage to biomolecules and counteracting protective mechanisms underlie the variability in UVA sensitivity among different bacterial species [64]. However, the reason of higher sensitivity of *S. oralis* and *S. sobrinus* to UV irradiation is unknown (Table 1). Further experiments are needed to understand the mechanistic basis for the variable susceptibility of oral bacteria to UVA.

In general, orthodontic patients are young, and oral care is a major problem for these patients. *S. mutans* and *S. sobrinus* are the most harmful cariogenic bacteria and TiO_2 coating have shown to be effective against them.

Bacteria form biofilms on the surface of the device. During biofilm formation, adherent bacteria produce a polymer matrix in which the community becomes embedded and biofilm bacteria are notoriously resistant to antimicrobial substances [65]. Once they are established on the exposed surface of a dental device, removal of biofilms can be extremely difficult. Effective methodology for cleaning of dental device is not well established. Application of photocatalyst is considered one of the potential strategy to overcome these problems. Therefore, further study is necessary for understanding the effects of TiO_2 on various organisms not only in vitro conditions but also in vivo and intraoral conditions.

With regard to flexural strength, there was no significant difference in bending strength even after irradiation for a long time. UV irradiated specimens fulfilled the requirements of the ISO 20795-2 standard for Fs testing (Figure 4A). Similarly, regarding strength modulus, there was no difference in bending strength even after irradiation for a long time (Figure 4B). These data imply that the resin can withstand irradiation for a long time to ensure a long-term clinical use of orthodontics. Even when irradiating for about 2 years, which is the recommended use period of the retainer, the durability was satisfactory. It was shown that clinical application is achievable.

Moreover, TiO_2-coating improved the hydrophilic properties of the surface of the denture base acrylic resin (Figure 5A,B). A previous study reported that the water contact angle of surfaces in TiO_2-coated resin was 68.1 $\pm$ 3.4 degrees [66]. However, TiO_2-coating makes the resin surface more hydrophilic, with a water contact angle of 25.4 $\pm$ 2.1 degrees (Figure 5). It has been reported that TiO_2 coating applied to acrylic resin inhibits the adhesion of *S. sanguinis* and *C. albicans* organisms [67,68]. In this study, enhancement in the hydrophilic properties of acrylic resin based orthodontic resin surface suppresses the adhesion of early colonizer, the subsequent adhesion of other microbes, which could reduce the total number of microbes adhering to orthodontic resin. Suppression of early colonizer could reduce further bacterial adhesion thereby reducing the risk of systemic disease. Moreover, improvement in the hydrophilic properties of orthodontic resin surface can suppress adhesion of other dirt such as food debris. Even without irradiation, the coat(+) group showed higher hydrophilicity making it easier to remove dirt.

We would like to establish the novel home care method for orthodontic retainer, with use of TiO_2-coating and UV irradiation. As one of the clinical applications, patients place the retainer under the UV lamp and they can also easily clean it at home. This cleaning methods is very simple. In addition, cleaning up the device can be carried out by a professional at the time of visit to the clinic. Our method can be applied not only to a retainer but also to other orthodontic appliances (expansion plate, functional orthodontic appliance), as well as to denture base and occlusal splint.

One of the important aspect of our method is biocompatibility. It has been reported that in animals the TiO_2-coated resin has no irritation to the oral mucosa, nor does it cause skin sensitization. Any elution of components from the coating has no deleterious effects on the tissues [69].

Overall, we demonstrate that the TiO_2-coated resin exposed to UVA irradiation shows great reduction of microbial counts when compared with uncoated and coated without UVA-exposed samples. In addition, the durability of the specimen showed a higher value than the required standard value, indicating that the effect of irradiation was small. In conclusion, the results of this preliminary study suggest that the antibacterial effect of TiO_2-coated resin can be beneficial in long-lasting orthodontic treatments.

5. Conclusions

The antimicrobial activity of the resin coated with TiO_2 was examined by bacterial count of the early colonizers and cariogenic bacteria under UV irradiation. The results of present study suggest that coating with the ultraviolet responsive photocatalyst TiO_2 is useful for antimicrobial properties of removable orthodontic resin based retainer.

Author Contributions: A.K., Y.N., T.O., T.S., R.N., T.H., H.K., Y.N., and N.H. conceived of and designed the experiments; A.K. and T.S. performed the experiments; A.K. and Y.N. analyzed the data; Y.N., T.O., R.N., and T.H. contributed materials/analysis tools; A.K., Y.N., T.O., and Y.N. wrote the manuscript.

Acknowledgments: The authors are grateful to Nihon Sotatu Co., for supplying the TiO_2 coating.

References

1. Littlewood, S.J.; Millett, D.T.; Doubleday, B.; Bearn, D.R.; Worthington, H.V. Retention procedures for stabilising tooth position after treatment with orthodontic braces. *Cochrane Database Syst. Rev.* **2006**, *51*, 94–95.
2. Batoni, G.; Pardini, M.; Giannotti, A.; Ota, F.; Giuca, M.R.; Gabriele, M.; Campa, M.; Senesi, S. Effect of removable orthodontic appliances on oral colonisation by mutans streptococci in children. *Eur. J. Oral Sci.* **2001**, *109*, 388–392. [CrossRef] [PubMed]
3. Bjerklin, K.; Gärskog, B.; Rönnerman, A. Proximal caries increment in connection with orthodontic treatment with removable appliances. *Br. J. Orthod.* **1983**, *10*, 21–24. [CrossRef] [PubMed]
4. Hibino, K.; Wong, R.W.; Hagg, U.; Samaranayake, L.P. The effects of orthodontic appliances on candida in the human mouth. *Int. J. Paediatr. Dent.* **2009**, *19*, 301–308. [CrossRef] [PubMed]
5. Kiyoko, T.; Kazuhiko, N.; Sonoko, M.; Atsuko, T.; Takashi, O. Clinical and microbiological evaluations of acute periodontitis in areas of teeth applied with orthodontic bands. *Pediatr. Dent. J.* **2005**, *15*, 212–218.
6. Kuroki, K.; Hayashi, T.; Sato, K.; Asai, T.; Okano, M.; Kominami, Y.; Takahashi, Y.; Kawai, T. Effect of self-cured acrylic resin added with an inorganic antibacterial agent on *Streptococcus mutans*. *Dent. Mater. J.* **2010**, *29*, 277–285. [CrossRef] [PubMed]
7. Madurantakam, P.; Kumar, S. Fixed and removable orthodontic retainers and periodontal health. *Evid. Based Dent.* **2017**, *18*, 103–104. [CrossRef] [PubMed]
8. Ramage, G.; Tomsett, K.; Wickes, B.L.; López-Ribot, J.L.; Redding, S.W. Denture stomatitis: A role for candida biofilms. *Oral Surg. Oral Med. Oral Pathol. Oral Radiol. Endodontol.* **2004**, *98*, 53–59. [CrossRef]
9. Turkoz, C.; Canigur Bavbek, N.; Kale Varlik, S.; Akca, G. Influence of thermoplastic retainers on *Streptococcus mutans* and *Lactobacillus* adhesion. *Am. J. Orthod. Dentofac. Orthop.* **2012**, *141*, 598–603. [CrossRef] [PubMed]
10. Zharmagambetova, A.; Tuleutayeva, S.; Akhmetova, S. Microbiological aspects of the orthodontic treatment. *Georgian Med. News* **2017**, *264*, 39–43.
11. Zingler, S.; Pritsch, M. Association between clinical and salivary microbial parameters during treatment with removable orthodontic appliances with or without use of fluoride mouth rinse. *Eur. J. Paediatr. Dent.* **2016**, *17*, 181–187. [PubMed]
12. Shay, K. Denture hygiene: A review and update. *J. Contemp. Dent. Pract.* **2000**, *1*, 28–41. [PubMed]
13. Song, W.S.; Lee, J.K.; Park, S.H.; Um, H.S.; Lee, S.Y.; Chang, B.S. Comparison of periodontitis-associated oral biofilm formation under dynamic and static conditions. *J. Periodontal Implant Sci.* **2017**, *47*, 219–230. [CrossRef] [PubMed]
14. Kolenbrander, P.E.; Andersen, R.N.; Blehert, D.S.; Egland, P.G.; Foster, J.S.; Palmer, R.J. Communication among oral bacteria. *Microbiol. Mol. Biol. Rev.* **2002**, *66*, 486–505. [CrossRef] [PubMed]
15. Teles, F.R.; Teles, R.P.; Sachdeo, A.; Uzel, N.G.; Song, X.Q.; Torresyap, G.; Singh, M.; Papas, A.; Haffajee, A.D.; Socransky, S.S. Comparison of microbial changes in early redeveloping biofilms on natural teeth and dentures. *J. Periodontol.* **2012**, *83*, 1139–1148. [CrossRef] [PubMed]
16. Nyvad, B.; Kilian, M. Microbiology of the early colonization of human enamel and root surfaces in vivo. *Scand. J. Dent. Res.* **1987**, *95*, 369–380. [CrossRef] [PubMed]
17. Verran, J.; Motteram, K.L. The effect of adherent oral streptococci on the subsequent adherence of candida albicans to acrylic in vitro. *J. Dent.* **1987**, *15*, 73–76. [CrossRef]
18. Da Silva, P.M.; Acosta, E.J.; Pinto Lde, R.; Graeff, M.; Spolidorio, D.M.; Almeida, R.S.; Porto, V.C. Microscopical analysis of candida albicans biofilms on heat-polymerised acrylic resin after chlorhexidine gluconate and sodium hypochlorite treatments. *Mycoses* **2011**, *54*, e712–e717. [CrossRef] [PubMed]
19. De Andrade, I.M.; Cruz, P.C.; da Silva, C.H.; de Souza, R.F.; Paranhos Hde, F.; Candido, R.C.; Marin, J.M.; de Souza-Gugelmin, M.C. Effervescent tablets and ultrasonic devices against candida and mutans streptococci in denture biofilm. *Gerodontology* **2011**, *28*, 264–270. [CrossRef] [PubMed]
20. De Freitas Fernandes, F.S.; Pereira-Cenci, T.; da Silva, W.J.; Ricomini Filho, A.P.; Straioto, F.G.; Cury, A.A.D.B. Efficacy of denture cleansers on *Candida* spp. Biofilm formed on polyamide and polymethyl methacrylate resins. *J. Prosthet. Dent.* **2011**, *105*, 51–58. [CrossRef]
21. De Souza, R.F.; de Freitas Oliveira Paranhos, H.; Lovato da Silva, C.H.; Abu-Naba'a, L.; Fedorowicz, Z.; Gurgan, C.A. Interventions for cleaning dentures in adults. *Cochrane Database Syst. Rev.* **2009**, CD007395. [CrossRef] [PubMed]

22. Dhamande, M.M.; Pakhan, A.J.; Thombare, R.U.; Ghodpage, S.L. Evaluation of efficacy of commercial denture cleansing agents to reduce the fungal biofilm activity from heat polymerized denture acrylic resin: An in vitro study. *Contemp. Clin. Dent.* **2012**, *3*, 168–172. [CrossRef] [PubMed]
23. Farhadian, N.; Usefi Mashoof, R.; Khanizadeh, S.; Ghaderi, E.; Farhadian, M.; Miresmaeili, A. *Streptococcus mutans* counts in patients wearing removable retainers with silver nanoparticles vs. those wearing conventional retainers: A randomized clinical trial. *Am. J. Orthod. Dentofac. Orthop.* **2016**, *149*, 155–160. [CrossRef] [PubMed]
24. Monteiro, D.R.; Gorup, L.F.; Takamiya, A.S.; de Camargo, E.R.; Filho, A.C.; Barbosa, D.B. Silver distribution and release from an antimicrobial denture base resin containing silver colloidal nanoparticles. *J. Prosthodont.* **2012**, *21*, 7–15. [CrossRef] [PubMed]
25. Oei, J.D.; Zhao, W.W.; Chu, L.; DeSilva, M.N.; Ghimire, A.; Rawls, H.R.; Whang, K. Antimicrobial acrylic materials with in situ generated silver nanoparticles. *J. Biomed. Mater. Res. B Appl. Biomater.* **2012**, *100*, 409–415. [CrossRef] [PubMed]
26. Regis, R.R.; Zanini, A.P.; Della Vecchia, M.P.; Silva-Lovato, C.H.; Oliveira Paranhos, H.F.; de Souza, R.F. Physical properties of an acrylic resin after incorporation of an antimicrobial monomer. *J. Prosthodont.* **2011**, *20*, 372–379. [CrossRef] [PubMed]
27. Shinonaga, Y.; Arita, K. Antibacterial effect of acrylic dental devices after surface modification by fluorine and silver dual-ion implantation. *Acta Biomater.* **2012**, *8*, 1388–1393. [CrossRef] [PubMed]
28. Sodagar, A.; Kassaee, M.Z.; Akhavan, A.; Javadi, N.; Arab, S.; Kharazifard, M.J. Effect of silver nano particles on flexural strength of acrylic resins. *J. Prosthodont. Res.* **2012**, *56*, 120–124. [CrossRef] [PubMed]
29. Sousa, F.A.; Paradella, T.C.; Koga-Ito, C.Y.; Jorge, A.O. Effect of sodium bicarbonate on candida albicans adherence to thermally activated acrylic resin. *Braz. Oral Res.* **2009**, *23*, 381–385. [CrossRef] [PubMed]
30. Vieira, A.P.; Senna, P.M.; Silva, W.J.; Del Bel Cury, A.A. Long-term efficacy of denture cleansers in preventing *Candida* spp. Biofilm recolonization on liner surface. *Braz. Oral Res.* **2010**, *24*, 342–348. [CrossRef] [PubMed]
31. Wady, A.F.; Machado, A.L.; Zucolotto, V.; Zamperini, C.A.; Berni, E.; Vergani, C.E. Evaluation of candida albicans adhesion and biofilm formation on a denture base acrylic resin containing silver nanoparticles. *J. Appl. Microbiol.* **2012**, *112*, 1163–1172. [CrossRef] [PubMed]
32. Wolff, M.S.; Larson, C. The cariogenic dental biofilm—Good, bad or just something to control? *Braz. Oral. Res.* **2009**, *23*, 31–38. [CrossRef] [PubMed]
33. Chandra, J.; Mukherjee, P.K.; Leidich, S.D.; Faddoul, F.F.; Hoyer, L.L.; Douglas, L.J.; Ghannoum, M.A. Antifungal resistance of candidal biofilms formed on denture acrylic in vitro. *J. Dent. Res.* **2001**, *80*, 903–908. [CrossRef] [PubMed]
34. Jagger, D.C.; Harrison, A. Denture cleaning the best approach. *Br. Dent. J.* **1995**, *178*, 413–417. [CrossRef] [PubMed]
35. Budtz-Jørgensen, E. Materials and methods for cleaning dentures. *J. Prosthet. Dent.* **1979**, *42*, 619–623. [CrossRef]
36. Fitjer, L.C.; Jonas, I.E.; Kappert, H.F. Corrosion susceptibility of lingual wire extensions in removable appliances. An in vitro study. *J. Orofac. Orthop.* **2002**, *63*, 212–226. [CrossRef] [PubMed]
37. Hong, G.; Murata, H.; Li, Y.; Sadamori, S.; Hamada, T. Influence of denture cleansers on the color stability of three types of denture base acrylic resin. *J. Prosthet. Dent.* **2009**, *10*, 205–213. [CrossRef]
38. Rantala, L.I.; Lastumäki, T.M.; Peltomäki, T.; Vallittu, P.K. Fatigue resistance of removable orthodontic appliancereinforced with glass fibre weave. *J. Oral Rehabil.* **2003**, *30*, 501–506. [CrossRef] [PubMed]
39. Yamada, Y.; Yamada, M.; Ueda, T.; Sakurai, K. Reduction of biofilm formation on titanium surface with ultraviolet-c pre-irradiation. *J. Biomater. Appl.* **2014**, *29*, 161–171. [CrossRef] [PubMed]
40. Tomomi, S.; Susumu, I.; Tsuyoshi, O.; Hiroyuki, K.; Yusuke, M.; Nobuhiro, H.; Yoshiki, N. Evaluation of antibacterial activity of visible light-responsive TiO_2-based photocatalyst coating on orthodontic materials against cariogenic bacteria. *Asian Pacfic. J. Dent.* **2016**, *16*, 15–22.
41. Fujishima, A.; Honda, K. Electrochemical photolysis of water at a semiconductor electrode. *Nature* **1972**, *238*, 37–38. [CrossRef] [PubMed]
42. Cho, M.; Chung, H.; Choi, W.; Yoon, J. Linear correlation between inactivation of *E. coli* and oh radical concentration in TiO_2 photocatalytic disinfection. *Water Res.* **2004**, *38*, 1069–1077. [CrossRef] [PubMed]
43. Choi, J.Y.; Chung, C.J.; Oh, K.T.; Choi, Y.J.; Kim, K.H. Photocatalytic antibacterial effect of TiO_2 film of tiag on streptococcus mutans. *Angle Orthod.* **2009**, *79*, 528–532. [CrossRef]

44. Choi, J.Y.; Kim, K.H.; Choy, K.C.; Oh, K.T.; Kim, K.N. Photocatalytic antibacterial effect of TiO_2 film formed on ti and tiag exposed to lactobacillus acidophilus. *J. Biomed. Mater. Res. B Appl. Biomater.* **2007**, *80*, 353–359. [CrossRef] [PubMed]
45. Ochiai, T.; Fujishima, A. Photoelectrochemical properties of TiO_2 photocatalyst and its applications for environmental purification. *J. Photochem. Photobiol. C Photochem. Rev.* **2012**, *13*, 247–262. [CrossRef]
46. Hoffmann, M.R.; Martin, S.T.; Choi, W. Environmental applications of semiconductor photocatalysis. *Chem. Rev.* **1995**, *95*, 69–96. [CrossRef]
47. Hosseinpour, S.; Tang, F.; Wang, F.; Livingstone, R.A.; Schlegel, S.J.; Ohto, T.; Bonn, M.; Nagata, Y.; Backus, E. Chemisorbed and physisorbed water at the TiO_2/water interface. *J. Phys. Chem. Lett.* **2017**, *8*, 2195–2199. [CrossRef] [PubMed]
48. Sunada, K.; Watanabe, T.; Hashimoto, K. Studies on photokilling of bacteria on TiO_2 thin film. *J. Photochem. Photobiol. A Chem.* **2003**, *156*, 227–233. [CrossRef]
49. Takeuchi, M.; Sakamoto, K.; Martra, G.; Coluccia, S.; Anpo, M. Mechanism of photoinduced superhydrophilicity on the TiO_2 photocatalyst surface. *J. Phys. Chem. B* **2005**, *109*, 15422–15428. [CrossRef] [PubMed]
50. Unosson, E.; Tsekoura, E.K.; Engqvist, H.; Welch, K. Synergetic inactivation of staphylococcus epidermidis and streptococcus mutansin a TiO_2/H_2O_2/uv system. *Biomatter* **2013**, *3*, e26727. [CrossRef] [PubMed]
51. ÖZyildiz, F.; Uzel, A.; Hazar, A.S.; GÜDen, M.; ÖLmez, S.; Aras, I.; Karaboz, İ. Photocatalytic antimicrobial effect of TiO_2 anatase thin-film–coated orthodontic arch wires on 3 oral pathogens. *Turkish J. Biol.* **2014**, *38*, 289–295. [CrossRef]
52. Uchimaru, M.; Sakai, T.; Moroi, R.; Shiota, S.; Shibata, Y.; Deguchi, M.; Sakai, H.; Yamashita, Y.; Terada, Y. Antimicrobial and antifungal effects of tissue conditioners containing a photocatalyst. *Dent. Mater. J.* **2011**, *30*, 691–699. [CrossRef] [PubMed]
53. Westas, E.; Hayashi, M.; Cecchinato, F.; Wennerberg, A.; Andersson, M.; Jimbo, R.; Davies, J.R. Bactericidal effect of photocatalytically-active nanostructured TiO_2 surfaces on biofilms of the early oral colonizer, streptococcus oralis. *J. Biomed. Mater. Res. A* **2017**, *105*, 2321–2328. [CrossRef] [PubMed]
54. Ahn, S.; Han, J.; Lim, B.; Lim, Y. Comparison of ultraviolet light-induced photocatalytic bactericidal effect on modified titanium implant surfaces. *Int. J. Oral Maxillofac. Implants* **2011**, *26*, 39–44. [PubMed]
55. Kayano, S.; Yoshihiko, K.; Kazuhito, H.; Akira, F. Batericidal and detoxification effects of TiO_2 film photocatalysts. *Environ. Sci. Technol.* **1998**, *32*, 726–728.
56. Saito, T.; Iwase, T.; Horie, J.; Morioka, T. Mode of photocatalytic bactericidal action of powdered semiconductor TiO_2 on mutans streptococci. *J. Photochem. Photobiol. B* **1992**, *14*, 369–379. [CrossRef]
57. Dongari, A.I.; Miyasaki, K.T. Sensitivity of actinobaciiius actinomycetemcomitans and haemophiius apiiropiiiius to oxicjative killing. *Oral Microbiol. Immunol.* **1991**, *6*, 363–372. [CrossRef] [PubMed]
58. Jagger, J. Near-uv radiation effects on microorganisms. *Photochem. Photobiol.* **1981**, *34*, 761–768. [CrossRef] [PubMed]
59. Maness, P.; Smolinski, S.; Blake, D.; Huang, Z.; Wolfrum, E.; Jacoby, W. Bactericidal activity of photocatalytic TiO_2 reaction: Toward an understanding of its killing mechanism. *Appl. Environ. Microbiol.* **1999**, *65*, 4094–4098. [PubMed]
60. Matallana-Surget, S.; Meador, J.; Joux, F.; Douki, T. Effect of the gc content of DNA on the distribution of uvb-induced bipyrimidinephotoproducts. *Photochem. Photobiol. Sci.* **2008**, *7*, 794–801. [CrossRef] [PubMed]
61. Arrieta, J.M.; Weinbauer, M.G.; Herndl, G.J. Interspecific variability in sensitivity to uv radiation and subsequent recovery in selected isolates of marine bacteria. *Appl. Environ. Microbiol.* **2000**, *66*, 1468–1473. [CrossRef] [PubMed]
62. Matallana-Surget, S.; Douki, T.; Cavicchioli, R.; Joux, F. Remarkable resistance to uvb of the marine bacterium photobacterium angustum explained by an unexpected role of photolyase. *Photoch. Photobio. Sci.* **2009**, *8*, 1313–1320. [CrossRef] [PubMed]
63. Santos, A.L.; Lopes, S.; Baptista, I.; Henriques, I.; Gomes, N.C.; Almeida, A.; Correia, A.; Cunha, A. Diversity in uv sensitivity and recovery potential among bacterioneuston and bacterioplankton isolates. *Lett. Appl. Microbiol.* **2011**, *52*, 360–366. [CrossRef] [PubMed]
64. Santos, A.L.; Oliveira, V.; Baptista, I.; Henriques, I.; Gomes, N.C.; Almeida, A.; Correia, A.; Cunha, A. Wavelength dependence of biological damage induced by uv radiation on bacteria. *Arch. Microbiol.* **2013**, *195*, 63–74. [CrossRef] [PubMed]

65. Gilbert, P.; Das, J.; Foley, I. Biofilm susceptibility to antimicrobials. *Adv. Dent. Res.* **1997**, *11*, 160–167. [CrossRef] [PubMed]
66. Kado, D.; Sakurai, K.; Sugiyama, T.; Ueda, T. Evaluation of cleanability of a titanium dioxide (TiO_2)-coated acrylic resin denture base. *Prosthodont. Res. Pract.* **2005**, *4*, 69–76. [CrossRef]
67. Arai, T.; Ueda, T.; Sugiyama, T.; Sakurai, K. Inhibiting microbial adhesion to denture base acrylic resin by titanium dioxide coating. *J. Oral Rehabil.* **2009**, *36*, 902–908. [CrossRef] [PubMed]
68. Obata, T.; Ueda, T.; Sakurai, K. Inhibition of denture plaque by TiO_2 coating on denture base resins in the mouth. *J. Prosthet. Dent.* **2017**, *118*, 759–764. [CrossRef] [PubMed]
69. Tsuji, M.; Ueda, T.; Sawaki, K.; Kawaguchi, M.; Sakurai, K. Biocompatibility of a titanium dioxide-coating method for denture base acrylic resin. *Gerodontology* **2016**, *33*, 539–544. [CrossRef] [PubMed]

4

Potential Causes of Titanium Particle and Ion Release in Implant Dentistry

Rafael Delgado-Ruiz [1,*] and Georgios Romanos [2,3]

1 Department of Prosthodontics and Digital Technology, School of Dental Medicine, Stony Brook University, New York, NY 11794, USA
2 Department of Periodontics, School of Dental Medicine, Stony Brook University, New York, NY 11794, USA; georgios.romanos@stonybrookmedicine.edu
3 Department of Oral Surgery and Implant Dentistry, Dental School, Johann Wolfgang Goethe University, 60323 Frankfurt, Germany
* Correspondence: rafael.delgado-ruiz@stonybrookmedicine.edu

Abstract: Implant surface characteristics, as well as physical and mechanical properties, are responsible for the positive interaction between the dental implant, the bone and the surrounding soft tissues. Unfortunately, the dental implant surface does not remain unaltered and changes over time during the life of the implant. If changes occur at the implant surface, mucositis and peri-implantitis processes could be initiated; implant osseointegration might be disrupted and bone resorption phenomena (osteolysis) may lead to implant loss. This systematic review compiled the information related to the potential sources of titanium particle and ions in implant dentistry. Research questions were structured in the Population, Intervention, Comparison, Outcome (PICO) framework. PICO questionnaires were developed and an exhaustive search was performed for all the relevant studies published between 1980 and 2018 involving titanium particles and ions related to implant dentistry procedures. Preferred Reporting Items for Systematic Reviews and Meta-Analyses (PRISMA) guidelines were followed for the selection and inclusion of the manuscripts in this review. Titanium particle and ions are released during the implant bed preparation, during the implant insertion and during the implant decontamination. In addition, the implant surfaces and restorations are exposed to the saliva, bacteria and chemicals that can potentially dissolve the titanium oxide layer and, therefore, corrosion cycles can be initiated. Mechanical factors, the micro-gap and fluorides can also influence the proportion of metal particles and ions released from implants and restorations.

Keywords: dental implants; titanium particles; wear; corrosion

---

1. Introduction

Titanium implants have been used for dental, orthopedic and other medical applications since the early 1980s [1,2]. Implant-related factors, such as the surface characteristics, material composition and chemistry, are responsible for the osseointegration. Specifically, the presence of a titanium oxide layer on the implant surface is considered crucial for the maintenance of the osseointegration and the prevention of the corrosion of the titanium surface [3]. The dental implant surface does not remain unaltered and, if changes occur at the implant surface, mucositis and peri-implantitis processes could be initiated; osseointegration might be disrupted, and bone resorption phenomena (osteolysis) may lead to implant loss [1–4]. Particularly, at the moment of implant insertion, the implant surface can incur changes in its chemical and topographic structures, which is sometimes irreversible [1] and also titanium particles of different sizes and characteristics can be released from the dental implant surface [5–9].

Subsequently, if the implant surface is altered, degraded or dissolved by the effects of acidic substances or an acidic environment, the titanium oxide layer can be lost, and corrosion phenomena can begin [10–14]. Furthermore, during functional loading, the combination of mechanical and chemical corrosion (fretting) between the implant surface and the adjacent bone can facilitate the release of more metal particles and ions and, if friction occurs between the internal implant walls and the prosthetic abutment, additional particles and ions can be released into the surrounding tissues [2–4,15]. Lastly, cleaning and disinfection of the implant surface with mechanical, physical or chemical methods have been shown to induce changes of different magnitudes at the implant and abutment, with subsequent titanium oxide layer loss, titanium particle or ion loss and corrosion initiation [16–20].

However, the sources of titanium particle or ions in implant dentistry procedures have not been studied in depth and methods for its reduction are currently unknown. Therefore, all the information related to the potential sources of titanium ions and particles and suggestions of methods for their control in implant dentistry is fundamental for the long-term survival of dental implants to improve clinical practice.

The purpose of this systematic review is to compile the information related to the potential sources of titanium particles and ions in dental implantology. Taken together, the findings of this review, including the percentages of particles, their characteristics, and detection methods, suggest ways for reducing titanium particle and ion release in implant dentistry.

2. Results

The initial search returned 635 articles. A total of 22 articles were removed because they were duplicates; the remaining 613 articles abstracts were read in full, and 378 articles were excluded because they did not fulfil the inclusion criteria. The full texts of the remaining 235 articles were read in full for eligibility, and 29 articles were removed because they presented reviews or expert opinions or were duplicated. Finally, 206 articles were included in this systematic review (Figure 1).

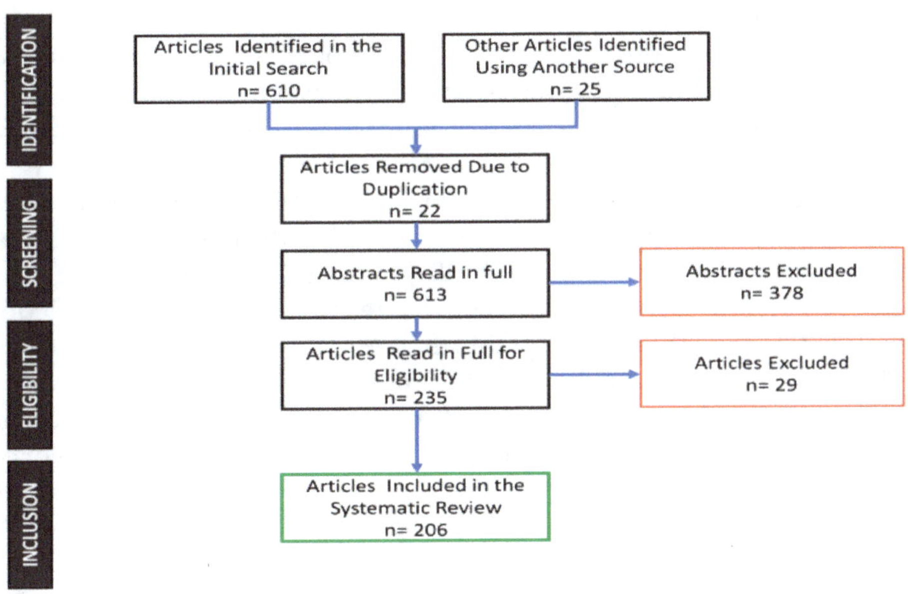

Figure 1. Preferred Reporting Items for Systematic Reviews (PRISMA) flow diagram of the screening and selection process.

The findings were grouped as follows: sources of titanium release during the surgical phase, during the prosthetic phase and during maintenance (Figure 2).

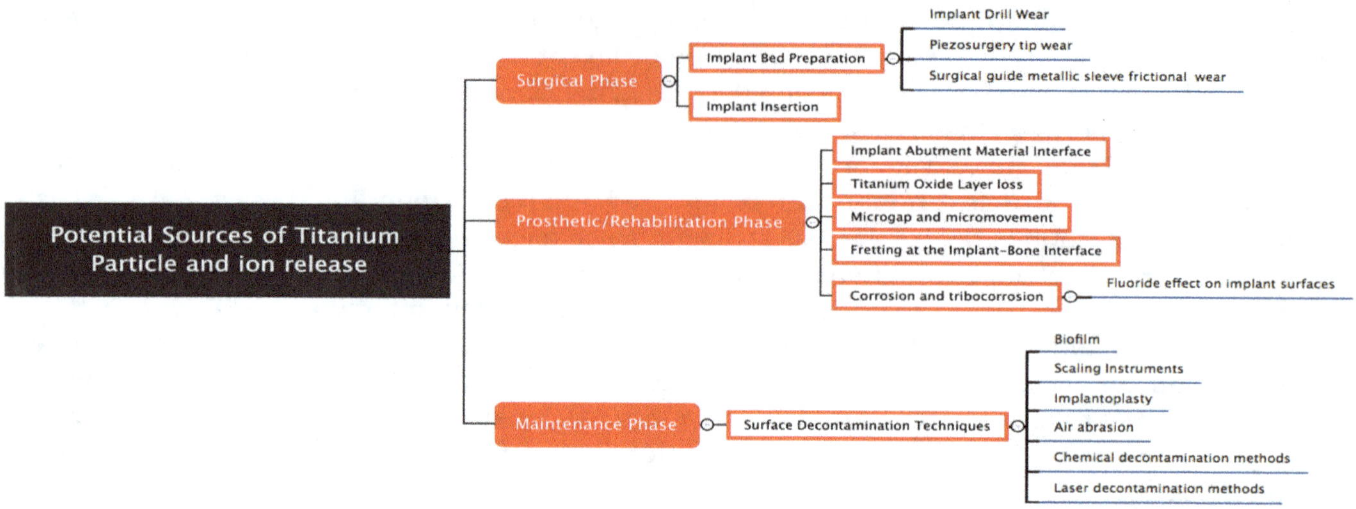

Figure 2. This systematic review found that titanium particles and ions can be released during the surgical, prosthetic and maintenance phases due to different causes during the life span of a dental implant. The rectangles filled in red are the three phases in implant dentistry procedures in which titanium particles and ions can be released. The rectangles with the red frame are procedures within the previous phases which resulted in titanium particles and ions release. The underlined sentences are the detailed sources or initiators of titanium particles and ions release.

2.1. Potential Causes of Titanium Particle Release during the Surgical Phase

2.1.1. Implant Bed Preparation

Bone-cutting instruments, when subjected to frictional forces, can suffer variable levels of metal attrition, wear and corrosion. Traces of different metallic elements have been observed after osteotomy in regional ganglions, kidneys and lungs [21,22]. In addition, it has been demonstrated that the irrigation liquid collected from the implant bed preparation contains metallic debris and ions. Rashad et al. [23] performed implant osteotomies with rotatory instruments and piezosurgery devices to detect drill deposits in bone or in the recovered irrigation liquid. After implant bed preparation, bone samples were examined by (Scanning Electron Microscope) SEM/energy dispersion X-ray spectroscopy (EDX), the irrigation liquid was collected and filtered with polycarbonate membranes with a specific pore size. The membranes were further analysed by SEM/EDX for the detection of metal content. The results showed different residual metals from the drills in the irrigation liquid (Ag, Si, Fe, Ti, V, Cu, Mn, Zr, Cr, Bi, Mg) for both osteotomy methods. The authors recommended the use of copious irrigation to reduce the metallic particle content in the implant bed area [23].

Implant drill bits and piezosurgery tips suffer characteristic patterns of wear after osteotomy procedures. Drills showed abrasive wear, plastic deformation, blunting, coating damage and material loss, mainly at the tip and cutting edges of the drill flank [24]. Meanwhile, piezosurgery showed abrasive wear of the tip and flanks and plastic deformation of the cutting point. The characteristics of the wear suffered by osteotomy instruments have been related to the drill material, drill and drill mechanical properties [24].

Carvalho et al. [25,26] demonstrated that substance loss, steel melting and condensation of particles detached from the active point increased proportionally to the number of uses; indeed, drills used 10 times showed 17.86% deformation and, drills used 50 times showed 33.97% deformation. These findings were also confirmed in drills used 50 or more times, on which increased areas of metal subtraction, the addition of loosened metal, and metal surface abrasion at the lateral surface of the cutting tip and drill edges were detected [27–29].

Another factor that seems to increase the wear of implant drills is the use of guided surgery techniques. Bone heating, drill deformation and roughness were evaluated after osteotomy with guided surgery and conventional osteotomy; greater drill deformation and wear were recorded after the 40th osteotomy in the guided surgery group produced by the drill friction against the metal sleeve and the bone [30].

Sterilization and irrigation also increase the release of metal particles and ions as well as drill wear. Allsobrook et al. [31] evaluated Straumann, Nobel Biocare and Neoss drills. The authors performed 50 osteotomies per drill. After 20 osteotomies, the drills suffered 30 μm to 100 μm of wear at the tip and edges and loss of the surface coating. Furthermore, analysis of corrosion after sterilization processes and irrigation with saline showed increased pitting corrosion of the drills after 20 cycles of sterilization [24,31,32]. Other authors also found that the autoclave sterilization of implant drills increased the surface corrosion of the drills and therefore the ion and particle release [25,33,34]. Similar results were obtained when implant drills with three different characteristics (smooth stainless steel drills, coated drills and smooth zirconia drills) were compared. After repeated drilling and sterilization, it was found that drills in all groups suffered wear, deformation, coating delamination and surface roughness changes [35].

The material of the drill seems to influence the amount of particle loosening of the drill surface. Zirconia drills showed less qualitative substrate loss than titanium drills when drilling 20 implant beds at a standard drilling speed of 800 rpm [36].

Remarks

During osteotomy procedures, surgical drills, implant drills and piezosurgery tips suffer deformation, surface wear, microfractures, delamination, and metal particle release (Figures 3–5). Additionally, sterilization of the cutting tools can initiate corrosion and can increase the particle and ion release. Sufficient irrigation, adequate suction of metallic debris, the use of single-use drills, adequate control of the number of sterilization procedures, inspection of cutting tool integrity, timely replacement of worn drills and the use of harder and more resistant cutting tools might reduce the deposition of metallic particles and ions released during implant bed preparation.

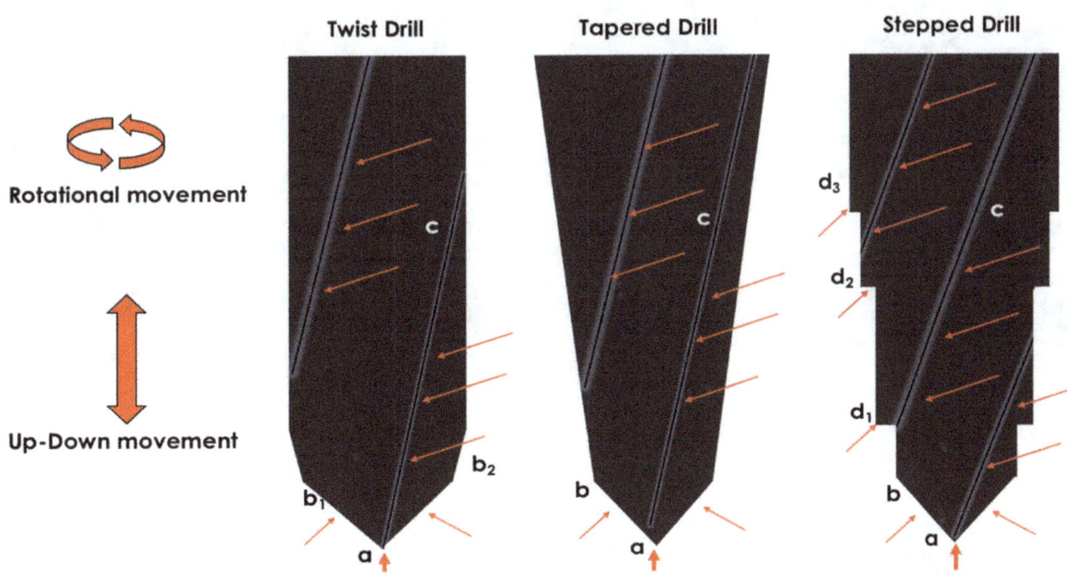

Figure 3. Areas of wear of implant drills. Different drill designs present wear and particle loosening at different levels under the effects of axial and rotational forces. Twist drills suffer deformation, blunting and delamination of the drill tip (a), tip angles (b1 and b2), and cutting blades (c). Tapered drills suffer deformation, blunting and delamination of the drill tip (a), tip angle (b), and cutting blades (c). Stepped drills suffer deformation, blunting and delamination of the drill tip (a), tip angles (b), cutting blades (c) and step angles (d1, d2, d3). Thin red arrows are showing the blade areas suffering wear as well as the tip angles. Thick arrows are showing the tip of the drills suffering wear and deformation.

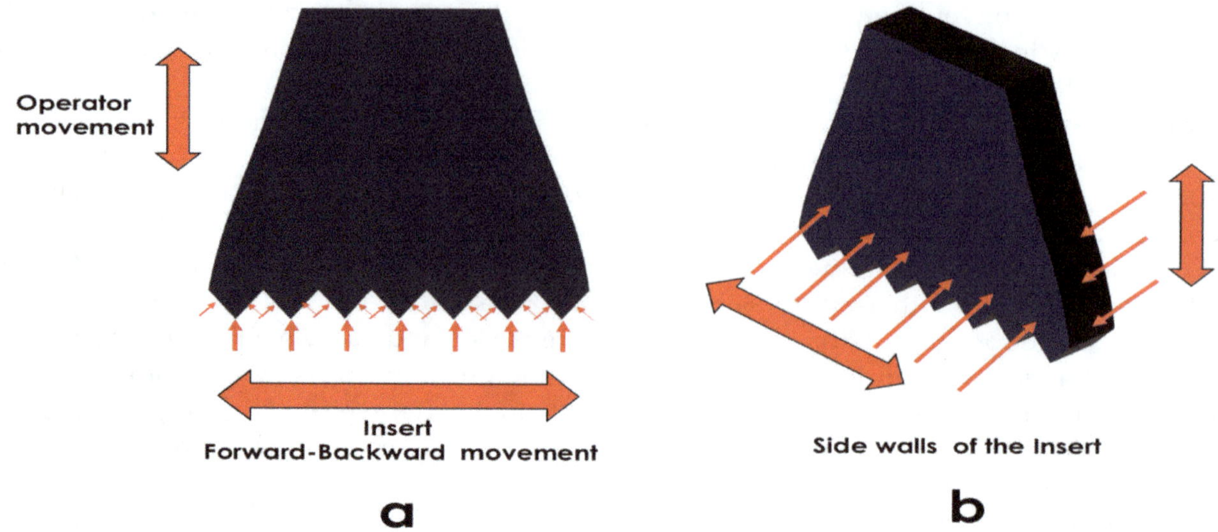

Figure 4. Areas of wear of piezosurgery inserts. The piezosurgery insert directions of movement: a vertical movement induced by the operator, and a minimal vertical displacement during the ultrasonic movement in conjunction with a horizontal component produced by oscillation of the tip. (**a**) The piezosurgery insert oscillates in a forward-backward movement. The insert tip and the sides of the tip suffer deformation, wear and particle detachment. (**b**) Additionally, the sidewalls and borders of the insert suffer deformation, wear and particle detachment. Short and long thing arrows are showing areas of angle and lateral wear and deformation. Thick arrows are showing the vertex of the tips suffering wear and deformation.

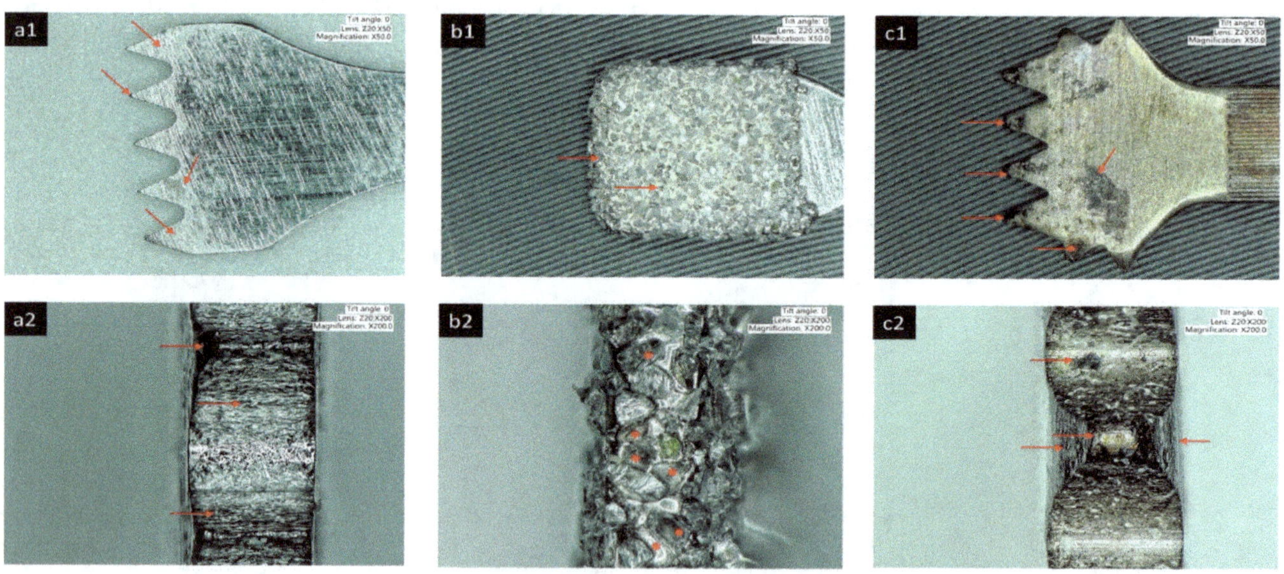

Figure 5. Piezosurgery tips used 1 time. The tips are made from different materials. (**a1**,**a2**) Stainless steel insert showing lateral wear of the active tip, abrasion and particle loosening at the flanks, deformation of the tip edges and material delamination. (**b1**,**b2**). Diamond-coated insert showing wear at the sides and empty spaces representing particle loosening. (**c1**,**c2**) Gold nitride-coated insert with several areas at the flanks, tips and sides of the tips showing excessive wear, particle delamination and deformation. The red arrows are showing the areas of wear, delamination and deformation suffered by piezosurgery inserts. The red asterisk is showing particle detachment from diamond coated piezosurgery inserts.

2.1.2. Implant Insertion

When the dental implant is inserted, frictional moments occur at the bone-implant interface and the initial mechanical interlocking results from interactions between the bone and the implant threads and walls [37]. As a consequence of implant insertion, microfractures and compression occur at the bone side and the implant surface is simultaneously subjected to a combination of torsional and frictional forces, which may alter the original implant surface. Wawrzinek et al. [38] described that shear forces originating from the friction of implants inserted against the surrounding bone tissue can produce a shifting of stresses at different locations along the implant surface related to the heterogeneity of the bone tissue (cortical or cancellous) and the implant geometry. Therefore, localized areas of stress concentration can appear and titanium particles can be released into the bone tissue [37]. A harder implant surface should be able to retain its characteristics more than a softer surface and should demonstrate increased abrasion resistance [39], however, the abrasive wear phenomena during implant insertion are influenced by additional factors that cannot be controlled simultaneously; these factors include the properties of the specimens, interactions with the environment and the experimental conditions [40–42].

Schliephake et al. [43] showed that the placement of self-tapping titanium implants abraded particles from the implant surface, as evidenced by deposits of these particles at the implant-bone interface. Seki et al. [44] and Kim et al. [45] revealed titanium particles in the tissue interposed between the bone and the titanium plate used for oral and maxillofacial fracture fixation. The authors speculated that the particles originated from two causes: first, the physical-mechanical removal of the oxidation layer during insertion; and second, the dissolution of the subjacent titanium into the surrounding tissues (corrosion), resulting in detection of the titanium particles and ions [44,45].

Different observations also showed that particles abraded from the implant surface ranged between 1.8–3.2 μm in diameter and were located at the bone surface and up to 100 μm inside the surrounding bone [5]. Other authors found titanium particles ranging widely in size from 20 nm to 20 μm at the implantation site concentrated at the cortical layer. Apparently, the process of implant insertion alone can release up to 0.5 mg of metallic debris at the implant-bone interface. Previous studies in orthopaedics have shown that aseptic osteolysis can be induced by 0.220 mg to 3.0 mg of titanium particles in the implant area as well as inside the medullary spaces [6]. In the case of titanium plasma-sprayed (TPS) implants, the particle dimensions decreased with increasing distance from the implant surface, probably due to gradual and passive dissolution, fretting and wear [7–9].

Martini et al. [46] found that titanium particles released from TPS implants can be present within 200–250 μm of the implant surface and some debris could be observed at 500 μm. It was speculated that detachment of titanium particles from the TPS implants resulted from the implant surface morphology, frictional forces during implant insertion and frictional forces between the titanium (Ti) coating and the pre-existing bone. These released metallic particles impeded bone formation and created gaps of 180–260 μm between the pre-existing bone and implant surface compared to non-TPS surfaces, which showed bone matrix on the implant surface after 14 days [47–49].

Wennerberg et al. [50] performed in vitro and in vivo studies to investigate the titanium concentration around titanium implants with different surface roughness inserted in rabbit tibias. They found that moderately rough surfaces (*Sa* 2.21 μm) presented more titanium release up to 400 μm from the implant surface than smooth surfaces (*Sa* < 1.43 μm). The authors recommended further chemical analysis of the implant surfaces to evaluate potential chemical changes at the implant surfaces and their biological consequences [51].

Mints et al. [52] compared acid-etched, anodized and machined implant surfaces after their insertion into bone blocks. They found that all the implants suffered surface damage, material removal from the implant surface, oxide layer breakdown, metal debris transportation (due to the insertion and friction) from the apical and middle third to the coronal area and cracks at the implant surface as result of the insertion process. The titanium debris ranged from nano- to microparticles; the nanoparticles were located in the coronal area and the microparticles were located in the mid and apical regions [52].

It seems that although almost all of an implant surface is exposed to wear and particle detachment during insertion, the tip of the threads and the lower flank of the threads are more exposed, while the apex microstructure is least exposed in conventional implant bed preparation [53]. It was also concluded that surfaces with subtractive modifications appeared to suffer less wear and particle loosening than surfaces with additive modifications and that re-establishment of the damaged TiO_2 layer was superior for surfaces with subtractive modifications [54].

Particles and ions released during titanium implant insertion can also be retained at the soft tissue level. Concentrations of specific metallic elements retained in the gingival cuff, surrounding the implant neck were detected in an analysis of histological sections processed with the laser ablation detection technique. The elemental mapping showed titanium from 0.4 mm up to 4 mm from the implant, with additional contents of aluminium and vanadium [55].

One in vitro study did not find metal particles released after the insertion and removal of sandblasted and acid-etched implants. The study was performed in polyurethane blocks with different densities and the methods of analysis were SEM observation of the implant surface and X-ray diffraction analysis. Albeit authors observed surface deformation, changes and wear, no traces of metals were observed in the samples [56]. Titanium particles and ions are not always detected; apparently, the irrigation of the surgical site could dilute and remove metallic particles and ions, thus reducing the overall metal content. However, the presence of measurable metals and ions in intraoperative fluid samples indicates that metal particles and ions are certainly released at the time of implantation [57].

The Food and Drug Administration (FDA), explained that variability in metals detection is possible given test interpretation differences, accuracy and precision of the detection method, variability in the test specimen, contamination by metal ions, variance between laboratories, interfering substances and lack of proficiency testing [58,59]. These factors should be considered in future comparisons of experiments.

Remarks

Implant insertion produces changes at the implant surface, as one or more of the following factors were observed: wear, deformation, particle delamination, scratches and cracks at the lower flank of the threads, thread tips and implant apex in different proportions. Released metallic particles with variable sizes and metallic ions can be located adjacent to the implant surface or can be displaced to other distant locations (Table 1). Factors, such as higher bone density, additive implant surfaces and lack of irrigation might lead to the detection of higher percentages of metallic particles and ions, while lower bone density, subtractive implant surfaces, and abundant irrigation might reduce the number of detectable metallic particles and ions produced during implant insertion. It is recommended to standardize the methods of metals particle and ion detection, as suggested by the FDA [59].

Table 1. Titanium/metal particles released during implant insertion. The table summarizes the particle size, locations and detection methods. The particles ranged from a few nanometers to micrometers in size.

Author and Year of Publication	Original Implant Surface	Animal Model and Area of Implant Insertion	Localization of the Metal Particles	Method of Detection	Metal Detected	Particle Size/Recovered Particle Weight	Particle Geometry
Schliephake et al. [43]	Titanium, machined	Minipig mandible	Peri-implant bone and implant surface	- Scanning Electron Microscopy (SEM) - Energy-Dispersive X-ray Spectroscopy (EDX)	Titanium particles	5–30 μm	Solid and leaf-like particles
			Lungs, liver and kidneys	- Flameless atomic absorption spectroscopy (FAAS)	Titanium concentration as ng/mg dry weight of the organ	Kidneys: 2.92 ± 0.69 ng/mg Liver: 11.5 ± 1.35 ng/mg Lungs: 135.7 ± 12.42 ng/mg	-
Tanaka et al. [5]	TPS	Dog mandible	Implant-bone interface and surrounding bone tissue	- SEM - Transmission Electron Microscopy (TEM) - X-ray microanalyzer - Electron diffraction	Titanium particles	1.8–3.2 μm	-
Martini et al. [46]	- TPS - TPS + coating of fluorohydroxyapatite	Mongrel sheep femoral and tibial diaphysis	- Surface of TPS implants - Inside the new bone - Inside the medullary spaces near the TPS surface	(EDS)	Titanium particles	-	-
Franchi et al. [47]	- Titanium, machined - TPS - Alumina oxide, sandblasted and acid-etched - Zirconium oxide, sandblasted + acid-etched	Sheep femur and tibia	- Peri-implant tissue - Inside the new bone - Near blood vessels of peri-implant connective tissue around TPS implants	SEM	Titanium granules	3–60 μm	-
Wennerberg et al. [50]	- Titanium, turned - Titanium, sandblasted	New Zealand rabbit tibia	- Titanium detection was related to the distance of evaluation	- X-ray fluorescence spectroscopy (SRXRF) - Secondary ion mass spectrometry (SIMS)	Titanium concentration as ng/mg dry weight of implant	Turned: 206.7 ± 25.2 ng/mg Sandblasted: 210 ± 35.2 ng/mg	-

Table 1. *Cont.*

Author and Year of Publication	Original Implant Surface	Animal Model and Area of Implant Insertion	Localization of the Metal Particles	Method of Detection	Metal Detected	Particle Size/Recovered Particle Weight	Particle Geometry
Meyer et al. [60]	- Titanium, sandblasted + acid-etched - TPS - Machined	Minipig mandible	- Titanium particles detected at the crestal bone	- SEM - EDS	- Titanium particles and nanoparticles	20 nm to a few microns	- Angular or round elongated particles - Large and oval-shaped particles
Flatebo et al. [55]	- Titanium, anodized	- Humans	- Titanium particles detected in the gingival mucosa around cover screws	- Laser ablation inductively coupled plasma mass spectrometry (LA-ICP-MS) - High-resolution optical darkfield microscopy (HR-ODM) - SEM	- Titanium particles - Titanium isotopes	140–2300 nm	-
Senna et al. [6]	- Titanium, anodized - Titanium, sandblasted + acid-etched	- In vitro bovine ribs	- Titanium particles detected along the implantation site bone walls and cortical layer - Implant surface damage	- SEM with backscattered electron detection (BSD)	- Titanium particles	10 nm to 20 µm	-
Deppe et al. [54]	- Titanium, sandblasted + acid-etched	- Human cadaver edentulous jaws	- Implant surface damage at the apical thread flanks	- SEM	- Areas of the implant surface with loose material, lack of surface characteristics (delamination)	-	-
Sridhar et al. [56]	- Titanium, sandblasted + acid-etched	- Polyurethane foam blocks with different densities	- No particles were detected	- Digital optical microscopy - SEM - X-ray diffraction (XRD)	-	-	-

Table 1. *Cont.*

Author and Year of Publication	Original Implant Surface	Animal Model and Area of Implant Insertion	Localization of the Metal Particles	Method of Detection	Metal Detected	Particle Size/Recovered Particle Weight	Particle Geometry
Deppe et al. [51]	- Four different implants with different surface treatments were compared - Titanium, sandblasted + acid-etched (Ankylos and Straumann) - Acid-etched (Frialit) - Titanium, anodized (Nobel)	- Porcine mandible	- Evaluation of the implant surface damage/changes	- 3D confocal microscopy	- Changes in the surface topography were detected along all the implant surfaces - Major changes were observed at the apical and cervical areas - -Significant destruction of the surface of anodized implants was recorded	-	-
Pettersson et al. [49]	- Titanium, machined implants - Titanium, anodized implants	- Pig jaw bone	- Peri-implant bone	- SEM for the evaluation of implant surface changes - Coupled plasma atomic emission spectroscopy (ICP-AES) for analysis of the released titanium particles	Titanium particles were detected	- Anodized titanium implant with parallel walls 2.80 ± 0.85 µg - Anodized titanium implant, slightly tapered 2.00 ± 0.56 µg - Machined titanium implant, slightly tapered 0.91 ± 0.36 µg	-

2.2. *Potential Causes of Titanium Particle and Ion Release in the Prosthetic Phase*

The implant-abutment interface involves the interaction of the internal walls of the implant connection and the surface of the abutment connection. The material properties, the magnitude, direction and duration of the forces, the composition and saliva pH and the microflora can all influence the amount of titanium particles and ions released from the implant-abutment interface into the surrounding environment [61–70].

2.2.1. Implant-Abutment Material Interface

Titanium and zirconia abutments induce different levels of wear to the implant connection. Klotz et al. [61] applied cyclic load of up to 1,000,000 cycles with forces from 20 N to 200 N to titanium and zirconia abutments connected to titanium implants. They found that implants with zirconia abutments suffered greater wear and more titanium particle release than implants with titanium abutments. The authors explained that these differences were produced because the hardness of the zirconia is approximately 10 times higher than the hardness of grade 4, commercially pure titanium (1600–2000 Vickers hardness (HV) for zirconia vs. 258 HV for titanium) [61,66,67].

The amount of wear at the implant-abutment connection was quantified by Stimmelmayr et al. [62], who demonstrated significantly more wear at the shoulder of implants connected to zirconia abutments (10.2 ± 1.5 μm) than that of implants connected to titanium abutments (0.7 ± 0.3 μm) [62]. When materials with different mechanical properties interact, more wear and deformation are expected in the weakest material. Indeed, the zirconia flexural strength is greater than 1000 MPa, and its elastic modulus is greater than 200 GPa, making it a more rigid material than titanium [63,64].

In similar studies comparing the zirconia abutment-titanium implant interface with the titanium-titanium interface, small regions of scratching and crushing after dynamic loading were observed in the titanium-titanium interface. In contrast, the zirconia-titanium implant interface was dramatically affected after dynamic loading. The interface between materials with very different Young's moduli could suffer wear, micro separations, and consequently, mechanical failure of the connection [65].

Furthermore, interactions between pure titanium and titanium alloys with greater hardness can result in more deformation and wear at the implant connection. For instance, an abutment made in titanium alloy (Ti6Al4V) is characterized by a mean hardness value of approximately 350–370 HV, while an implant synthesized from commercially pure titanium has a hardness of approximately 200–280 HV. Consequently, plastic deformation and wear often occur within implant connection surfaces, resulting in loosening of the joint and a reduction in its mechanical integrity [68–70].

Remarks

Implant-abutment connection wear is influenced by the characteristics of the coupled materials. The combination of an implant with an abutment (harder or softer) will result in wear of the weakest involved material and potentially in metallic particle release. The released particles can remain inside the connection area (thus increasing the frictional wear) or can be displaced to adjacent tissues, potentially favoring a foreign body reaction.

It is recommended to utilize materials with similar hardness and mechanical properties to reduce the wear of the abutment and the inner walls of the implant at the implant-abutment connection.

2.2.2. Microgap and Micromovement

The mismatch between implant and abutment components (micro-gap) can be increased by micromotion phenomena under functional loading, which could result in increased friction, microleakage, material wear, titanium particle release and screw loosening [68,71–80]. Braian et al. [71] evaluated the horizontal micro-gap between abutments and implants with external and internal hexagonal connections. They found the smallest micro-gap for prefabricated gold abutments (less than

50 μm) placed on implants with external hexagon compared to prefabricated plastic cylinders (less than 130 μm) placed on implants with internal hexagonal connections.

Meanwhile, Morse taper connections with no or minimal micro-gap and titanium abutments instead of zirconium abutments can reduce the wear and micromovement at the implant-abutment interface [72–74]. Conical connections also showed micro-gaps. Fatigue changes of conical connections were evaluated after functional loading by SEM and EDX. The results showed that the micro-gap between dental implant-abutment assemblies with conical connections exists prior to cyclic loading, that titanium and metallic particles (ranging from 2 μm to 80 μm in diameter) were released within the interface and outside the interface and that the effects of the wear and the micro-gap increased with the number of cycles [75].

The physicochemical and microscopic characteristics of different implant-abutment configurations were evaluated, and without exception, defects from 0.5 to 5.6 μm were present in all the samples. Therefore, the original micro-gap between the parts can lead to micromotion and wear, the release of more particles, the penetration of oral fluids and bacteria into the connection, the initiation of corrosion, as well as potential late failures [68,76–80].

Remarks

The micro-gap potentially exists in all implant-abutment connections, given unavoidable discrepancies in the fabrication process. Its dimensions are variable and it has been demonstrated that smaller micro-gaps are present in Morse and conical connections and that larger micro-gaps exist in external connections than internal connections. Larger micro-gaps result in increased micromovements, which under functional loading can increase the friction between the parts, the wear and the particle release. In addition, under functional loading, saliva and bacteria will flow, producing an additional effect, along with the displacement of titanium particles to peri-implant tissues and peri-implant bacteria to the gap of the implant-abutment connection. The presence of saliva, bacteria and their sub-products and the wear and the corrosion initiation of the metallic parts inside the implant-abutment connection might induce mechanical (screw loosening, corrosion, fatigue, fracture) and biological (mucositis, peri-implantitis) implant failures.

Therefore, it is recommended to use internal connections and Morse or conical connections that possess smaller micro-gaps. Additionally, implant companies should provide information about the micro-gap that exists in their implant-abutment connections to clinicians.

2.2.3. Titanium Oxide Layer Loss

When the titanium implant surface is exposed to air, a stable titanium oxide film is spontaneously formed at the implant surface. This thin layer (1.5–10 nm thickness) is formed due to the high affinity of Ti for oxygen [81,82]. The oxide layer protects the bulk material from reactive species and consists of TiO_2 coexisting with other titanium oxides, such as TiO and Ti_2O_3 [83,84]. The resistance to corrosion of titanium implants originates in this titanium oxide layer [85–87].

Once the oxide layer is formed (passivation), it can be altered and damaged by various environmental and functional factors and in the event of damage, the oxide layer can spontaneously reform under normal physiological conditions (re-passivation) [86]. Examples of environmental and functional factors that can alter the oxide layer are abnormal cyclic loads (overloading or continued loading), micromotion of the implant, micromovement of the implant-abutment interface, acidic environments and the combined effects of these factors [88]. Continued attack of the implant surface by these factors can result in permanent breakdown of the oxide film, leaving exposed the bulk metal to electrolytes. Varying pH conditions can turn the implant environment into a more acidic environment and active dissolution of metallic ions can occur (corrosion) [89–91].

Regarding the effects of an acidic environment on the integrity of the titanium oxide layer and bulk titanium, metabolites, such as lactic acid can induce the depletion of oxygen sources required for re-passivation, thus hindering the capability of the titanium surface to reform the oxide layer [11,89,91–97]. Therefore, metallic Ti ions are released into the surrounding tissues. Simultaneously, metallic debris is also loosened from the weakened implant surfaces exacerbating inflammatory conditions and facilitating further surface corrosion [11,89,91–97].

Saliva also plays a role in the corrosion of dental implants [98]. The dental implant interface is exposed continuously to saliva via the gingival sulcus. Saliva can act as a weak electrolyte, and the oral cavity can simulate an electrochemical cell facilitating dissolution of the oxide layer. Further electrochemical corrosion of titanium and its alloys may lead to crevice corrosion and ultimately the release of corrosion products [90,99,100].

Remarks

The titanium oxide layer appears on the implant surface as soon as the implant comes into contact with air, and although the titanium oxide layer has the capability to regrow (re-passivation), the action of continued wear, exposure to chemicals, bacteria and their sub-products, and the presence of an acidic environment can deteriorate and degrade the titanium oxide layer. To preserve the oxide layer integrity, the use of non-aggressive chemicals to disinfect the titanium surface and reduce the bacterial content and environmental acidity is recommended.

2.2.4. Corrosion

Degradation of the implant surface in the human body can be induced by two main events, i.e., wear (a mechanical degradation producing particles) and corrosion (a chemical degradation that mainly produces soluble metal ions) [101]. The term "corrosion" is generally used for metals and consists of material degradation induced by actions of the environment [102–104].

Over time and by the effects of implant function, the implant surface can experience corrosion and can release ions and particulate debris [4,105]. The metallic debris released from titanium implants can be present in various forms, including nanometric and micrometric particles, colloidal and ionic forms (bonded to proteins) [106,107], organic forms (iron-storage complexes), inorganic metal oxides and salts [106].

In the oral cavity, fluctuations in temperature, pH, oxygen, bacteria and food decomposition are attacking continuously the implant surface [91]. The TiO_2 layer is disrupted, and ions and debris generated by the physicochemical degradation of the surface are removed [108]. Through the abrasion produced by food, liquids and toothbrushes, the cycle continues [109].

Factors that can alter the corrosion resistance of the titanium surface are inflammation of the surrounding tissues (which can produce local acidification) and the acidic environment created by lactic acid released by bacteria [94,110]. The lipopolysaccharide (LPS) of gram-negative bacteria can increase the inflammation of peri-implant tissues by its marked effects on macrophages, lymphocytes, fibroblasts, and osteoblasts [111,112]. LPS chains attack the oxide film of the titanium surface (by adsorption phenomena), inducing voids in the oxide film. The Ti surface is exposed and ion exchange between the exposed surface (metal ions, M^+) and the saliva (electrons, e^-) initiates the corrosion process [113].

Furthermore, the interactions between the current flows of the dental implant and the prosthetic superstructures (produced by the differences in the electric potential of the materials) can create crevice, pitting and galvanic corrosion and the subsequent dissolution of the pure metal and alloy components [100]. Under mechanical loading, the corrosion resistance of the metal alloy decreases in different proportions, with cast and machined titanium having the most passive current density at a given potential and chromium-nickel alloys having the most active critical current density values. High-gold-content alloys have excellent corrosion resistance, and palladium alloys have a low critical current density due to the presence of gallium [114].

Chromium-cobalt framework and implant interactions were analysed in vitro, and the results showed that both the implants and the frameworks suffered active degradation processes, ions of all the materials were released and leakage of cobalt ions was greater than the leakage of titanium and chromium ions. In addition, the surfaces of the implants and frameworks became rougher after exposure to saliva [115]. These differences in percentages could be explained by the nature of metallic elements (crystalline structure, surface energy, solubility and exposed area) [116,117] and the quantity and duration of exposure [118]. Ion leakage will occur for all solid surfaces in contact with liquids until the solubility constant is reached [93].

Corrosion could occur also at the intraosseous portion of the implant surrounded by bone. This occurs by a phenomenon in which two surfaces (the implant surface and bone) under mechanical loading can have an oscillatory relative motion of a small, amplitude (fretting) [93], in which chemical reactions are prevalent. This type of corrosion is characterized by particle removal, oxide formation and increased abrasion, which increase the wear of the implant surface [119].

2.2.5. Tribocorrosion

This mechanism involves a combination of tribological (wear and fretting) and corrosive (chemical or electrochemical) events and is influenced by variations in mechanical contact conditions (loading and relative velocity) and in the nature of the environment (pH, humidity and biochemistry) [120–122].

Revathi et al. [120] described the sequence of tribocorrosion as follows: a given load is applied between two surfaces; in the presence of lubricant particles, the load will allow a sliding movement that will produce oxide layer fractures, microcracks, diffusion and re-passivation, wear debris release and finally material dissolution through five types of corrosion, i.e., microbial, galvanic, uniform, crevice and fretting corrosion [121].

Specifically, for titanium implants and the salivary pH, the titanium showed inferior performance in tribocorrosion at pH 6.0, which manifested as greater weight loss and increased cracking [113]. The normal pH of saliva ranges between 6.3 and 7.0 [11,123], various conditions can lower the pH of saliva to below 6.0 (infection, food, oral hygiene products, age, periodontitis, smoking, systemic disease and salivary gland radiation) [123], favoring the corrosion process [124–126]; under these simultaneous actions, the total material loss may be significantly greater than that under mechanical wear or corrosion individually [127].

2.2.6. Fluoride and Titanium Corrosion

Fluoride is one of the main methods for dental caries prevention and is present in many toothpastes and gels. Its percentages range from 0.1 to 2.0 wt%. At these concentrations, fluoride can reduce the corrosion resistance of metallic implants [128]. Apparently, the presence of fluoride ions in the electrolytic environment of the oral cavity attacks the titanium oxide layer and facilitates its dissolution [129].

The interaction between fluoride and titanium surface was described by Kaneko et al. [130]; the oxide film reacts in the presence of fluoride solutions by forming complexes of molecules on the implant surface (titanium fluoride, titanium oxide fluoride and sodium titanium fluoride). These soluble molecules replace the titanium oxide film, allowing corrosion initiation [130]. Once the titanium oxide film is lost, the compound films formed on the surface will undergo rapid dissolution. The rate of dissolution depends on the formation of a new oxide compound at the metal oxide interface, the flow of electrons to fill the metal or oxygen vacancies in the film, the generation or consumption of vacancies at the oxide/electrolyte interface and the chemical or electrochemical dissolution process itself [10–13].

The effect of the time of immersion of titanium implants with different surface treatments (sandblasted and acid-etched, micro-sanded with calcium phosphate and acid-etching, saline solution and saliva) on the percentage of metallic particle and ion release were evaluated by Barbieri et al. [14]. Different time points were selected, and mass spectrometry was used for the detection of particles and ions in the solution. The authors found that all implant surfaces released titanium, nickel and vanadium after seven days and that these percentages increased in proportional to the elapsed time until the sixth month [14].

Remarks

Fluoride ions have the capability to bond to the titanium oxide layer and create compounds that dissolve easily in acidic media, thereby facilitating titanium or metal dissolution and particle and ion release. Although the behavior of fluoride in vitro may vary slightly compared to that in clinical settings (based on the buffer capability of food and saliva), the noxious effect of fluoride on titanium corrosion cannot be denied. It is recommended to utilize non-fluoride rinses or gels for daily care and use alternative (non-acidic) substances in patients with titanium dental implants.

2.3. *Potential Causes of Titanium Particle and Ion Release during the Maintenance Phase*

The maintenance phase of dental implants and restorations involves the control of biological (i.e., biofilm and plaque) and mechanical risk factors. There are no defined protocols for dental implant maintenance, cleaning or disinfection, and apparently, all existing methods have negative effects of different magnitudes on the implant surface.

2.3.1. Biofilms

The extraosseous surface of dental implants (i.e., polished neck) and restorations (i.e., abutments, metal frameworks) will develop a biofilm once exposed to the oral cavity environment [131,132]. Different surface characteristics, such as chemistry, energy and topography, can influence biofilm formation [133,134].

The first step in biofilm formation is the adsorption of a layer of organic molecules (i.e., salivary proteins) to the material surface [133]. The subsequent step is the adhesion of cells and bacteria mediated by membrane binding sites, such as glucan-binding sites or specific protein-binding sites, such as those for proline-rich proteins [134]. Then, different bacterial populations attach to the pellicle, allowing accumulation of the biofilm, which depends on additional surface characteristics, such as the surface tension. These steps were demonstrated in experimental studies showing that the initial retention of microorganisms to surfaces was strongly related to the forces required for mechanical removal and to the energy of the exposed surface [135].

Within the oral cavity, there is a continuous introduction and removal of microorganisms and nutrients; for these microorganisms to survive they must be adhered to soft or hard tissues to resist, shear forces [135,136]. Bacterial adhesion to soft tissues is reduced by the turnover of the oral epithelia, however, hard, solid structures (teeth, dentures, implants) provide non-shedding surfaces, which allow the formation of thicker and more stable biofilms [137]. In general, established biofilms maintain equilibrium with the host, but uncontrolled accumulation or metabolism of bacteria on hard surfaces can cause dental caries, gingivitis, periodontitis, peri-implantitis and stomatitis [137].

Oral bacteria will adsorb, organize and group on exposed surfaces, forming plaques. These microenvironments of bacteria and their sub-products require efficient removal from the contaminated surface. The main problem associated with plaque removal from an implant surface is potential damage to the surface, which can be permanent [138,139].

Therefore, methods of implant surface detoxification and plaque and calculus removal causing little or no damage to the surface should be preferred. Current methods used for the decontamination of implant surfaces include mechanical instruments, chemical agents and lasers [140]. Different advantages, disadvantages and limitations have been correlated with these methods, thus, there is no defined gold standard for implant surface decontamination [141].

2.3.2. Scaling Instruments

Non-metal instruments (plastic and Teflon tips) were found to cause minimal damage to both smooth and rough titanium surfaces. Meanwhile, hard instruments (metallic) cause major damage to smooth and rough surfaces [16–20,142,143]. Burs seemed to be the instruments of choice if the smoothening of a rough surface was required, but they led to increased metal particle release [16].

Non-metal instruments and rubber cups were shown to be adequate for smooth and rough implant surfaces, air abrasives should be preferred if the surface integrity must be maintained. However, these approaches involve two events that alter the original surface: first, the release of titanium particles produced by the cleaning method; and second, the deposition of instrumentation materials, and residues of the air-abrasive (cleaning powders) [17].

Instruments used for the mechanical cleaning of the implant surface, such as metal curettes and conventional sonic and ultrasonic scalers can damage the implant surface (particle release, modification of the original surface topography and chemical changes). Meanwhile, non-metal instruments and air abrasives produce less damage and fewer alterations to the surface but have been associated with incomplete plaque removal and the generation of sub-products [16]. If the surface roughness is modified, biofilm formation or cell re-attachment can also be influenced, thus altering the healing process [17].

Hallmon et al. [18] and Homiak et al. [19] also found that after multiple uses, plastic curettes changed the structure of the titanium surface. Similarly, Cross-Poline et al. [20] studied the effects of instrumentation on titanium surfaces. They found that the surfaces changed compared to the original control surfaces and observed both particle detachment from the surface and traces of instrumentation materials on the treated surface [20].

The most external areas of the implant are more exposed to damage and deformation than internal areas during mechanical instrumentation. Augthun et al. [142] found roughening of the original implant surface at the implant thread edges after the use of a steel curette for 60 s. Differences can be expected given the multiple factors that influence the extent of surface damage, i.e., the number of strokes, the pressure, the number of treatments and the cleaning instrument [143].

2.3.3. Implantoplasty

This procedure aims to reduce the adherence of plaque by eliminating the contaminated titanium surface, removing inaccessible areas below the contaminated threads, and smoothing the surface topography, thus facilitating implant cleaning [144]. The most efficient drills for implantoplasty regarding the smoothness of the surface achieved were conical carbide drills (Ra < 1 μm) compared with round carbide drills (Ra > 1 μm) [18,145].

Intentionally changing the implant surface by implantoplasty with diamond burs and polishing devices was evaluated; originally, smooth titanium surfaces suffered severe damage and increased surface roughness, together with metallic traces and deposits on the titanium surfaces [146]. When performing implantoplasty, titanium or metallic particles are released, and extraordinary care must be taken to completely remove all titanium particle deposits from the surrounding tissue [147]. Carbide and diamond burs for implantoplasty were compared in vitro; the burs were used alone and in sequence. The original roughness of titanium implants with TPS and SLA surfaces were compared with that of the surfaces after implantoplasty, and both drills changed the roughness of both surfaces [148]. Implantoplasty can reduce bacterial adhesion (through reducing the surface roughness and eliminating non-cleansable areas), but some risks exist with this treatment, including high temperatures, released particles, implant surface damage, implant diameter reduction and implant fracture [149].

Implants immersed in acrylic blocks, were treated by implantoplasty with one of the following methods: diamond burs and silicone polishers; diamond burs and Arkansas stones; diamond drill short sequence; diamond drill short sequence and silicone polishers; diamond drill complete sequence; and diamond drill complete sequence and silicone polishers [150]. The authors found that all methods reduced the surface roughness, but pollution of the operative field was observed in the groups using silicone polishers. The authors concluded that the use of diamond burs and Arkansas stones resulted in a smoother surface with less debris and recommended studies investigating the bio-toxicity of the different types of debris that can be generated during implantoplasty procedures [150].

One potential drawback of implantoplasty procedures is that titanium particles removed from a contaminated implant surface are also contaminated and may not be fully removed from the surrounding environment, which could disseminate bacteria into the surrounding tissues [151].

Remarks

Implantoplasty is the implant surface decontamination procedure releasing relatively more titanium and metal debris. The surface topography is completely modified after implantoplasty, and the external geometry of the implant is removed (using different drills) to facilitate decontamination. A second procedure (polishing) is performed to reduce the surface roughness. As a consequence, particles of different sizes (nanometric and micrometric) and weights are released. It is recommended to use sufficient irrigation during and after the implantoplasty procedure, as well as powerful surgical suction that will be useful for removing released particles from the peri-implant tissues.

2.3.4. Air-Abrasion

Air-abrasion or polishing is a mechanical method for cleaning teeth and implants surfaces. The method uses powders with different particle sizes contained in a waterjet [152,153] that can remove contaminants and clean and polish the surface [154]. Low-abrasive powders (glycine and erythritol) are used in the waterjet, and a specially designed subgingival nozzle allows application to contaminated implant areas [155–157].

The cleaning efficiency of the air-abrasion method was investigated by Tastepe et al. [158]. The authors applied air-abrasion to the simulated subgingival area of titanium implant surfaces in 48 titanium discs. The most efficient decontamination was obtained when the parameters of cleaning were adjusted as follows: application of higher air pressure (while avoiding air emphysema), better insertion of the nozzle tip into the subgingival area, increased movement of the nozzle tip in the subgingival area (up-down, rotation, and slow upward movements) and sufficient water flow [158].

Ronay et al. [159] compared three implant surface debridement methods: curettes, ultrasonic scaling and air-powder abrasion. The authors found that air-abrasion cleaned more surface area than the other methods and did not alter the titanium surface [159]. Duarte et al. [160] evaluated bacterial adhesion on smooth and rough surfaces after decontamination with one of the following procedures: erbium-doped:yttrium, aluminium, and garnet (Er:YAG) laser, metal and plastic curettes and air-powder abrasion. They found that smooth implant surface roughness was increased when metal curettes were used, and rough surfaces showed reduced roughness and bacterial adhesion when metal curettes followed by air-abrasion were used; the authors did not evaluate the presence of metallic debris [160].

Kreisler et al. [161] compared Er:YAG laser and an air-powder system to remove *Porphyromonas gingivalis* from titanium plates. After the surface treatment, fibroblasts were incubated on the specimens, and the proliferation rate was evaluated. They found that both treatments (laser and air powder) supported comparable cell growth, but the air-powder treatment produced slight changes on the implant surface, whereas the laser-treated surfaces remained unchanged [162]. Apparently, in air-abrasion, the optimal air pressure for decontaminating a surface without causing significant alterations is 60–90 psi for 60 s [163].

Remarks

Air-abrasion methods with soft powders seem to provide adequate decontamination of titanium discs and titanium implant surfaces. The surfaces treated with this method show minimal or no titanium particle release when the air pressure is adequate (60–90 psi) and sufficient water flow is provided. To reach subgingival areas, specially designed tips are required. This method is apparently safe for dental implant surfaces.

2.3.5. Chemical Decontamination Methods

Chemical methods can be used alone or in combination with mechanical methods for more efficient implant surface decontamination. Chemical methods reduce bacterial adhesion and eliminate bacterial toxins or sub-products present at the implant surface. Among these chemicals are citric acid, tetracycline, saline, chlorhexidine, hydrogen peroxide, tetracycline and doxycycline [164–167]. Usually, a carrier (cotton swab) is immersed or soaked in the chemical solution and applied to the implant surface with a rubbing movement to clean all the contaminated implant surfaces [168].

Wheelis et al. [168] observed that the combination of rubbing, treatment with a carbon dioxide laser, and any of the following chemicals produced different levels of surface corrosion: citric acid, 15% hydrogen peroxide, chlorhexidine gluconate, tetracycline, doxycycline, sodium fluoride and peroxyacetic acid. Surface corrosion and pitting were presented when more acidic solutions were used ($pH < 3$); mildly acidic solutions caused surface discoloration, and neutral solutions did not cause signs of corrosion. However, EDS-analysis of all cotton swabs showed the presence of titanium particles [168].

This findings can be explained as follows: acidic solutions ($pH < 3$) and/or solution with high fluoride concentrations (greater than 0.2%) disrupt the oxide layer on the titanium surface and may inhibit re-passivation (resulting in corrosion), causing localized dissolution of the bulk titanium (pitting), discoloration and the release of ions and metallic debris into the surrounding medium [92,96,129,169–173].

Chemicals for decontamination have also been used in combinations; Wiedmer et al. [174] used combinations of hydrogen peroxide and titanium oxide (H_2O_2 + TiO_2) compared to H_2O_2 alone and chlorhexidine (CHX) for the decontamination of titanium surfaces contaminated with *Staphylococcus epidermidis* biofilms. The authors found that surface treatment with a H_2O_2 + TiO_2 suspension was superior to that with H_2O_2 and CHX for the decontamination of dental implants. This antimicrobial effect is produced by the chemical interaction of TiO_2 particles with H_2O_2, producing ROS (hydroperoxyl and hydroxyl radicals) and rupturing the bacterial membrane. Unfortunately, its effects on the titanium oxide layer have not been confirmed [174].

Among chemical methods, the application of citric acid is considered slightly superior to that of saline for biofilm removal from titanium surfaces [175,176]. However, studies showed that citric acid at a 40% concentration applied by rubbing to the titanium surface induced changes in the topography and potentially increased the surface roughness; because of its acidic nature, it also potentially dissolves the titanium oxide layer [96,177–179].

Ungvari et al. [180], compared three chemical cleaning methods (3% H_2O_2 for 5 min; saturated citric acid at pH 1 for 1 min, and chlorhexidine gel at 0.12% for 5 min). After treatment, the samples were evaluated by atomic force microscopy (AFM) and X-ray photoelectron spectroscopy (XPS). AFM showed a slight increase in the surface roughness but did not reveal differences in roughness among the groups, and XPS confirmed the presence of an intact TiO_2 layer on all the surfaces, thus demonstrating that these chemicals applied under these conditions will not damage the titanium oxide layer of the titanium surface [180].

Remarks

Chemical methods facilitate the removal of plaque, elimination of bacteria and reduction of toxins deposited on the implant surface. As a consequence of their pH, some chemical methods can damage the titanium oxide layer and produce corrosion of the titanium surface. When applying chemical substances to an implant surface, the friction removes existing corrosion products, releasing titanium particles from the implant surface and leaving the bulk titanium exposed.

Among the chemical decontamination methods, it seems that saline, chlorhexidine, hydrogen peroxide and saturated citric acid (less than 1 min) produce minimal alterations on the implant surface. There is a lack of information about the effects of tetracycline and doxycycline on titanium particle release from implant surfaces.

2.3.6. Laser Decontamination Methods

The antimicrobial activity of laser light is based on its photothermal effects [181] and its capability to denature proteins [182], and these effects on titanium surfaces are related to the wavelength and operation settings.

When the CO_2-laser beam is directed onto a titanium implant surface, the laser light is reflected by rougher surfaces [183].

Different power settings for CO_2 lasers might have different impacts on the titanium surface. The effect of laser irradiation on four titanium surfaces at a power of 1.0 W and 4.0 W with 50 pulses per second (pps) and energies from 15.2 to 60.8 Joules per pulse with a laser beam diameter of 200 μm was compared and surface alterations were found both macroscopically (dark spots) and microscopically (melted and glazed Ti) at power outputs above 2 W [183–186]. Shibli et al. [187], who evaluated the effects of laser decontamination of the surface of failed titanium implants. A CO_2-laser at a power of 1.2 W and energy of 40 J for 40 s at a distance of 30 mm from the implant surface was used. No alterations in the implant surface were detected by SEM or EDS analysis [187].

Also Park et al. [188,189] showed that the CO_2-laser at a low power (1.0 or 2.0 W) did not alter the implant surface, regardless of implant type, while at of 3.5 and 5 W, the laser produced surface alterations and gas. Romanos et al. [190] evaluated the effects of CO_2 lasers for the treatment of peri-implantitis and concluded that the application of a CO_2 laser does not alter the implant surface, decreases bacterial contamination, and enhances osseointegration. Finally, Stuebinger et al. [191] compared different lasers for titanium surface decontamination. The CO_2 laser at a power of 2, 4 and 6 W for 10 s in continuous-wave mode did not modify surfaces [191–193].

Schmage et al. [194] compared 10 methods for the surface decontamination of titanium discs. An Er:YAG laser was used in pulsed mode at a distance of 2 mm from the implant surface and the authors found that it produced slight surface damage and only partial bacteria removal. Unfortunately, laser energy, power pulse rate were not reported [194].

The Er:YAG-laser can induce different effects on different implant surfaces. Shin et al. [195] evaluated the effect of Er:YAG-laser irradiation on the microscopic structure and surface roughness of different implant surfaces. Titanium implants with anodized and SLA surfaces were irradiated with an Er:YAG-laser with a 60, 100, 120 and 140 mJ/pulse at 10 Hz. No significant surface changes were observed in SLA surface implants, but severe changes were observed in anodic-oxidized implants with only 100 mJ/pulse irradiation [195].

Er:YAG-lasers seem to be safe for titanium surface at a power of 1 W. Park et al. [189] used higher powers of 1, 2, 3, 4 and 5 W at 20 pulses per second on pure titanium discs (machined and anodized). They observed that 2, 3, 4 and 5 W of power generated melting, coagulation and microfractures of the titanium surface in proportion to the used power.

The time of laser exposure and the energy applied are also responsible for the alterations observed in different titanium implant surfaces. Settings of 100 mJ/pulse, 10 Hz and 1 min preserve the titanium surface structure [196,197]. Meanwhile, higher energies and longer times produce surface melting, particle loosening, and surface fractures on hydroxyapatite (HA)-coated surfaces and TiO_2 surfaces [198,199]. Finally, Takagi et al. [200] analysed the efficacy of implant decontamination (calcified deposit removal) and the surface alterations of treatment with erbium lasers (Er:YAG and Er,Cr:YSGG), cotton pellets and titanium curettes. The authors found that Er:YAG and Er,Cr:YSGG lasers at 40 mJ/pulse (ED 14.2 J/cm^2/pulse) and 20 Hz with water spray in non-contact mode were superior to cotton pellets or titanium curettes and the surfaces suffered minimal damage [200].

Romanos et al. [201] analyzed the effect of a diode laser (980 nm) with different power settings applied to titanium discs in continuous-wave mode in comparison with an Nd:YAG laser. Castro et al [202] also showed intact titanium surfaces after treatment with the diode laser but extensive melting and damage after irradiation with the Nd:YAG laser [201,202].

Gonçalves et al. [203] used a 980-nm diode laser with continuous emission for 5 min at 2.5 and at 3 W to irradiate implants contaminated with *P. gingivalis* and *E. faecalis* and evaluated the bacteria reduction and the changes to the implant surfaces. The authors demonstrated that while the used parameters did not change the treated surfaces, 3 W was 100% effective for surface decontamination [203]. The thermal effects of diode lasers (810 nm and 980 nm) when used at low energy (1 W) in pulsed mode with air/water cooling maintained the temperature below the critical threshold of 47 °C [204–206].

Remarks on Laser-Assisted Decontamination Methods

Lasers used for titanium surface decontamination produce titanium surface alterations depending on the laser energy, radiation time and titanium surface characteristics. There are no studies measuring titanium particles released during or after laser decontamination. The changes in the titanium surface induced by lasers are mainly produced by the temperature increase at the irradiated spot. Each laser behaves differently on rough or machined surfaces. In general, surfaces that reflect the laser (machined surfaces) produce smaller local temperature increases but can affect the surrounding areas. On the other hand, surfaces that absorb the laser (rough surfaces) show significant implant temperature increments. Safe operation settings for each laser and surface should be carefully evaluated before the laser decontamination of implant surfaces to avoid thermal damage and surface changes. To reduce the surface damage during laser decontamination, it is recommended to use pulsed mode, short periods of irradiation, cooling with proper air-water ratios and low energies. This section may be divided by subheadings. It should provide a concise and precise description of the experimental results, their interpretation as well as the experimental conclusions that can be drawn.

3. Materials and Methods

PICO questionnaires were developed and problems, interventions, comparisons and outcomes were organized for the surgical, prosthetic and maintenance phases in implant dentistry procedures (Table 2). An exhaustive search of the literature was performed in PubMed, Medline and Google Scholar for all the relevant studies in the literature published between 1980 and 2018 involving titanium particles and ions related to dental implants and implant dentistry procedures. The following search keywords were used in this systematic review.

Table 2. PICO questions used for preparation of the systematic review to identify sources and aetiological factors for titanium particle and ion release.

P (Probelem)	Subgroup		P (Population)	I (Interventions)	C (Comparisons)	O (Outcomes)
The potential sources of titanium particle and ion release are not known or compiled in the literature	Surgical phase	Implant bed preparation	Experimental, animal and human studies	Bone drilling	Implant drills and other implant bed preparation methods	- Metal content in the adjacent bone or soft tissues after implant bed preparation - Tool wear, damage and corrosion
		Implant placement	Experimental, animal and human studies	Implant Insertion	Implant after Insertion	- Implant surface, alterations after insertion - Metal content in the adjacent bone or soft tissues after implant insertion
		Implant removal	Experimental, animal and human studies	Bone drilling	Other methods for implant removal	- Metal content in the adjacent bone or soft tissues after implant removal - Implant surface alterations and corrosion evaluated after implant removal
	Prosthetic phase	Implant abutment connection	Experimental, animal and human studies	Functional load at the implant abutment connection	Type of connection, misfit gap material	- Implant connection frictional damage - Corrosion and particle/ion release at the implant-abutment connection - Metal content in the adjacent bone or soft tissues
	Maintenance phase	Implant cleaning and decontamination techniques	Experimental, animal and human studies	Implant cleaning, disinfection and polishing	Scaling Ultrasonication Rubber cups and brushes Air-polishing Lasers Cleaning and antibacterial substances	- Metal content in the adjacent bone or soft tissues after implant cleaning, decontamination or polishing - Implant surface alterations and corrosion evaluated after implant cleaning disinfection and polishing

3.1. For the Surgical Phase

Implant bed preparation AND titanium particles; OR implant bed preparation AND metal release; OR bone drilling AND titanium particles; OR bone drilling and metal release; metal debris AND drills; OR implant drill AND wear; OR implant drill and corrosion; OR implant drill and damage; OR bone piezosurgery AND titanium particles/ions; OR osteotomy and metal particles/ions; OR osteotomy and metal debris.

Implant insertion AND metal ions; implant insertion AND titanium ions; Implant insertion AND titanium particles; OR implant insertion and implant surface alterations; OR implant insertion AND titanium release; implant insertion and metal release; OR implant insertion AND titanium particles detachment; OR implant insertion and metal debris; OR implant insertion AND bone contamination; OR implant insertion and bone metal content; implant insertion and tissue metal content.

Implant removal AND metal ions release; implant removal and titanium release; Implant removal AND titanium particles; implant removal and surface alterations; OR implant removal AND metal release; OR Implant removal and particles dislodgement; OR implant removal and metal debris.

3.2. For the Prosthetic Phase

Implant abutment connection AND wear; OR implant abutment connection and deformation; OR implant abutment connection AND titanium particles; implant abutment connection AND ions release; OR implant abutment connection AND corrosion; OR implant abutment connection material AND wear; OR implant abutment connection misfit; implant abutment connection misfit AND wear; dental Implants AND fretting corrosion.

3.3. For the Maintenance Phase

Implant decontamination AND wear; OR implant decontamination and corrosion; OR fluoride AND titanium corrosion; OR chlorhexidine AND titanium corrosion; OR implant scaling AND titanium wear; OR implant surface polishing AND particles release; implant surface polishing AND titanium findings in soft tissues; implant surface polishing AND titanium particles in bone; OR chemical decontamination AND implant surface OR laser decontamination AND implant surface OR laser decontamination AND titanium particles OR laser decontamination AND titanium ions.

Two investigators (RD and GR) performed the initial searches using the keyword combinations; the titles that appeared in the search containing the keywords were reviewed and these fulfilling the inclusion criteria were included for abstract review. The abstracts of the articles were read in full, and those fulfilling the inclusion criteria were included for full-text review and data extraction.

In the case of a disagreement between reviewers, a third investigator (JLC) was included for a final decision regarding the inclusion or exclusion of the articles.

The inclusion criteria were determined as follows: experimental, animal and human studies published in the English language that analyzed titanium particle or ion release in the surgical, prosthetic/restorative or maintenance phase in implant dentistry. The titanium/metal particles released during implant insertion, particle size, location and detection methods were compiled (Table 3).

The exclusion criteria were as follows: articles in languages other than English, reviews, other systematic reviews and expert opinions as well as duplicated articles were excluded.

Table 3. Titanium/metal particles released during implant insertion. The table summarizes the particle size, locations and detection methods. The particles ranged from a few nanometers to micrometers in size.

Author and Year of Publication	Original Implant Surface	Animal Model and Area of Implant Insertion	Localization of the Metal Particles	Method of Detection	Metal Detected	Particle Size/Recovered Particle Weight	Particle Geometry
Schliephake et al. [43]	Titanium, machined	Minipig mandible	Peri-implant bone and implant surface	- Scanning Electron Microscopy (SEM) - Energy-Dispersive X-ray Spectroscopy (EDX)	Titanium particles	5–30 µm	Solid and leaf-like particles
			Lungs, liver and kidneys	- Flameless atomic absorption spectroscopy (FAAS)	Titanium concentration as ng/mg dry weight of the organ	Kidneys: 2.92 ± 0.69 ng/mg Liver: 11.5 ± 1.35 ng/mg Lungs: 135.7 ± 12.42 ng/mg	-
Tanaka et al. [5]	TPS	Dog mandible	Implant-bone interface and surrounding bone tissue	- SEM - Transmission Electron Microscopy (TEM) - X-ray microanalyzer - Electron diffraction	Titanium particles	1.8–3.2 µm	-
Martini et al. [46]	- TPS - TPS + coating of fluorohydroxyapatite	Mongrel sheep femoral and tibial diaphysis	- Surface of TPS implants - Inside the new bone - Inside the medullary spaces near the TPS surface	(EDS)	Titanium particles	-	-
Franchi et al. [47]	- Titanium, machined - TPS - Alumina oxide, sandblasted and acid-etched - Zirconium oxide, sandblasted + acid-etched	Sheep femur and tibia	- Peri-implant tissue - Inside the new bone - Near blood vessels of peri-implant connective tissue around TPS implants	SEM	Titanium granules	3–60 µm	-
Wennerberg et al. [50]	- Titanium, turned - Titanium, sandblasted	New Zealand rabbit tibia	- Titanium detection was related to the distance of evaluation	- X-ray fluorescence spectroscopy (SRXRF) - Secondary ion mass spectrometry (SIMS)	- Titanium concentration as ng/mg dry weight of implant	Turned: 206.7 ± 25.2 ng/mg Sandblasted: 210 ± 35.2 ng/mg	-
Meyer et al. [60]	- Titanium, sandblasted + acid-etched - TPS - Machined	Minipig mandible	- Titanium particles detected at the crestal bone	- SEM - EDS	- Titanium particles and nanoparticles	20 nm to a few microns	- Angular or round elongated particles - Large and oval-shaped particles

Table 3. *Cont.*

Author and Year of Publication	Original Implant Surface	Animal Model and Area of Implant Insertion	Localization of the Metal Particles	Method of Detection	Metal Detected	Particle Size/Recovered Particle Weight	Particle Geometry
Flatebo et al. [55]	- Titanium, anodized	- Humans	- Titanium particles detected in the gingival mucosa around cover screws	- Laser ablation inductively coupled plasma mass spectrometry (LA-ICP-MS) - High-resolution optical darkfield microscopy (HR-ODM) - SEM	- Titanium particles - Titanium isotopes	140–2300 nm	-
Senna et al. [6]	- Titanium, anodized - Titanium, sandblasted + acid-etched	- In vitro bovine ribs	- Titanium particles detected along the implantation site bone walls and cortical layer - Implant surface damage	- SEM with backscattered electron detection (BSD)	- Titanium particles	10 nm to 20 μm	-
Deppe et al. [54]	- Titanium, sandblasted + acid-etched	- Human cadaver edentulous jaws	- Implant surface damage at the apical thread flanks	- SEM	- Areas of the implant surface with loose material, lack of surface characteristics (delamination)	-	-
Sridhar et al. [56]	- Titanium, sandblasted + acid-etched	- Polyurethane foam blocks with different densities	- No particles were detected	- Digital optical microscopy - SEM - X-ray diffraction (XRD)	-	-	-
Deppe et al. [51]	- Four different implants with different surface treatments were compared - Titanium, sandblasted + acid-etched (Ankylos and Straumann) - Acid-etched (Frialit) - Titanium, anodized (Nobel)	- Porcine mandible	- Evaluation of the implant surface damage/changes	- 3D confocal microscopy	- Changes in the surface topography were detected along all the implant surfaces - Major changes were observed at the apical and cervical areas - Significant destruction of the surface of anodized implants was recorded	-	-

Table 3. *Cont.*

Author and Year of Publication	Original Implant Surface	Animal Model and Area of Implant Insertion	Localization of the Metal Particles	Method of Detection	Metal Detected	Particle Size/Recovered Particle Weight	Particle Geometry
Pettersson et al. [49]	- Titanium, machined implants - Titanium, anodized implants	- Pig jaw bone	- Peri-implant bone	- SEM for the evaluation of implant surface changes - Coupled plasma atomic emission spectroscopy (ICP-AES) for analysis of the released titanium particles	Titanium particles were detected	- Anodized titanium implant with parallel walls 2.80 ± 0.85 µg - Anodized titanium implant, slightly tapered 2.00 ± 0.56 µg - Machined titanium implant, slightly tapered 0.91 ± 0.36 µg	-

4. Conclusions

Dental implants have revolutionized the dentistry profession, and titanium dental implants have demonstrated their utility and safety for more than 40 years. However, over time, it has become evident that debris and sub-products can be generated during the life of the implant.

Titanium particles and ions can also be released from metallic instruments used for implant bed preparation, from the implant surfaces during insertion and from the implant-abutment interface during insertion and functional loading. In addition, the implant surfaces and restorations are exposed to the environment, saliva, bacteria and chemicals that can potentially dissolve the titanium oxide layer. If these agents attack continuously, the implant surface can permanently lose its titanium oxide layer.

The formation of soluble compounds on the titanium surface will alter the implant surface chemistry and facilitate the dissolution and degradation of exposed bulk titanium, resulting in the initiation of corrosion cycles. Implant maintenance procedures can potentially alter implant surfaces and produce titanium debris that will be released into the peri-implant tissues.

Multiple variables, such as the bone density, mechanical overloading and the use of fluorides, can also influence the proportion of metal particles and ions released from implants and restorations. The complex oral environment can also change with age and the use of medications, and these factors have not yet been studied.

This review provides, for the first time, a summary of the potential sources of titanium particles and ion release in implant dentistry and, based on the findings, suggests methods for reducing this release. The long-term local and systemic effects of titanium particles and ions released into the oral environment and their potential effects on cells, tissues and organs remain unknown due to the rapid evolution and variability of new implant surfaces, new implant-abutment connections and new restorative materials.

Author Contributions: Conceptualization: R.D.-R., G.R.; Data Curation and Resources: R.D.-R., G.R.; Formal Analysis: R.D.-R., G.R.; Funding Acquisition and Research: R.D.-R., G.R.: Methodology: R.D.-R., G.R.; R.D.-R., G.R.; Writing—original draft: R.D.-R., G.R.; Writing—review & editing: R.D.-R., G.R.; Visualization and Methodology: R.D.-R., G.R.; Supervision: R.D.-R., G.R.

Acknowledgments: The authors thank Jose Luis Calvo-Guirado for helping in solving disagreement regarding the inclusion or exclusion or articles for this systematic review.

References

1. Staroveski, T.; Brezak, D.; Udiljak, T. Drill wear monitoring in cortical bone drilling. *Med. Eng. Phys.* **2015**, *37*, 560–566. [CrossRef] [PubMed]
2. Ferguson, A.B.; Laing, P.G.; Hodge, E.S. The ionization of metal implants in living tissues. *J. Bone Jt. Surg.* **1960**, *42*, 77–90. [CrossRef]
3. Ferguson, A.B.; Akahoshi, Y.; Laing, P.G.; Hodge, E.S. Characteristics of trace ion release from embedded metal implants in the rabbit. *J. Bone Jt. Surg.* **1962**, *44*, 317–336. [CrossRef]
4. Meachim, G.; Williams, D.F. Changes in nonosseous tissue adjacent to titanium implants. *J. Biomed. Mater. Res.* **1973**, *7*, 555–572. [CrossRef] [PubMed]
5. Tanaka, N.; Ichinose, S.; Kimijima, Y.; Mimura, M. Investigation of titanium leak to bone tissue surrounding dental titanium implant: Electron microscopic findings and analysis by electron diffraction. *Med. Electron Microsc.* **2000**, *33*, 96–101. [CrossRef] [PubMed]
6. Senna, P.; Cury, A.A.D.; Kates, S.; Meirelles, L. Surface damage on dental implants with release of loose particles after insertion into bone. *Clin. Implant Dent. Relat. Res.* **2015**, *17*, 681–692. [CrossRef] [PubMed]
7. Bianco, P.D.; Ducheyne, P.; Cuckler, J.M. Titanium serum and urine levels in rabbits with a titanium implant in the absence of wear. *Biomaterials* **1996**, *17*, 1937–1942. [CrossRef]

8. Browne, M.; Gregson, P.J. Effect of mechanical surface pretreatment on metal ion release. *Biomaterials* **2000**, *21*, 385–392. [CrossRef]
9. Ferguson, A.B. Metals in living tissues. *Surg. Clin. N. Am.* **1960**, *40*, 521–529. [CrossRef]
10. Frateur, I.; Cattarin, S.; Musiani, M.; Tribollet, B. Electrodissolution of Ti and p-Si in acidic fluoride media: Formation ratio of oxide layers from electrochemical impedance spectroscopy. *J. Electroanal. Chem.* **2000**, *482*, 202–210. [CrossRef]
11. Mabilleau, G.; Bourdon, S.; Joly-Guillou, M.L.; Filmon, R.; Baslé, M.F.; Chappard, D. Influence of fluoride, hydrogen peroxide and lactic acid on the corrosion resistance of commercially pure titanium. *Acta Biomater.* **2006**, *2*, 121–129. [CrossRef] [PubMed]
12. Siirila, H.S.; Kononen, M. The effect of oral topical fluorides on the surface of commercially pure titanium. *Int. J. Oral Maxillofac. Implant.* **1991**, *6*, 50–54.
13. Toumelin-Chemla, F.; Rouelle, F.; Burdairon, G. Corrosive properties of fluoride-containing odontologic gels against titanium. *J. Dent.* **1996**, *24*, 109–115. [CrossRef]
14. Barbieri, M.; Mencio, F.; Papi, P.; Rosella, D.; di Carlo, S.; Valente, T.; Pompa, G. Corrosion behavior of dental implants immersed into human saliva: Preliminary results of an in vitro study. *Eur. Rev. Med. Pharmacol. Sci.* **2017**, *21*, 3543–3548. [PubMed]
15. Woodman, J.L.; Jacobs, J.J.; Galante, J.O.; Urban, R.M. Metal ion release from titanium-based prosthetic segmental replacements of long bones in baboons: A long-term study. *J. Orthop. Res.* **1984**, *1*, 421–430. [CrossRef] [PubMed]
16. Louropoulou, A.; Slot, D.E.; van der Weijden, F.A. Titanium surface alterations following the use of different mechanical instruments: A systematic review. *Clin. Oral Implants Res.* **2012**, *23*, 643–658. [CrossRef] [PubMed]
17. Ruhling, A.; Kocher, T.; Kreusch, J.; Plagmann, H.C. Treatment of subgingival implant surfaces with TeflonR-coated sonic and ultrasonic scaler tips and various implant curettes. An in vitro study. *Clin. Oral Implant. Res.* **1994**, *5*, 19–29. [CrossRef]
18. Hallmon, W.W.; Waldrop, T.C.; Meffert, R.M.; Wade, B.W. A comparative study of the effects of metallic, nonmetallic, and sonic instrumentation on titanium abutment surfaces. *Int. J. Oral Maxillofac. Implant.* **1996**, *11*, 96–100. [CrossRef]
19. Homiak, A.W.; Cook, P.A.; DeBoer, J. Effect of hygiene instrumentation on titanium abutments: A scanning electron microscopy study. *J. Prosthet. Dent.* **1992**, *67*, 364–369. [CrossRef]
20. Cross-Poline, G.N.; Shaklee, R.L.; Stach, D.J. Effect of implant curettes on titanium implant surfaces. *Am. J. Dent.* **1997**, *10*, 41–45. [PubMed]
21. Bertoldi, C.; Pradelli, J.M.; Consolo, U.; Zaffe, D. Release of elements from retrieved maxillofacial plates and screws. *J. Mater. Sci. Mater. Med.* **2005**, *16*, 857–861. [CrossRef] [PubMed]
22. Thomas, P.; Bandl, W.-D.; Maier, S.; Summer, B.; Przybilla, B. Hypersensitivity to titanium osteosynthesis with impaired fracture healing, eczema, and T-cell hyperresponsiveness in vitro: Case report and review of the literature. *Contact Dermat.* **2006**, *55*, 199–202. [CrossRef] [PubMed]
23. Rashad, A.; Sadr-Eshkevari, P.; Weuster, M.; Schmitz, I.; Prochnow, N.; Maurer, P. Material attrition and bone micromorphology after conventional and ultrasonic implant site preparation. *Clin. Oral Implant. Res.* **2013**, *24*, 110–114. [CrossRef] [PubMed]
24. Ercoli, C.; Funkenbusch, P.D.; Lee, H.J.; Moss, M.E.; Graser, G.N. The influence of drill wear on cutting efficiency and heat production during osteotomy preparation for dental implants: A study of drill durability. *Int. J. Oral Maxillofac. Implant.* **2004**, *19*, 335–349.
25. Carvalho, A.C.; Queiroz, T.P.; Okamoto, R.; Margonar, R.L.; Garcia, I.R., Jr.; Filho, O.M. Evaluation of bone heating, immediate bone cell viability, and wear of high-resistance drills after the creation of implant osteotomies in rabbit tibias. *Int. J. Oral Maxillofac. Implant.* **2011**, *26*, 1193–1201.
26. De-Melo, J.F.; Gjerdet, N.R.; Erichsen, E.S. Metal release from cobalt-chromium partial dentures in the mouth. *Acta Odontol. Scand.* **1983**, *41*, 71–74. [CrossRef] [PubMed]
27. Queiroz, T.P.; Souza, F.Á.; Okamoto, R.; Margonar, R.; Pereira-Filho, V.A.; Garcia, I.R.; Vieira, E.H. Evaluation of immediate bone-cell viability and of drill wear after implant osteotomies: Immunohistochemistry and scanning electron microscopy analysis. *J. Oral Maxillofac. Surg.* **2008**, *66*, 1233–1240. [CrossRef] [PubMed]

28. Hochscheidt, C.J.; Shimizu, R.H.; Andrighetto, A.R.; Pierezan, R.; Thomé, G.; Salatti, R. Comparative analysis of cutting efficiency and surface maintenance between different types of implant drills. *Implant Dent.* **2017**, *26*, 723–729. [CrossRef] [PubMed]
29. Gupta, V.; Pandey, P.M. In-situ tool wear monitoring and its effects on the performance of porcine cortical bone drilling: A comparative in-vitro investigation. *Mech. Adv. Mater. Mod. Process.* **2017**, *3*, 1–7. [CrossRef]
30. Dos Santos, P.L.; Queiroz, T.P.; Margonar, R.; de Souza Carvalho, A.C.; Betoni, W., Jr.; Rezende, R.R.; dos Santos, P.H.; Garcia, I.R., Jr. Evaluation of bone heating, drill deformation, and drill roughness after implant osteotomy: Guided surgery and classic drilling procedure. *Int. J. Oral Maxillofac. Implant.* **2014**, *29*, 51–58. [CrossRef] [PubMed]
31. Allsobrook, O.F.L.; Leichter, J.; Holborow, D.; Swain, M. Descriptive study of the longevity of dental implant surgery drills. *Clin. Implant Dent. Relat. Res.* **2011**, *13*, 244–254. [CrossRef] [PubMed]
32. Chacon, G.E.; Bower, D.L.; Larsen, P.E.; McGlumphy, E.A.; Beck, F.M. Heat production by 3 implant drill systems after repeated drilling and sterilization. *J. Oral Maxillofac. Surg.* **2006**, *64*, 265–269. [CrossRef] [PubMed]
33. Cooley, R.L.; Marshall, T.D.; Young, J.M.; Huddleston, A.M. Effect of sterilization on the strength and cutting efficiency of twist drills. *Quintessence Int.* **1990**, *21*, 919–923. [PubMed]
34. Harris, B.H.; Kohles, S.S. Effects of mechanical and thermal fatigue on dental drill performance. *Int. J. Oral Maxillofac. Implant.* **2001**, *16*, 819–826.
35. Mendes, G.C.B.; Padovan, L.E.M.; Ribeiro-Júnior, P.D.; Sartori, E.M.; Valgas, L.; Claudino, M. Influence of implant drill materials on wear, deformation, and roughness after repeated drilling and sterilization. *Implant Dent.* **2014**, *23*, 188–194. [CrossRef] [PubMed]
36. Sartori, E.M.; Shinohara, É.H.; Ponzoni, D.; Padovan, L.E.M.; Valgas, L.; Golin, A.L. Evaluation of deformation, mass loss, and roughness of different metal burs after osteotomy for osseointegrated implants. *J. Oral Maxillofac. Surg.* **2012**, *70*, e608–e621. [CrossRef] [PubMed]
37. Guan, H.; van Staden, R.C.; Johnson, N.W.; Loo, Y.-C. Dynamic modelling and simulation of dental implant insertion process—A finite element study. *Finite Elem. Anal. Des.* **2011**, *47*, 886–897. [CrossRef]
38. Wawrzinek, C.; Sommer, T.; Fischer-Brandies, H. Microdamage in cortical bone due to the overtightening of orthodontic microscrews. *J. Orofac. Orthop.* **2008**, *69*, 121–134. [CrossRef] [PubMed]
39. Cvijović-Alagić, I.; Cvijović, Z.; Mitrović, S.; Panić, V.; Rakin, M. Wear and corrosion behaviour of Ti–13Nb–13Zr and Ti–6Al–4V alloys in simulated physiological solution. *Corros. Sci.* **2011**, *53*, 796–808. [CrossRef]
40. Hokkirigawa, K.; Kato, K. An experimental and theoretical investigation of ploughing, cutting and wedge formation during abrasive wear. *Tribol. Int.* **1988**, *21*, 51–57. [CrossRef]
41. Ni, W.; Cheng, Y.-T.; Lukitsch, M.J.; Weiner, A.M.; Lev, L.C.; Grummon, D.S. Effects of the ratio of hardness to Young's modulus on the friction and wear behavior of bilayer coatings. *Appl. Phys. Lett.* **2004**, *85*, 4028–4030. [CrossRef]
42. Rigney, D.A. Some thoughts on sliding wear. *Wear* **1992**, *152*, 187–192. [CrossRef]
43. Schliephake, H.; Reiss, G.; Urban, R.; Neukam, F.W.; Guckel, S. Metal release from titanium fixtures during placement in the mandible: An experimental study. *Int. J. Oral Maxillofac. Implant.* **1993**, *8*, 502–511.
44. Seki, Y.; Bessho, K.; Sugatani, T.; Kageyama, T.; Inui, M.; Tagawa, T. Clinicopathological study on titanium miniplates. *J. Oral Maxillofac. Surg.* **1994**, *40*, 892–896. [CrossRef]
45. Kim, Y.-K.; Yeo, H.-H.; Lim, S.-C. Tissue response to titanium plates: A transmitted electron microscopic study. *J. Oral Maxillofac. Surg.* **1997**, *55*, 322–326. [CrossRef]
46. Martini, D.; Fini, M.; Franchi, M.; Pasquale, V.D.; Bacchelli, B.; Gamberini, M.; Tinti, A.; Taddei, P.; Giavaresi, G.; Ottani, V.; et al. Detachment of titanium and fluorohydroxyapatite particles in unloaded endosseous implants. *Biomaterials* **2003**, *24*, 1309–1316. [CrossRef]
47. Franchi, M.; Bacchelli, B.; Martini, D.; Pasquale, V.D.; Orsini, E.; Ottani, V.; Fini, M.; Giavaresi, G.; Giardino, R.; Ruggeri, A. Early detachment of titanium particles from various different surfaces of endosseous dental implants. *Biomaterials* **2004**, *25*, 2239–2246. [CrossRef] [PubMed]
48. Geis-Gerstorfer, J.; Sauer, K.H.; Passler, K. Ion release from Ni-Cr-Mo and Co-Cr-Mo casting alloys. *Int. J. Prosthodont.* **1991**, *4*, 152–158. [PubMed]

49. Pettersson, M.; Pettersson, J.; Thorén, M.M.; Johansson, A. Release of titanium after insertion of dental implants with different surface characteristics—An ex vivo animal study. *Acta Biomater. Odontol. Scand.* **2017**, *3*, 63–73. [CrossRef] [PubMed]
50. Wennerberg, A.; Ide-Ektessabi, A.; Hatkamata, S.; Sawase, T.; Johansson, C.; Albrektsson, T.; Martinelli, A.; Sodervall, U.; Odelius, H. Titanium release from implants prepared with different surface roughness. An in vitro and in vivo study. *Clin. Oral Implant. Res.* **2004**, *15*, 505–512. [CrossRef] [PubMed]
51. Deppe, H.; Wolff, C.; Bauer, F.; Ruthenberg, R.; Sculean, A.; Mücke, T. Dental implant surfaces after insertion in bone: An in vitro study in four commercial implant systems. *Clin. Oral Implant. Res.* **2018**, *22*, 1593–1600. [CrossRef] [PubMed]
52. Mints, D.; Elias, C.; Funkenbusch, P.; Meirelles, L. Integrity of implant surface modifications after insertion. *Int. J. Oral Maxillofac. Implant.* **2014**, *29*, 97–104. [CrossRef] [PubMed]
53. Salerno, M.; Itri, A.; Frezzato, M.; Rebaudi, A. Surface microstructure of dental implants before and after insertion: An in vitro study by means of scanning probe microscopy. *Implant Dent.* **2015**, *24*, 248–255. [CrossRef] [PubMed]
54. Deppe, H.; Grünberg, C.; Thomas, M.; Sculean, A.; Benner, K.-U.; Bauer, F.J.M. Surface morphology analysis of dental implants following insertion into bone using scanning electron microscopy: A pilot study. *Clin. Oral Implant. Res.* **2015**, *26*, 1261–1266. [CrossRef] [PubMed]
55. Flatebø, R.S.; Høl, P.J.; Leknes, K.N.; Kosler, J.; Lie, S.A.; Gjerdet, N.R. Mapping of titanium particles in peri-implant oral mucosa by laser ablation inductively coupled plasma mass spectrometry and high-resolution optical darkfield microscopy. *J. Oral Pathol. Med.* **2011**, *40*, 412–420. [CrossRef] [PubMed]
56. Sridhar, S.; Wilson, T.G.; Valderrama, P.; Watkins-Curry, P.; Chan, J.Y.; Rodrigues, D.C. In vitro evaluation of titanium exfoliation during simulated surgical insertion of dental implants. *J. Oral Implantol.* **2016**, *42*, 34–40. [CrossRef] [PubMed]
57. Cundy, W.J.; Mascarenhas, A.R.; Antoniou, G.; Freeman, B.J.C.; Cundy, P.J. Local and systemic metal ion release occurs intraoperatively during correction and instrumented spinal fusion for scoliosis. *J. Child. Orthop.* **2015**, *9*, 39–43. [CrossRef] [PubMed]
58. Sampson, B.; Hart, A. Clinical usefulness of blood metal measurements to assess the failure of metal-on-metal hip implants. *Ann. Clin. Biochem.* **2012**, *49*, 118–131. [CrossRef] [PubMed]
59. USFDA. *FDA Executive Summary Memorandum. Metal-On-Metal Hip Implant Systems*; USFDA: Washington, DC, USA, 2012.
60. Meyer, U.; Bühner, M.; Büchter, A.; Kruse-Lösler, B.; Stamm, T.; Wiesmann, H.P. Fast element mapping of titanium wear around implants of different surface structures. *Clin. Oral Implant. Res.* **2006**, *17*, 206–211. [CrossRef] [PubMed]
61. Klotz, M.W.; Taylor, T.D.; Goldberg, A.J. Wear at the titanium-zirconia implant-abutment interface: A pilot study. *Int. J. Oral Maxillofac. Implant.* **2011**, *26*, 970–975.
62. Stimmelmayr, M.; Edelhoff, D.; Güth, J.-F.; Erdelt, K.; Happe, A.; Beuer, F. Wear at the titanium–titanium and the titanium–zirconia implant–abutment interface: A comparative in vitro study. *Dent. Mater.* **2012**, *28*, 1215–1220. [CrossRef] [PubMed]
63. Aboushelib, M.N.; Kleverlaan, C.J.; Feilzer, A.J. Evaluation of a high fracture toughness composite ceramic for dental applications. *J. Prosthodont.* **2008**, *17*, 538–544. [CrossRef] [PubMed]
64. Elias, C.N.; Fernandes, D.J.; Resende, C.R.S.; Roestel, J. Mechanical properties, surface morphology and stability of a modified commercially pure high strength titanium alloy for dental implants. *Dent. Mater.* **2015**, *31*, e1–e13. [CrossRef] [PubMed]
65. Cavusoglu, Y.; Akça, K.; Gürbüz, R.; Cehreli, M.C. A pilot study of joint stability at the zirconium or titanium abutment/titanium implant interface. *Int. J. Oral Maxillofac. Implant.* **2014**, *29*, 338–343. [CrossRef] [PubMed]
66. Yüzügüllü, B.; Avci, M. The implant-abutment interface of alumina and zirconia abutments. *Clin. Implant Dent. Relat. Res.* **2008**, *10*, 113–121. [CrossRef] [PubMed]
67. Beuer, F.; Korczynski, N.; Rezac, A.; Naumann, M.; Gernet, W.; Sorensen, J.A. Marginal and internal fit of zirconia based fixed dental prostheses fabricated with different concepts. *Clin. Cosmet. Investig. Dent.* **2010**, *2*, 5–11. [CrossRef] [PubMed]
68. Gratton, D.G.; Aquilino, S.A.; Stanford, C.M. Micromotion and dynamic fatigue properties of the dental implant–abutment interface. *J. Prosthet. Dent.* **2001**, *85*, 47–52. [CrossRef] [PubMed]

69. Quek, H.C.; Tan, K.B.; Nicholls, J.I. Load fatigue performance of four implant-abutment interface designs: Effect of torque level and implant system. *Int. J. Oral Maxillofac. Implant.* **2008**, *23*, 253–262.
70. Seetoh, Y.L.; Tan, K.B.; Chua, E.K.; Quek, H.C.; Nicholls, J.I. Load fatigue performance of conical implant-abutment connections. *Int. J. Oral Maxillofac. Implant.* **2011**, *26*, 797–806.
71. Braian, M.; Bruyn, H.; Fransson, H.; Christersson, C.; Wennerberg, A. Tolerance measurements on internal- and external-hexagon implants. *Int. J. Oral Maxillofac. Implant.* **2014**, *29*, 846–852. [CrossRef] [PubMed]
72. Rack, T.; Zabler, S.; Rack, A.; Riesemeier, H.; Nelson, K. An in vitro pilot study of abutment stability during loading in new and fatigue-loaded conical dental implants using synchrotron-based radiography. *Int. J. Oral Maxillofac. Implant.* **2013**, *28*, 44–50. [CrossRef] [PubMed]
73. Karl, M.; Taylor, T. Parameters determining micromotion at the implant-abutment interface. *Int. J. Oral Maxillofac. Implant.* **2014**, *29*, 1338–1347. [CrossRef] [PubMed]
74. Alqutaibi, A.Y.; Aboalrejal, A.N. Microgap and micromotion at the implant abutment interface cause marginal bone loss around dental implant but more evidence is needed. *J. Evid. Based Dent. Pract.* **2018**, *18*, 171–172. [CrossRef] [PubMed]
75. Blum, K.; Wiest, W.; Fella, C.; Balles, A.; Dittmann, J.; Rack, A.; Maier, D.; Thomann, R.; Spies, B.C.; Kohal, R.J.; et al. Fatigue induced changes in conical implant–abutment connections. *Dent. Mater.* **2015**, *31*, 1415–1426. [CrossRef] [PubMed]
76. Pereira, J.; Morsch, C.; Henriques, B.; Nascimento, R.; Benfatti, C.; Silva, F.; López-López, J.; Souza, J. Removal torque and biofilm accumulation at two dental implant–abutment joints after fatigue. *Int. J. Oral Maxillofac. Implant.* **2016**, *31*, 813–819. [CrossRef] [PubMed]
77. Prado, A.; Pereira, J.; Henriques, B.; Benfatti, C.; Magini, R.; López-López, J.; Souza, J. Biofilm affecting the mechanical integrity of implant-abutment joints. *Int. J. Prosthodont.* **2016**, *29*, 381–383. [CrossRef] [PubMed]
78. Lopes, P.A.; Carreiro, A.F.P.; Nascimento, R.M.; Vahey, B.R.; Henriques, B.; Souza, J.C.M. Physicochemical and microscopic characterization of implant-abutment joints. *Eur. J. Dent.* **2018**, *12*, 100–104. [CrossRef] [PubMed]
79. Tsuge, T.; Hagiwara, Y.; Matsumura, H. Marginal fit and microgaps of implant-abutment interface with internal anti-rotation configuration. *Dent. Mater. J.* **2008**, *27*, 29–34. [CrossRef] [PubMed]
80. Binon, P.P. The effect of implant/abutment hexagonal misfit on screw joint stability. *Int. J. Prosthodont.* **1996**, *9*, 149–160. [PubMed]
81. Kuromoto, N.K.; Simão, R.A.; Soares, G.A. Titanium oxide films produced on commercially pure titanium by anodic oxidation with different voltages. *Mater. Charact.* **2007**, *58*, 114–121. [CrossRef]
82. Rodriguez, L.L.; Sundaram, P.A.; Rosim-Fachini, E.; Padovani, A.M.; Diffoot-Carlo, N. Plasma electrolytic oxidation coatings on γTiAl alloy for potential biomedical applications. *J. Biomed. Mater. Res. Part B Appl. Biomater.* **2014**, *102*, 988–1001. [CrossRef] [PubMed]
83. Gittens, R.A.; Scheideler, L.; Rupp, F.; Hyzy, S.L.; Geis-Gerstorfer, J.; Schwartz, Z.; Boyan, B.D. A review on the wettability of dental implant surfaces II: Biological and clinical aspects. *Acta Biomater.* **2014**, *10*, 2907–2918. [CrossRef] [PubMed]
84. Khanlou, H.M.; Ang, B.C.; Barzani, M.M.; Silakhori, M.; Talebian, S. Prediction and characterization of surface roughness using sandblasting and acid etching process on new non-toxic titanium biomaterial: Adaptive-network-based fuzzy inference System. *Neural Comput. Appl.* **2015**, *26*, 1751–1761. [CrossRef]
85. Long, M.; Rack, H.J. Titanium alloys in total joint replacement—A materials science perspective. *Biomaterials* **1998**, *19*, 1621–1639. [CrossRef]
86. Addison, O.; Davenport, A.J.; Newport, R.J.; Kalra, S.; Monir, M.; Mosselmans, J.F.W.; Proops, D.; Martin, R.A. Do 'passive' medical titanium surfaces deteriorate in service in the absence of wear? *J. R. Soc. Interface* **2012**, *9*, 3161–3164. [CrossRef] [PubMed]
87. Abey, S.; Mathew, M.T.; Lee, D.J.; Knoernschild, K.L.; Wimmer, M.A.; Sukotjo, C. Electrochemical behavior of titanium in artificial saliva: Influence of pH. *J. Oral Implantol.* **2014**, *40*, 3–10. [CrossRef] [PubMed]
88. Mathew, M.T.; Abbey, S.; Hallab, N.J.; Hall, D.J.; Sukotjo, C.; Wimmer, M.A. Influence of pH on the tribocorrosion behavior of CpTi in the oral environment: Synergistic interactions of wear and corrosion. *J. Biomed. Mater. Res. Part B Appl. Biomater.* **2012**, *100B*, 1662–1671. [CrossRef] [PubMed]
89. Souza, J.C.M.; Henriques, M.; Oliveira, R.; Teughels, W.; Celis, J.P.; Rocha, L.A. Do oral biofilms influence the wear and corrosion behavior of titanium? *Biofouling* **2010**, *26*, 471–478. [CrossRef] [PubMed]

90. Chaturvedi, T.P. An overview of the corrosion aspect of dental implants (titanium and its alloys). *Indian J. Dent. Res.* **2009**, *20*, 91–98. [CrossRef] [PubMed]
91. Mouhyi, J.; Ehrenfest, D.M.D.; Albrektsson, T. The peri-implantitis: Implant surfaces, microstructure, and physicochemical aspects. *Clin. Implant Dent. Relat. Res.* **2012**, *14*, 170–183. [CrossRef] [PubMed]
92. Bhola, R.; Bhola, S.M.; Mishra, B.; Olson, D.L. Corrosion in titanium dental implants/ prostheses—A review. *Trends Biomater. Artif. Organs* **2011**, *25*, 34–46.
93. Reclaru, L.; Meyer, J.M. Study of corrosion between a titanium implant and dental alloys. *J. Dent.* **1994**, *22*, 159–168. [CrossRef]
94. Souza, J.C.M.; Ponthiaux, P.; Henriques, M.; Oliveira, R.; Teughels, W.; Celis, J.-P.; Rocha, L.A. Corrosion behaviour of titanium in the presence of Streptococcus mutans. *J. Dent.* **2013**, *41*, 528–534. [CrossRef] [PubMed]
95. Souza, J.C.M.; Barbosa, S.L.; Ariza, E.A.; Henriques, M.; Teughels, W.; Ponthiaux, P.; Celis, J.-P.; Rocha, L.A. How do titanium and Ti6Al4V corrode in fluoridated medium as found in the oral cavity? An in vitro study. *Mater. Sci. Eng. C* **2015**, *47*, 384–393. [CrossRef] [PubMed]
96. Rodrigues, D.; Valderrama, P.; Wilson, T.; Palmer, K.; Thomas, A.; Sridhar, S.; Adapalli, A.; Burbano, M.; Wadhwani, C. Titanium corrosion mechanisms in the oral environment: A retrieval study. *Materials* **2013**, *6*, 5258–5274. [CrossRef] [PubMed]
97. Olmedo, D.G.; Tasat, D.R.; Duffo, G.; Guglielmotti, M.B.; Cabrini, R.L. The issue of corrosion in dental implants: A review. *Acta Odontol. Latinoam.* **2009**, *22*, 3–9. [PubMed]
98. Nikolopoulou, F. Saliva and dental implants. *Implant Dent.* **2006**, *15*, 372–376. [CrossRef] [PubMed]
99. Henry, P.J. Clinical experiences with dental implants. *Adv. Dent. Res.* **1999**, *13*, 147–152. [CrossRef] [PubMed]
100. Gittens, R.A.; Olivares-Navarrete, R.; Tannenbaum, R.; Boyan, B.D.; Schwartz, Z. Electrical implications of corrosion for osseointegration of titanium implants. *J. Dent. Res.* **2011**, *90*, 1389–1397. [CrossRef] [PubMed]
101. Jacobs, J.J.; Gilbert, J.L.; Urban, R.M. Corrosion of metal orthopaedic implants. *J. Bone Jt. Surg.* **1998**, *80*, 268–282. [CrossRef]
102. Geis-Gerstorfer, J. In vitro corrosion measurements of dental alloys. *J. Dent.* **1994**, *22*, 247–251. [CrossRef]
103. Branemark, P.I.; Hansson, B.O.; Adell, R.; Breine, U.; Lindstrom, J.; Hallen, O.; Ohman, A. Osseointegrated implants in the treatment of the edentulous jaw. Experience from a 10-year period. *Scand. J. Plast. Reconstr. Surg. Suppl.* **1997**, *16*, 1–132.
104. Adell, R.; Lekholm, U.; Rockler, B.; Brånemark, P.I. A 15-year study of osseointegrated implants in the treatment of the edentulous jaw. *Int. J. Oral Surg.* **1981**, *10*, 387–416. [CrossRef]
105. Galante, J.O.; Lemons, J.; Spector, M.; Wilson, P.D.; Wright, T.M. The biologic effects of implant materials. *J. Orthop. Res.* **1991**, *9*, 760–775. [CrossRef] [PubMed]
106. Hallab, N.J.; Mikecz, K.; Vermes, C.; Skipor, A.; Jacobs, J.J. Orthopaedic implant related metal toxicity in terms of human lymphocyte reactivity to metal-protein complexes produced from cobalt-base and titanium-base implant alloy degradation. *Mol. Cell. Biochem.* **2001**, *222*, 127–136. [CrossRef] [PubMed]
107. Hallab, N.J.; Jacobs, J.J.; Skipor, A.; Black, J.; Mikecz, K.; Galante, J.O. Systemic metal-protein binding associated with total joint replacement arthroplasty. *J. Biomed. Mater. Res.* **2000**, *49*, 353–361. [CrossRef]
108. Correa, C.B.; Pires, J.R.; Fernandes-Filho, R.B.; Sartori, R.; Vaz, L.G. Fatigue and fluoride corrosion on Streptococcus mutansadherence to titanium-based implant/component surfaces. *J. Prosthodont.* **2009**, *18*, 382–387. [CrossRef] [PubMed]
109. Fathi, M.H.; Salehi, M.; Saatchi, A.; Mortazavi, V.; Moosavi, S.B. In vitro corrosion behavior of bioceramic, metallic, and bioceramic–metallic coated stainless steel dental implants. *Dent. Mater.* **2003**, *19*, 188–198. [CrossRef]
110. Yu, F.; Addison, O.; Baker, S.J.; Davenport, A.J. Lipopolysaccharide inhibits or accelerates biomedical titanium corrosion depending on environmental acidity. *Int. J. Oral Sci.* **2015**, *7*, 179–186. [CrossRef] [PubMed]
111. Simon, B.I.; Goldman, H.M.; Ruben, M.P.; Baker, E. The role of endotoxin in periodontal disease. I. A reproducible, quantitative method for determining the amount of endotoxin in human gingival exudate. *J. Periodontol.* **1969**, *40*, 695–701. [CrossRef] [PubMed]
112. Casarin, R.C.V.; Ribeiro, É.P.; Mariano, F.S.; Nociti, F.H., Jr.; Casati, M.Z.; Gonçalves, R.B. Levels of aggregatibacter actinomycetemcomitans, Porphyromonas gingivalis, inflammatory cytokines and species-specific immunoglobulin G in generalized aggressive and chronic periodontitis. *J. Periodontal. Res.* **2010**, *45*, 635–642. [CrossRef] [PubMed]

113. Mathew, M.T.; Barão, V.A.; Yuan, J.C.-C.; Assunção, W.G.; Sukotjo, C.; Wimmer, M.A. What is the role of lipopolysaccharide on the tribocorrosive behavior of titanium? *J. Mech. Behav. Biomed. Mater.* **2012**, *8*, 71–85. [CrossRef] [PubMed]
114. Gil, F.J.; Canedo, R.; Padros, A.; Baneres, M.V.; Arano, J.M. Fretting corrosion behaviour of ball-and-socket joint on dental implants with different prosthodontic alloys. *Biomed. Mater. Eng.* **2003**, *13*, 27–34. [PubMed]
115. Hjalmarsson, L.; Smedberg, J.I.; Wennerberg, A. Material degradation in implant-retained cobalt-chrome and titanium frameworks. *J. Oral Rehabil.* **2010**, *38*, 61–71. [CrossRef] [PubMed]
116. Wataha, J.C. Biocompatibility of dental casting alloys: A review. *J. Prosthet. Dent.* **2000**, *83*, 223–234. [CrossRef]
117. Brune, D. Metal release from dental biomaterials. *Biomaterials* **1986**, *7*, 163–175. [CrossRef]
118. Wataha, J.C.; Malcolm, C.T.; Hanks, C.T. Correlation between cytotoxicity and the elements released by dental casting alloys. *Int. J. Prosthodont.* **1995**, *8*, 9–14. [PubMed]
119. Sarkar, N.; Fuys, R.; Stanford, J.W. Applications of electrochemical techniques to characterize the corrosion of dental alloys. In *Corrosion and Degradation of Implant Materials*; Syrett, B.C., Acharya, A., Eds.; ASTM: West Conshohocken, PA, USA, 1979; pp. 277–294.
120. Revathi, A.; Borrás, A.D.; Muñoz, A.I.; Richard, C.; Manivasagam, G. Degradation mechanisms and future challenges of titanium and its alloys for dental implant applications in oral environment. *Mater. Sci. Eng. C* **2017**, *76*, 1354–1368. [CrossRef] [PubMed]
121. Mathew, M.T.; Pai, P.S.; Pourzal, R.; Fischer, A.; Wimmer, M.A. Significance of tribocorrosion in biomedical applications: Overview and current status. *Adv. Tribol.* **2009**, *2009*, 1–12. [CrossRef]
122. Landolt, D.; Mischler, S.; Stemp, M. Electrochemical methods in tribocorrosion: A critical appraisal. *Electrochim. Acta* **2001**, *46*, 3913–3929. [CrossRef]
123. Licausi, M.P.; Muñoz, A.I.; Borrás, V.A. Influence of the fabrication process and fluoride content on the tribocorrosion behaviour of Ti6Al4V biomedical alloy in artificial saliva. *J. Mech. Behav. Biomed. Mater.* **2013**, *20*, 137–148. [CrossRef] [PubMed]
124. Dodds, M.W.J.; Johnson, D.A.; Yeh, C.-K. Health benefits of saliva: A review. *J. Dent.* **2005**, *33*, 223–233. [CrossRef] [PubMed]
125. Cruz, H.V.; Souza, J.C.M.; Henriques, M.; Rocha, L.A. Tribocorrosion and bio-tribocorrosion in the oral environment: The case of dental implants. In *Biomedical Tribology*; Davim, J.P., Ed.; Nova Science Publishers: New York, NY, USA, 2011; pp. 1–33.
126. Souza, J.C.M.; Henriques, M.; Teughels, W.; Ponthiaux, P.; Celis, J.-P.; Rocha, L.A. Wear and corrosion interactions on titanium in oral environment: Literature review. *J. Bio-Tribo-Corros.* **2015**, *1*, 13. [CrossRef]
127. Mischler, S. Triboelectrochemical techniques and interpretation methods in tribocorrosion: A comparative evaluation. *Tribol. Int.* **2008**, *41*, 573–583. [CrossRef]
128. Schiff, N.; Grosgogeat, B.; Lissac, M.; Dalard, F. Influence of fluoride content and pH on the corrosion resistance of titanium and its alloys. *Biomaterials* **2002**, *23*, 1995–2002. [CrossRef]
129. Huang, H.-H. Effects of fluoride concentration and elastic tensile strain on the corrosion resistance of commercially pure titanium. *Biomaterials* **2002**, *23*, 59–63. [CrossRef]
130. Kaneko, K.; Yokoyama, K.I.; Moriyama, K.; Asaoka, K.; Sakai, J.I.; Nagumo, M. Delayed fracture of beta titanium orthodontic wire in fluoride aqueous solutions. *Biomaterials* **2003**, *24*, 2113–2120. [CrossRef]
131. Ratner, B.D.; Johnston, A.B.; Lenk, T.J. Biomaterial surfaces. *J. Biomed. Mater. Res.* **1987**, *21*, 59–89. [CrossRef] [PubMed]
132. Smith, D.C.; Pilliar, R.M.; Chernecky, R. Dental implant materials. I. Some effects of preparative procedures on surface topography. *J. Biomed. Mater. Res.* **1991**, *25*, 1045–1068. [CrossRef] [PubMed]
133. Christersson, C.E.; Dunford, R.G.; Glantz, P.O.; Baier, R.E. Effect of critical surface tension on retention of oral microorganisms. *Scand. J. Dent. Res.* **1989**, *97*, 247–256. [CrossRef] [PubMed]
134. Teughels, W.; van Assche, N.; Sliepen, I.; Quirynen, M. Effect of material characteristics and/or surface topography on biofilm development. *Clin. Oral Implant. Res.* **2006**, *17*, 68–81. [CrossRef] [PubMed]
135. Ma, Y.; Lassiter, M.O.; Banas, J.A.; Galperín, M.Y.; Taylor, K.G.; Doyle, R.J. Multiple glucan-binding proteins of Streptococcus sobrinus. *J. Bacteriol.* **1996**, *178*, 1572–1577. [CrossRef] [PubMed]
136. Steinberg, D.; Eyal, S. Early formation of Streptococcus sobrinus biofilm on various dental restorative materials. *J. Dent.* **2001**, *30*, 47–51. [CrossRef]

137. Zitzmann, N.U.; Abrahamsson, I.; Berglundh, T.; Lindhe, J. Soft tissue reactions to plaque formation at implant abutments with different surface topography. An experimental study in dogs. *J. Clin. Periodontol.* **2002**, *29*, 456–461. [CrossRef] [PubMed]
138. Dmytiyk, J.J.; Fox, S.C.; Moriarty, J.D. The effects of scaling titanium implant surfaces with metal and plastic instruments on cell attachment. *J. Periodontol.* **1990**, *61*, 491–496. [CrossRef] [PubMed]
139. Fox, S.C.; Moriarty, J.D.; Kusy, R.P. The effects of scaling a titanium implant surface with metal and plastic instruments: An in vitro study. *J. Periodontol.* **1990**, *61*, 485–490. [CrossRef] [PubMed]
140. Schou, S.; Berglundh, T.; Lang, N.P. Surgical treatment of peri-implantitis. *Int. J. Oral Maxillofac. Implant.* **2004**, *19*, 140–149.
141. Claffey, N.; Clarke, E.; Polyzois, I.; Renvert, S. Surgical treatment of peri-implantitis. *J. Clin. Periodontol.* **2008**, *35*, 316–332. [CrossRef] [PubMed]
142. Augthun, M.; Tinschert, J.; Huber, A. In vitro studies on the effect of cleaning methods on different implant surfaces. *J. Periodontol.* **1998**, *69*, 857–864. [CrossRef] [PubMed]
143. Brookshire, F.V.G.; Nagy, W.W.; Dhuru, V.B.; Ziebert, G.J.; Chada, S. The qualitative effects of various types of hygiene instrumentation on commercially pure titanium and titanium alloy implant abutments: An in vitro and scanning electron microscope study. *J. Prosthet. Dent.* **1997**, *78*, 286–294. [CrossRef]
144. Meier, R.M.; Pfammatter, C.; Zitzmann, N.U.; Filippi, A.; Kuhl, S. Surface quality after implantoplasty. *Schweiz. Monatsschr. Zahnmed.* **2012**, *122*, 714–724. [PubMed]
145. Ramaglia, L.; di Lauro, A.E.; Morgese, F.; Squillace, A. Profilometric and standard error of the mean analysis of rough implant surfaces treated with different instrumentations. *Implant Dent.* **2006**, *15*, 77–82. [CrossRef] [PubMed]
146. Barbour, M.E.; O'Sullivan, D.J.; Jenkinson, H.F.; Jagger, D.C. The effects of polishing methods on surface morphology, roughness and bacterial colonisation of titanium abutments. *J. Mater. Sci. Mater. Med.* **2007**, *18*, 1439–1447. [CrossRef] [PubMed]
147. Schwarz, F.; Sahm, N.; Iglhaut, G.; Becker, J. Impact of the method of surface debridement and decontamination on the clinical outcome following combined surgical therapy of peri-implantitis: A randomized controlled clinical study. *J. Clin. Periodontol.* **2011**, *38*, 276–284. [CrossRef] [PubMed]
148. Rimondini, L.; Simoncini, F.C.; Carrassi, A. Micro-morphometric assessment of titanium plasma-sprayed coating removal using burs for the treatment of peri-implant disease. *Clin. Oral Implant. Res.* **2000**, *11*, 129–138. [CrossRef]
149. Valderrama, P.; Wilson, T.G., Jr. Detoxification of implant surfaces affected by peri-implant disease: An overview of surgical methods. *Int. J. Dent.* **2013**, *2013*, 740680. [CrossRef] [PubMed]
150. Ramel, C.F.; Lüssi, A.; Özcan, M.; Jung, R.E.; Hämmerle, C.H.F.; Thoma, D.S. Surface roughness of dental implants and treatment time using six different implantoplasty procedures. *Clin. Oral Implant. Res.* **2016**, *27*, 776–781. [CrossRef] [PubMed]
151. Rosen, P.; Qari, M.; Froum, S.; Dibart, S.; Chou, L. A pilot study on the efficacy of a treatment algorithm to detoxify dental implant surfaces affected by peri-implantitis. *Int. J. Periodontics Restor. Dent.* **2018**, *38*, 261–267. [CrossRef] [PubMed]
152. Moëne, R.; Décaillet, F.; Andersen, E.; Mombelli, A. Subgingival plaque removal using a new air-polishing device. *J. Periodontol.* **2010**, *81*, 79–88. [CrossRef] [PubMed]
153. Kozlovsky, A.; Soldinger, M.; Sperling, I. The effectiveness of the air-powder abrasive device on the tooth and periodontium: An overview. *Clin. Prev. Dent.* **1989**, *11*, 7–11. [PubMed]
154. Atkinson, D.R.; Cobb, C.M.; Killoy, W.J. The effect of an air-powder abrasive system on in vitro root surfaces. *J. Periodontol.* **1984**, *55*, 13–18. [CrossRef] [PubMed]
155. Petersilka, G.J.; Bell, M.; Haberlein, I.; Mehl, A.; Hickel, R.; Flemmig, T.F. In vitro evaluation of novel low abrasive air polishing powders. *J. Clin. Periodontol.* **2003**, *30*, 9–13. [CrossRef] [PubMed]
156. Petersilka, G.J.; Tunkel, J.; Barakos, K.; Heinecke, A.; Häberlein, I.; Flemmig, T.F. Subgingival plaque removal at interdental sites using a low-abrasive air polishing powder. *J. Periodontol.* **2003**, *74*, 307–311. [CrossRef] [PubMed]
157. Petersilka, G.J.; Steinmann, D.; Haberlein, I.; Heinecke, A.; Flemmig, T.F. Subgingival plaque removal in buccal and lingual sites using a novel low abrasive air-polishing powder. *J. Clin. Periodontol.* **2003**, *30*, 328–333. [CrossRef] [PubMed]

158. Tastepe, C.S.; Lin, X.; Donnet, M.; Wismeijer, D.; Liu, Y. Parameters that improve cleaning efficiency of subgingival air polishing on titanium implant surfaces: An in vitro study. *J. Periodontol.* **2017**, *88*, 407–414. [CrossRef] [PubMed]
159. Ronay, V.; Merlini, A.; Attin, T.; Schmidlin, P.R.; Sahrmann, P. In vitro cleaning potential of three implant debridement methods. Simulation of the non-surgical approach. *Clin. Oral Implant. Res.* **2017**, *28*, 151–155. [CrossRef] [PubMed]
160. Duarte, P.M.; Reis, A.F.; de Freitas, P.M.; Ota-Tsuzuki, C. Bacterial adhesion on smooth and rough titanium surfaces after treatment with different instruments. *J. Periodontol.* **2009**, *80*, 1824–1832. [CrossRef] [PubMed]
161. Kreisler, M.; Al Haj, H.; d'Hoedt, B. Clinical efficacy of semiconductor laser application as an adjunct to conventional scaling and root planing. *Lasers Surg. Med.* **2005**, *37*, 350–355. [CrossRef] [PubMed]
162. Kreisler, M.; Kohnen, W.; Christoffers, A.-B.; Götz, H.; Jansen, B.; Duschner, H.; D'Hoedt, B. In vitro evaluation of the biocompatibility of contaminated implant surfaces treated with an Er:YAG laser and an air powder system. *Clin. Oral Implant. Res.* **2005**, *16*, 36–43. [CrossRef] [PubMed]
163. Razzoog, M.E.; Koka, S. In vitro analysis of the effects of two air-abrasive prophylaxis systems and inlet air pressure on the surface of titanium abutment cylinders. *J. Prosthodont.* **1994**, *3*, 103–107. [CrossRef] [PubMed]
164. Finnegan, M.; Linley, E.; Denyer, S.P.; McDonnell, G.; Simons, C.; Maillard, J.Y. Mode of action of hydrogen peroxide and other oxidizing agents: Differences between liquid and gas forms. *J. Antimicrob. Chemother.* **2010**, *65*, 2108–2115. [CrossRef] [PubMed]
165. Gosau, M.; Hahnel, S.; Schwarz, F.; Gerlach, T.; Reichert, T.E.; Burgers, R. Effect of six different peri-implantitis disinfection methods on in vivo human oral biofilm. *Clin. Oral Implant. Res.* **2010**, *21*, 866–872. [CrossRef]
166. Waal, Y.C.M.; Raghoebar, G.M.; Meijer, H.J.A.; Winkel, E.G.; van Winkelhoff, A.J. Implant decontamination with 2% chlorhexidine during surgical peri-implantitis treatment: A randomized, double-blind, controlled trial. *Clin. Oral Implant. Res.* **2014**, *26*, 1015–1023. [CrossRef] [PubMed]
167. Valderrama, P.; Gonzalez, M.G.; Cantu, M.G.; Wilson, T.G. Detoxification of implant surfaces affected by peri-implant disease: An overview of non-surgical methods. *Open Dent. J.* **2014**, *8*, 77–84. [CrossRef] [PubMed]
168. Wheelis, S.E.; Gindri, I.M.; Valderrama, P.; Wilson, T.G.; Huang, J.; Rodrigues, D.C. Effects of decontamination solutions on the surface of titanium: Investigation of surface morphology, composition, and roughness. *Clin. Oral Implant. Res.* **2016**, *27*, 329–340. [CrossRef] [PubMed]
169. Könönen, M.H.O.; Lavonius, E.T.; Kivilahti, J.K. SEM observations on stress corrosion cracking of commercially pure titanium in a topical fluoride solution. *Dent. Mater.* **1995**, *11*, 269–272. [CrossRef]
170. Rodrigues, D.C.; Urban, R.M.; Jacobs, J.J.; Gilbert, J.L. In vivo severe corrosion and hydrogen embrittlement of retrieved modular body titanium alloy hip-implants. *J. Biomed. Mater. Res. Part B Appl. Biomater.* **2009**, *88*, 206–219. [CrossRef] [PubMed]
171. Sartori, R.; Correa, C.B.; Marcantonio, E., Jr.; Vaz, L.G. Influence of a fluoridated medium with different pHs on commercially pure titanium-based implants. *J. Prosthodont.* **2009**, *18*, 130–134. [CrossRef] [PubMed]
172. Muguruma, T.; Iijima, M.; Brantley, W.A.; Yuasa, T.; Kyung, H.-M.; Mizoguchi, I. Effects of sodium fluoride mouth rinses on the torsional properties of miniscrew implants. *Am. J. Orthod. Dentofac. Orthop.* **2011**, *139*, 588–593. [CrossRef] [PubMed]
173. Toniollo, M.B.; Galo, R.; Macedo, A.P.; Rodrigues, R.C.S.; Ribeiro, R.F.; Mattos, M.D.G. Effect of fluoride sodium mouthwash solutions on cpTI: Evaluation of physicochemical properties. *Braz. Dent. J.* **2012**, *23*, 496–501. [CrossRef] [PubMed]
174. Wiedmer, D.; Petersen, F.C.; Lönn-Stensrud, J.; Tiainen, H. Antibacterial effect of hydrogen peroxide-titanium dioxide suspensions in the decontamination of rough titanium surfaces. *Biofouling* **2017**, *33*, 451–459. [CrossRef] [PubMed]
175. Ntrouka, V.I.; Slot, D.E.; Louropoulou, A.; van der Weijden, F. The effect of chemotherapeutic agents on contaminated titanium surfaces: A systematic review. *Clin. Oral Implant. Res.* **2011**, *22*, 681–690. [CrossRef] [PubMed]
176. Ntrouka, V.; Hoogenkamp, M.; Zaura, E.; van der Weijden, F. The effect of chemotherapeutic agents on titanium-adherent biofilms. *Clin. Oral Implants Res.* **2011**, *22*, 1227–1234. [CrossRef] [PubMed]
177. Ramesh, D.; Sridhar, S.; Siddiqui, D.A.; Valderrama, P.; Rodrigues, D.C. Detoxification of titanium implant surfaces: Evaluation of surface morphology and bone-forming cell compatibility. *J. Bio-Tribo-Corros.* **2017**, *3*, 1–13. [CrossRef]

178. Oliveira, M.N.; Schunemann, W.V.H.; Mathew, M.T.; Henriques, B.; Magini, R.S.; Teughels, W.; Souza, J.C.M. Can degradation products released from dental implants affect peri-implant tissues? *J. Periodontal Res.* **2018**, *53*, 1–11. [CrossRef] [PubMed]
179. Souza, J.G.S.; Cordeiro, J.M.; Lima, C.V.; Barão, V.A.R. Citric acid reduces oral biofilm and influences the electrochemical behavior of titanium: An in situ and in vitro study. *J. Periodontol.* **2018**. [CrossRef] [PubMed]
180. Ungvari, K.; Pelsoczi, I.K.; Kormos, B.; Oszko, A.; Rakonczay, Z.; Kemeny, L.; Radnai, M.; Nagy, K.; Fazekas, A.; Turzo, K. Effects on titanium implant surfaces of chemical agents used for the treatment of peri-implantitis. *J. Biomed. Mater. Res. B Appl. Biomater.* **2010**, *94*, 222–229. [CrossRef] [PubMed]
181. Soukos, N.S.; Mulholland, S.E.; Socransky, S.S.; Doukas, A.G. Photodestruction of human dental plaque bacteria: Enhancement of the photodynamic effect by photomechanical waves in an oral biofilm model. *Lasers Surg. Med.* **2003**, *33*, 161–168. [CrossRef] [PubMed]
182. Kreisler, M.; Kohnen, W.; Marinello, C.; Schoof, J.; Langnau, E.; Jansen, B.; d'Hoedt, B. Antimicrobial efficacy of semiconductor laser irradiation on implant surfaces. *Int. J. Oral Maxillofac. Implant.* **2003**, *18*, 706–711.
183. Cohen, M.I.; Epperson, J.P. Application of lasers to microelectronic fabrication. In *Electron Beam and Laser Beam Technology*; Marton, L., El-Kareh, A.B., Eds.; Academic Press: New York, NY, USA, 1968; pp. 139–186.
184. Wilson, M. Photolysis of oral bacteria and its potential use in the treatment of caries and periodontal disease. *J. Appl. Bacteriol.* **1993**, *75*, 299–306. [CrossRef] [PubMed]
185. Hall, R.R. The healing of tissues incised by a carbon-dioxide laser. *Br. J. Surg.* **1971**, *58*, 222–225. [CrossRef] [PubMed]
186. Kreisler, M.; Gotz, H.; Duschner, H. Effect of Nd:YAG, Ho:YAG, Er: YAG, CO2, and GaAIAs laser irradiation on surface properties of endosseous dental implants. *Int. J. Oral Maxillofac. Implant.* **2002**, *17*, 202–211.
187. Shibli, J.A.; Theodoro, L.H.; Haypek, P.; Garcia, V.G.; Marcantonio, E. The effect of CO2 laser irradiation on failed implant surfaces. *Implant. Dent.* **2004**, *13*, 342–351. [CrossRef] [PubMed]
188. Park, C.-Y.; Kim, S.-G.; Kim, M.-D.; Eom, T.-G.; Yoon, J.-H.; Ahn, S.-G. Surface properties of endosseous dental implants after NdYAG and CO2 laser treatment at various energies. *J. Oral Maxillofac. Surg.* **2005**, *63*, 1522–1527. [CrossRef] [PubMed]
189. Park, J.H.; Heo, S.J.; Koak, J.Y.; Kim, S.K.; Han, C.H.; Lee, J.H. Effects of laser irradiation on machined and anodized titanium disks. *Int. J. Oral Maxillofac. Implant.* **2012**, *27*, 265–272.
190. Romanos, G.; Ko, H.-H.; Froum, S.; Tarnow, D. The use of CO2 laser in the treatment of peri-implantitis. *Photomed. Laser Surg.* **2009**, *27*, 381–386. [CrossRef] [PubMed]
191. Stuebinger, S.; Etter, C.; Miskiewicz, M.; Homann, F.; Saldamli, B.; Wieland, M.; Sader, R. Surface alterations of polished and sandblasted and acid-etched titanium implants after Er:YAG, carbon dioxide, and diode laser irradiation. *Int. J. Oral Maxillofac. Implant.* **2010**, *25*, 104–111.
192. Aoki, A.; Ando, Y.; Watanabe, H.; Ishikawa, I. In vitro studies on laser scaling of subgingival calculus with an erbium:YAG laser. *J. Periodontol.* **1994**, *65*, 1097–1106. [CrossRef] [PubMed]
193. Ishikawa, I.; Aoki, A.; Takasaki, A.A. Clinical application of erbium: YAG laser in periodontology. *J. Int. Acad. Periodontol.* **2008**, *10*, 22–30. [PubMed]
194. Schmage, P.; Thielemann, J.; Nergiz, I.; Scorziello, T.M.; Pfeiffer, P. Effects of 10 cleaning instruments on four different implant surfaces. *Int. J. Oral Maxillofac. Implant.* **2012**, *27*, 308–317.
195. Shin, S.-I.; Min, H.-K.; Park, B.-H.; Kwon, Y.-H.; Park, J.-B.; Herr, Y.; Heo, S.-J.; Chung, J.-H. The effect of Er:YAG laser irradiation on the scanning electron microscopic structure and surface roughness of various implant surfaces: An in vitro study. *Lasers Med. Sci.* **2011**, *26*, 767–776. [CrossRef] [PubMed]
196. Galli, C.; Macaluso, G.M.; Elezi, E.; Ravanetti, F.; Cacchioli, A.; Gualini, G.; Passeri, G. The effects of Er:YAG laser treatment on titanium surface profile and osteoblastic cell activity: An in vitro study. *J. Periodontol.* **2011**, *82*, 1169–1177. [CrossRef] [PubMed]
197. Taniguchi, Y.; Aoki, A.; Mizutani, K.; Takeuchi, Y.; Ichinose, S.; Takasaki, A.A.; Schwarz, F.; Izumi, Y. Optimal Er:YAG laser irradiation parameters for debridement of microstructured fixture surfaces of titanium dental implants. *Lasers Med. Sci.* **2013**, *28*, 1057–1068. [CrossRef] [PubMed]
198. Shin, S.-I.; Lee, E.-K.; Kim, J.-H.; Lee, J.-H.; Kim, S.-H.; Kwon, Y.-H.; Herr, Y.; Chung, J.-H. The effect of Er:YAG laser irradiation on hydroxyapatite-coated implants and fluoride-modified TiO_2-blasted implant surfaces: A microstructural analysis. *Lasers Med. Sci.* **2013**, *28*, 823–831. [CrossRef] [PubMed]

199. Ayobian-Markazi, N.; Karimi, M.; Safar-Hajhosseini, A. Effects of Er:YAG laser irradiation on wettability, surface roughness, and biocompatibility of SLA titanium surfaces: An in vitro study. *Lasers Med. Sci.* **2015**, *30*, 561–566. [CrossRef] [PubMed]
200. Takagi, T.; Aoki, A.; Ichinose, S.; Taniguchi, Y.; Tachikawa, N.; Shinoki, T.; Meinzer, W.; Sculean, A.; Izumi, Y. Effective removal of calcified deposits on microstructured titanium fixture surfaces of dental implants with erbium lasers. *J. Periodontol.* **2018**, *89*, 680–690. [CrossRef] [PubMed]
201. Romanos, G.E.; Everts, H.; Nentwig, G.H. Effects of diode and Nd:YAG laser irradiation on titanium discs: A scanning electron microscope examination. *J. Periodontol.* **2000**, *71*, 810–815. [CrossRef] [PubMed]
202. Castro, G.L.; Gallas, M.; Núñez, I.R.; Borrajo, J.L.L.; Álvarez, J.C.; Varela, L.G. Scanning electron microscopic analysis of diode laser-treated titanium implant surfaces. *Photomed. Laser Surg.* **2007**, *25*, 124–128. [CrossRef] [PubMed]
203. Gonçalves, F.; Zanetti, A.L.; Zanetti, R.V.; Martelli, F.S.; Avila-Campos, M.J.; Tomazinho, L.F.; Granjeiro, J.M. Effectiveness of 980-mm diode and 1064-nm extra-long-pulse neodymium-doped yttrium aluminum garnet lasers in implant disinfection. *Photomed. Laser Surg.* **2010**, *28*, 273–280. [CrossRef] [PubMed]
204. Leja, C.; Geminiani, A.; Caton, J.; Romanos, G.E. Thermodynamic effects of laser irradiation of implants placed in bone: An in vitro study. *Lasers Med. Sci.* **2013**, *28*, 1435–1440. [CrossRef] [PubMed]
205. Geminiani, A.; Caton, J.G.; Romanos, G.E. Temperature change during non-contact diode laser irradiation of implant surfaces. *Lasers Med. Sci.* **2012**, *27*, 339–342. [CrossRef] [PubMed]
206. Giannelli, M.; Lasagni, M.; Bani, D. Thermal effects of $\lambda = 808$ nm GaAlAs diode laser irradiation on different titanium surfaces. *Lasers Med. Sci.* **2015**, *30*, 2341–2352. [CrossRef] [PubMed]

5

Effects of Three Calcium Silicate Cements on Inflammatory Response and Mineralization-Inducing Potentials in a Dog Pulpotomy Model

Chung-Min Kang [1,2,†], Jiwon Hwang [1,†], Je Seon Song [1,3], Jae-Ho Lee [1,3], Hyung-Jun Choi [1,3] and Yooseok Shin [3,4,*]

1 Department of Pediatric Dentistry, College of Dentistry, Yonsei University, Seoul, 03722, Korea; zezu7@yuhs.ac (C.-M.K.); kntdent@naver.com (J.H.); songjs@yuhs.ac (J.S.S.); leejh@yuhs.ac (J.-H.L.); choihj88@yuhs.ac (H.-J.C.)

2 Department of Pharmacology, College of Medicine, Yonsei University, Seoul 03722, Korea

3 Oral Science Research Center, College of Dentistry, Yonsei University, Seoul 03722, Korea

4 Department of Conservative Dentistry, College of Dentistry, Yonsei University, 50-1 Yonseiro, Seodaemun-Gu, Seoul 03722, Korea

* Correspondence: densys@yuhs.ac

† These authors contributed equally to this work.

Abstract: This beagle pulpotomy study compared the inflammatory response and mineralization-inducing potential of three calcium silicate cements: ProRoot mineral trioxide aggregate (MTA) (Dentsply, Tulsa, OK, USA), OrthoMTA (BioMTA, Seoul, Korea), and Endocem MTA (Maruchi, Wonju, Korea). Exposed pulp tissues were capped with ProRoot MTA, OrthoMTA, or Endocem MTA. After 8 weeks, we extracted the teeth, then performed hematoxylin-eosin and immunohistochemical staining with osteocalcin and dentin sialoprotein. Histological evaluation comprised a scoring system with eight broad categories and analysis of calcific barrier areas. We evaluated 44 teeth capped with ProRoot MTA (n = 15), OrthoMTA (n = 18), or Endocem MTA (n = 11). Most ProRoot MTA specimens formed continuous calcific barriers; these pulps contained inflammation-free palisading patterns in the odontoblastic layer. Areas of the newly formed calcific barrier were greater with ProRoot MTA than with Endocem MTA (p = 0.006). Although dentin sialoprotein was highly expressed in all three groups, the osteocalcin expression was reduced in the OrthoMTA and Endocem MTA groups. ProRoot MTA was superior to OrthoMTA and Endocem MTA in all histological analyses. ProRoot MTA and OrthoMTA resulted in reduced pulpal inflammation and more complete calcific barrier formation, whereas Endocem MTA caused a lower level of calcific barrier continuity with tunnel defects.

Keywords: calcium silicate cements; pulpal response; mineralization; calcific barrier; inflammation; odontoblastic layer

---

1. Introduction

Vital pulp therapy consists of apexogenesis, pulpotomy, pulpal debridement, indirect pulp capping, and direct pulp capping [1]. The aim of these treatments includes maintenance of vitality and preservation of the remaining pulp to enable adequate healing of the pulp-dentin complex [2,3]. These procedures offer a more conservative approach to root canal therapy for traumatic and cariously exposed pulps [4,5]. ProRoot mineral trioxide aggregate (PMTA) (Dentsply, Tulsa, OK, USA) has been recognized as an appropriate material for vital pulp therapy, and has provided higher clinical success rates in a long-term study [6].

Although PMTA possesses bioactive and antibacterial activities with high sealing properties [7–10], it has some drawbacks such as a prolonged setting time, discoloration potential, and difficult handling properties [11]. Recently, calcium silicate cement development has helped to overcome these disadvantages in the search for bioactive dental materials. These include OrthoMTA (OMTA; BioMTA) and Endocem MTA (EMTA; Maruchi, Wonju, Korea).

OMTA contains lower concentrations of heavy metals for greater biocompatibility [12] and has a low expansion rate and a good sealing ability [13]. According to the manufacturer, OMTA prevents microleakage by forming a layer of hydroxyapatite that acts as an interface between the material and the canal wall [14]. Moreover, it has been reported to create a favorable environment for bacterial entombment through intratubular mineralization [15]. Clinical studies reported that both PMTA and OMTA had high success rates in pulpotomy and partial pulpotomy when used in primary and permanent teeth [16,17]. However, OMTA showed lower biocompatibility compared with PMTA in an in vitro study [18]. EMTA has been introduced as an MTA-derived pozzolan cement. EMTA has a short setting time (around 4 min) without the addition of a chemical accelerator because it uses a pozzolanic reaction [19]. It is convenient to handle based on its adequate consistency and washout resistance [20]. Indeed, EMTA demonstrated good biocompatibility, osteogenicity, and odontogenic effects similar to PMTA in an in vitro study [19].

Despite the increased use of various calcium silicate cements in vital pulp therapy, their effects after pulpotomy in an in vivo animal model have not yet been investigated. In addition, most studies have had short durations of approximately 4 weeks. Accordingly, the present study aimed to evaluate and compare levels of calcific barrier formation, inflammation reaction, and hard tissue barrier formation histologically following the application of PMTA, OMTA, and EMTA for 8 weeks in a beagle pulpotomy model. The null hypothesis is that there is no significant difference in inflammatory response and mineralization-inducing potentials among the three materials; both OMTA and EMTA have similar biologic effects to PMTA.

2. Materials and Methods

2.1. Animal Model

The present study used a beagle dog pulpotomy model. The inclusion criteria were non-damaged dentition and healthy periodontium. The teeth of two dogs were numbered and randomly divided into three groups with a table of random sampling numbers; the three calcium silicate material groups are shown in Table 1. We performed animal selection, control, the surgical operation, and preparation as per the procedures approved by the Yonsei University Health System's Institutional Animal Care and Use Committee (certification #2013-0317-4). These experiments were performed in accordance with the National Institutes of Health Guide for the Care and Use of Laboratory Animals.

Table 1. The chemical compositions of the calcium silicate cements tested in this study.

Materials	Composition	Setting Time
PMTA	Tricalcium silicate Tricalcium aluminate Dicalcium silicate Tetracalcium aluminoferrite Gypsum Free calcium oxide Bismuth oxide	Initial setting time: 78 min (±5 min) Final setting time: 261 min (±21 min)
OMTA	Tricalcium silicate Dicalcium silicate Tricalcium aluminate Tetracalcium aluminoferrite Free calcium oxide Bismuth oxide	Initial setting time: 180 min Final setting time: 360 min (±21 min)

Table 1. *Cont.*

Materials	Composition	Setting Time
EMTA	Calcium oxide Silicon dioxide Bismuth oxide Aluminum oxide H_2O/CO_2 Magnesium oxide Sulfur trioxide Ferrous oxide Titanium dioxide	Initial setting time: 2 min (±30 s) Final setting time: 4 min (±30 s)

PMTA, ProRoot MTA® (Dentsply Tulsa, OK, USA); OMTA, Ortho MTA® (BioMTA, Seoul, Korea); EMTA, Endocem MTA® (Maruchi, Wonju, Korea).

2.2. Surgical Procedure

We performed all operations in a clean, sterilized room. We administered intravascular injections of tiletamine/zolazepam (Zoletile® 5 mg/kg; Virbac Korea, Seoul, Korea) and xylazine (Rompun® 0.2 mg/kg; Bayer Korea, Seoul, Korea), and used the inhalational anesthetic isoflurane (Gerolan®, Choongwae Pharmaceutical, Seoul, Korea) for general anesthesia induction. To prevent infection, we injected enfloxacin (5 mg/kg) subcutaneously immediately before and after the operation. We administered amoxicillin clavulanate (12.5 mg/kg) orally for 5 to 7 days after the operation.

2.3. Pulpotomy Procedure

We used lidocaine hydrochloride (2%) with 1:100,000 epinephrine (Kwangmyung Pharmaceutical, Seoul, Korea) for local anesthesia. After forming a cavity on the occlusal surface using a high-speed carbide bur #330 (H7 314 008, Brasseler, Lemgo, Germany), we mechanically exposed the pulp. We removed the crown of the pulp at the level of the cementoenamel junction and stopped bleeding by injecting sterile saline and applying slight pressure with sterile cotton pellets. We applied the MTA to the top of the cut pulp as per the manufacturer's guidelines in each group. When we applied the MTA to the pulp area, we used cotton balls soaked in saline. We performed the final cavity restoration using the self-curing glass ionomer cement Ketac-Molar (3M ESPE; St. Paul, MN, USA). Eight weeks after the operation, we euthanized the dogs by over-sedation.

2.4. Histological Analysis

We extracted the teeth with forceps and removed one-third of the root using a high-speed bur. We fixed the specimens in 10% neutral-buffered formalin (Sigma-Aldrich, St. Louis, MO, USA) for 48 h, and demineralized them in ethylenediaminetetraacetic acid (EDTA; pH 7.4; Fisher Scientific, Houston, TX, USA) for 6 weeks before embedding them in paraffin. For each specimen, we created 3-μm continuous sections in the buccolingual direction and stained them subsequently with hematoxylin and eosin (HE). We used InnerView 2.0 software (InnerView Co., Seongnam-si, Gyeonggi-do, Korea) for image analysis. Five observers blinded to the group allocations examined the specimens. We evaluated the specimens for calcific barrier formation, dental pulp inflammation, and odontoblastic cell layer formation with a scoring system reported in a previous study [21–23] (Table 2). We adopted the score agreed upon by at least three of the five observers who were blinded to specimen grouping. In addition, we measured the area of the newly formed hard tissue using ImageJ version 1.48 (National Institute of Health, Bethesda, MD, USA).

2.5. Immunohistochemistry

For immunohistochemistry (IHC), we deparaffinized 3-μm cross-sections with xylene, rehydrated them, and rinsed them with distilled water. For antigen retrieval, we used protease K (Dako North America Inc., Carpinteria, CA, USA) for osteocalcin (OC) and dentin sialoprotein (DSP) staining.

To activate endogenous peroxidase, we added 3% hydrogen peroxide, while preventing non-specific binding by incubating sections in 5% bovine serum albumin (Sigma-Aldrich). Subsequently, we incubated sections overnight with the following primary antibodies: anti-OC antibody (rabbit polyclonal, Ab109112, 1:10,000; Abcam, Cambridge, UK) or anti-DSP antibody (rabbit polyclonal, sc-33586, 1:500; Santa Cruz Biotechnology, Santa Cruz, CA, USA). Subsequently, we applied EnVision + System-Horseradish peroxidase (HRP)-Labeled Polymer anti-rabbit (K4003, Dako) for 20 min. After developing color using the labeled streptavidin biotin kit (Dako) as per the manufacturer's guidelines, we counterstained the sections with Gill's hematoxylin (Sigma-Aldrich).

Table 2. Scores used during the histological analysis of calcific barriers and dental pulp.

Scores	Calcific Barrier Continuity
1	Complete calcific barrier formation
2	Partial/incomplete calcific barrier formation extending to more than one-half of the exposure site but not completely closing the exposure site
3	Initial calcific barrier formation extending to no more than one-half of the exposure site
4	No calcific barrier formation
Scores	**Calcific barrier morphology**
1	Dentin or dentin-associated with irregular hard tissue
2	Only irregular hard tissue deposition
3	Only a thin layer of hard tissue deposition
4	No hard tissue deposition
Scores	**Tubules in calcific barrier**
1	No tubules present
2	Mild (tubules present in less than 30% of the calcific barrier)
3	Moderate to severe (tubules present in more than 30% of the calcific barrier)
4	No hard tissue deposition
Scores	**Inflammation intensity**
1	Absent or very few inflammatory cells
2	Mild (an average of <10 inflammatory cells)
3	Moderate (an average of 10–25 inflammatory cells)
4	Severe (an average >25 inflammatory cells)
Scores	**Inflammation extensity**
1	Absent
2	Mild (inflammatory cells next to the dentin bridge or area of pulp exposure only)
3	Moderate (inflammatory cells observed in one-third or more of the coronal pulp or in the mid pulp)
4	Severe (all of the coronal pulp is infiltrated or necrotic)
Scores	**Inflammation type**
1	No inflammation
2	Chronic inflammation
3	Acute and chronic inflammation
4	Acute inflammation
Scores	**Dental pulp congestion**
1	No congestion
2	Mild (enlarged blood vessels next to the dentin bridge or area of pulp exposure only)
3	Moderate (enlarged blood vessels observed in one-third or more of the coronal pulp or in the mid pulp)
4	Severe (all of the coronal pulp is infiltrated with blood cells)
Scores	**Odontoblastic cell layer**
1	Complete palisading cell pattern
2	Partial/incomplete palisading cell pattern
3	Presence of odontoblast-like cells only
4	Absent

2.6. Statistical Analysis

We performed statistical analyses using SPSS version 23 software (SPSS, Chicago, IL, USA). To analyze the area of the newly formed calcific barrier, we applied a one-way analysis of variance (ANOVA) (significance at $p < 0.05$) and the post hoc Scheffé test (Bonferroni correction; $p < 0.017$).

3. Results

The present study used two male beagle dogs aged 18–24 months that weighed approximately 12 kg. We selected 60 teeth from the two dogs. Among the 60 teeth, we excluded five teeth from the PMTA group, two from the OMTA group, and nine from the EMTA group that failed during tooth removal or specimen production; we evaluated only 44 specimens in the final analysis. Eventually, we analyzed the PMTA (n = 15), OMTA (n = 18), and EMTA (n = 11) specimens histologically.

3.1. Calcific Barrier Formation

Most specimens in the PMTA group formed a complete calcific barrier, while some in the OMTA and EMTA groups produced a partially discontinuous calcific barrier (Figure 1 and Table 3). We observed no calcific barrier in only one specimen from the EMTA group (Figure 2B). In addition, the PMTA group produced hard tissue most similar to the dentin, while we observed a partially irregular or thinly formed calcific layer in the OMTA and EMTA groups. Although three groups contained calcific barriers with low tubule formation (Figure 2D), moderate to severe tubule formation in calcific barrier was found in an OMTA specimen (Figure 2C). We compared the areas of the formed calcific barriers; the calcific barrier in the PMTA group was the widest, followed by those in the OMTA and EMTA groups. There was a statistically significant difference between the PMTA and EMTA groups ($p = 0.006$; Figure 3E). When the calcific barriers were standardized with coronal pulpal width according to tooth type, PMTA also had a significantly higher area than EMTA ($p = 0.0114$; Figure 3F).

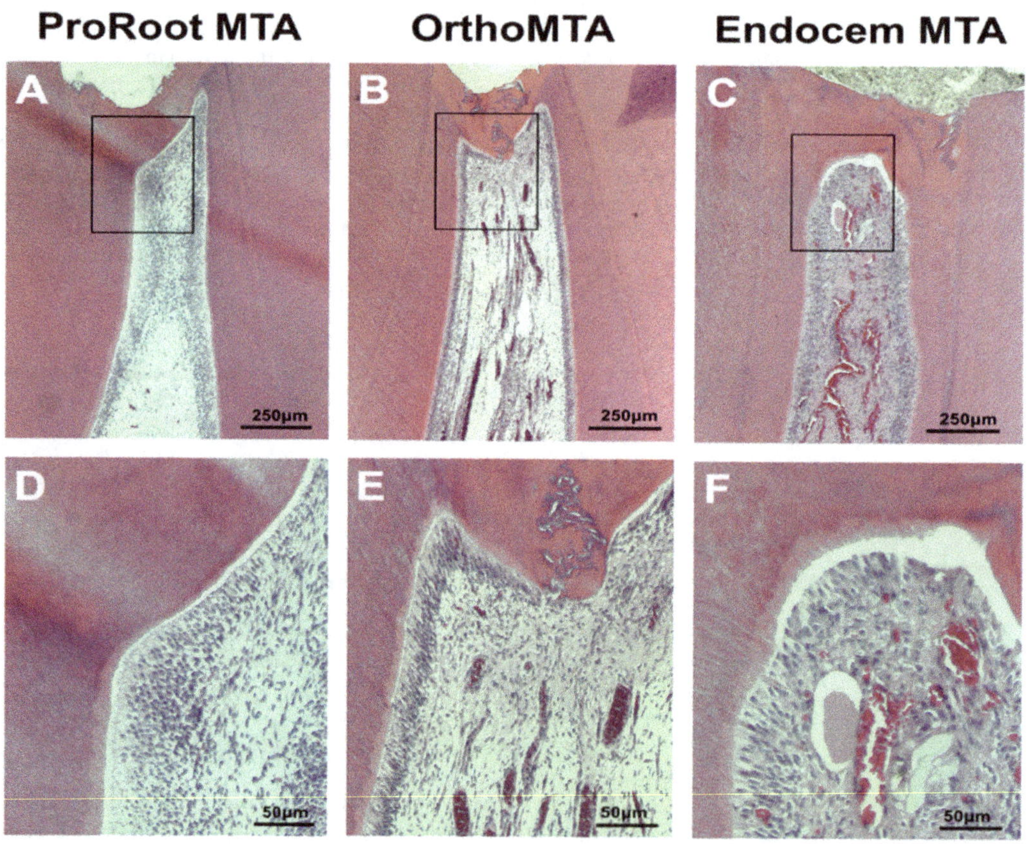

Figure 1. Hematoxylin-eosin staining for the evaluation of the histomorphologic characteristics of the newly formed calcific barrier (CB) after 8 weeks. Most PMTA and OMTA specimens formed continuous CBs and the pulps contained palisading patterns in the odontoblastic layer that were free from inflammation. However, EMTA specimens showed less favorable odontoblastic layer formation ((**A–C**): scale bars = 250 μm, (**D–F**): scale bars = 50 μm).

Table 3. Score percentages for calcific barriers.

Groups	Calcific Barrier Continuity (%)			
	1	2	3	4
PMTA	100 (15/15) *	-	-	-
OMTA	66.67 (12/18)	16.67 (3/18)	16.67 (3/18)	-
EMTA	45.45 (5/11)	18.18 (2/11)	27.27 (3/11)	9.09 (1/11)
Groups	**Calcific Barrier Morphology (%)**			
	1	**2**	**3**	**4**
PMTA	86.67 (13/15)	13.33 (2/15)	-	-
OMTA	38.89 (7/18)	27.78 (5/18)	33.33 (6/18)	-
EMTA	45.45 (5/11)	18.18 (2/11)	27.27 (3/11)	9.09 (1/11)
Groups	**Tubules in Calcific Barrier (%)**			
	1	**2**	**3**	**4**
PMTA	60 (9/15)	33.33 (5/15)	6.67 (1/15)	-
OMTA	61.11 (11/18)	27.78 (5/18)	11.11 (2/18)	-
EMTA	63.64 (7/11)	18.18 (2/11)	9.09 (1/11)	9.09 (1/11)

PMTA, ProRoot MTA®; OMTA, Ortho MTA®; EMTA, Endocem MTA®. * (number of teeth receiving the score/total number of teeth evaluated).

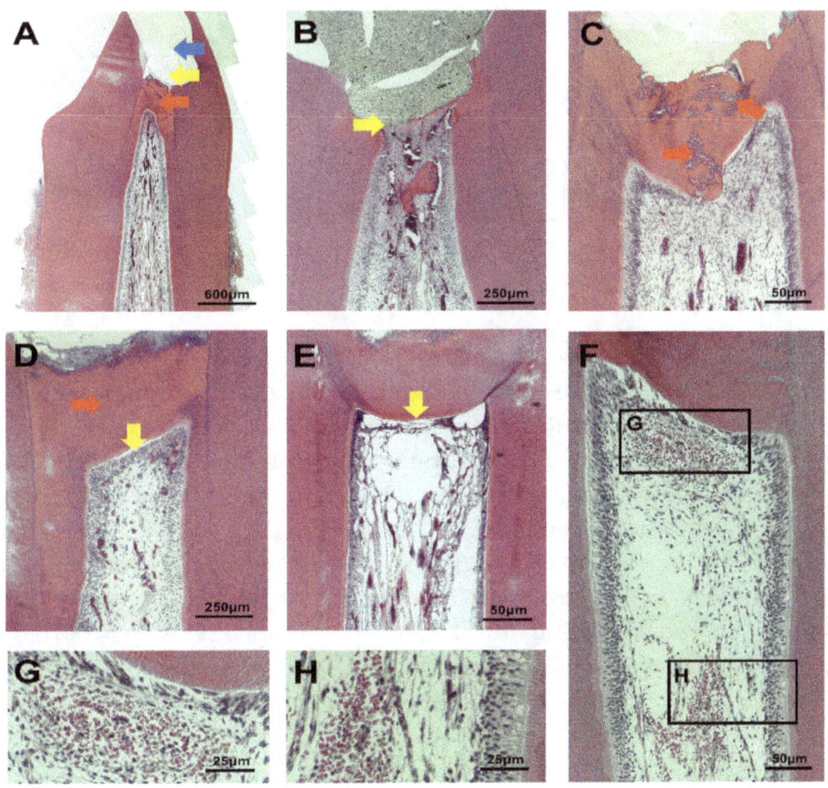

Figure 2. (**A**) An example of a pulpotomy procedure. The site of pulpotomy (yellow arrow) was an upper part of the calcific barrier (red arrow). MTA was filled in the pulp exposure area, but the material is not visible due to partial loss during specimen processing (blue arrow); (**B**) An EMTA specimen without a calcific barrier (yellow arrow). This corresponds to score 4 in the calcific barrier continuity category; (**C**) Moderate to severe tubule formation in calcific barrier of an OMTA specimen (red arrow); (**D**) A PMTA specimen with complete calcific barrier formation and no tubule in barrier (red arrow). It also has complete palisading cell pattern in odontoblastic cell layer (yellow arrow); (**E**) An EMTA specimen with absent odontoblastic cell layer under calcific barrier. This corresponds to score 4 in the odontoblastic cell layer category; (**F–H**) Inflammatory cells that are observed in coronal and middle pulps.

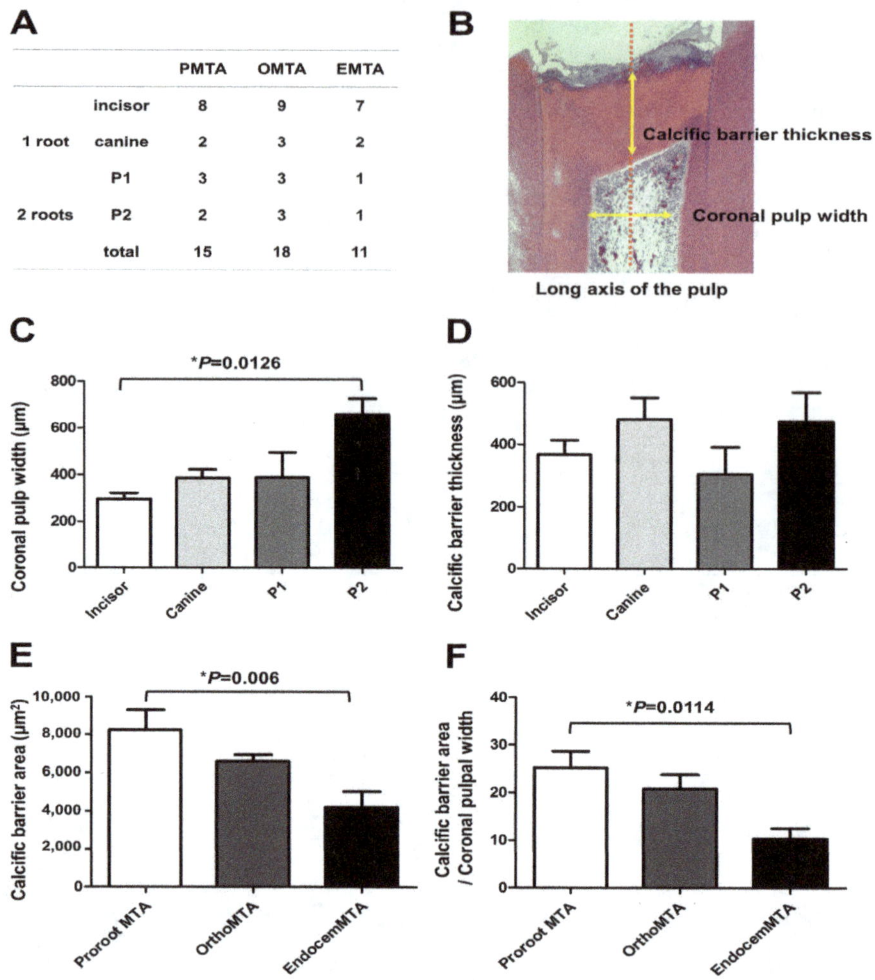

Figure 3. The area of the newly formed calcific barrier for each material after 8 weeks. (**A**) The distributions of tooth types among the three test groups; (**B**) An example measuring coronal pulpal width and calcific barrier thickness; Although the thickness of the calcific barriers did not vary according to tooth type (**C**); the width of the coronal pulp differed by tooth type ($p = 0.0126$) (**D**). Thus, the area of the calcific barrier was calculated by dividing by the horizontal width of the coronal pulp. The bars represent the mean ± the standard deviation; (**E**) In the PMTA group, the calcific barrier is widest, followed by those in the OMTA and EMTA groups. There is a statistically significant difference between the PMTA and EMTA groups ($p = 0.006$); (**F**) When the calcific barriers were standardized by coronal pulpal width, PMTA also had a significantly higher area than EMTA ($p = 0.0114$). We performed statistical analyses with a one-way ANOVA and the post hoc Scheffé test. The number of specimens is $n = 15$ in the PMTA group, $n = 18$ in the OMTA group, and $n = 11$ in the EMTA group.

3.2. Pulpal Reaction

We observed mononuclear inflammatory cells in 26.67% of the specimens from the PMTA group, 44.44% from the OMTA group, and 63.64% from the EMTA group (Table 4). When we compared the extent of inflammation among the groups, inflammation was mild or almost absent in the PMTA and OMTA groups. In 9% of the EMTA specimens, we observed inflammatory cells in one-third or more of the coronal pulp or middle pulp. While there was almost no acute inflammation in any group, a few cases demonstrated chronic inflammation exclusively. The pulpal congestion reaction was mild in the PMTA group and most severe in the EMTA group. We observed no pulpal congestion above the moderate level in any of the three groups.

Table 4. Score percentages for inflammatory responses.

Groups	Inflammation Intensity (%)			
	1	2	3	4
PMTA	73.33 (11/15) *	26.67 (4/15)	-	-
OMTA	55.56 (10/18)	44.44 (8/18)	-	-
EMTA	36.36 (4/11)	63.64 (7/11)	-	-
Groups	**Inflammation Extensity (%)**			
	1	**2**	**3**	**4**
PMTA	73.33 (11/15)	26.67 (4/15)	-	-
OMTA	55.56 (10/18)	44.44 (8/18)	-	-
EMTA	36.36 (4/11)	54.55 (6/11)	9.09 (1/11)	-
Groups	**Inflammation Type (%)**			
	1	**2**	**3**	**4**
PMTA	73.33 (11/15)	26.67 (4/15)	-	-
OMTA	55.56 (10/18)	44.44 (8/18)	-	-
EMTA	36.36 (4/11)	63.64 (7/11)	-	-
Groups	**Dental Pulp Congestion (%)**			
	1	**2**	**3**	**4**
PMTA	40 (6/15)	53.33 (8/15)	6.67 (1/15)	-
OMTA	27.78 (5/18)	61.11 (11/18)	11.11 (2/18)	-
EMTA	18.18 (2/11)	63.64 (7/11)	18.18 (2/11)	-

* (number of teeth receiving the score/total number of teeth evaluated).

3.3. Odontoblastic Cell Layer

In the PMTA group, a complete palisading cell pattern was visible in 60% of the specimens, with 26.67% showing Partial/incomplete palisading cell pattern (Table 5). The OMTA and EMTA groups showed less favorable results compared with the PMTA group: all OMTA specimens showed an odontoblastic cell layer. In contrast, approximately 9.09% of the EMTA group specimens showed no odontoblastic cell layer.

Table 5. Score percentages for the odontoblastic cell layer.

Groups	Odontoblastic Cell Layer (%)			
	1	2	3	4
PMTA	60 (9/15) *	26.67 (4/15)	13.33 (4/15)	-
OMTA	33.33 (6/18)	50 (9/18)	16.67 (3/18)	-
EMTA	45.45 (5/11)	18.18 (2/11)	27.27 (3/11)	9.09 (1/11)

* (number of teeth receiving the score/total number of teeth evaluated).

3.4. Immunohistochemistry

DSP and OC staining indicated hard tissue formation in all three groups. The DSP was highly expressed in all three groups, which indicated odontogenic differential potential (Figure 4A–F). Although OC was also expressed in all three groups, its expression was relatively less in the EMTA group (Figure 4G–L).

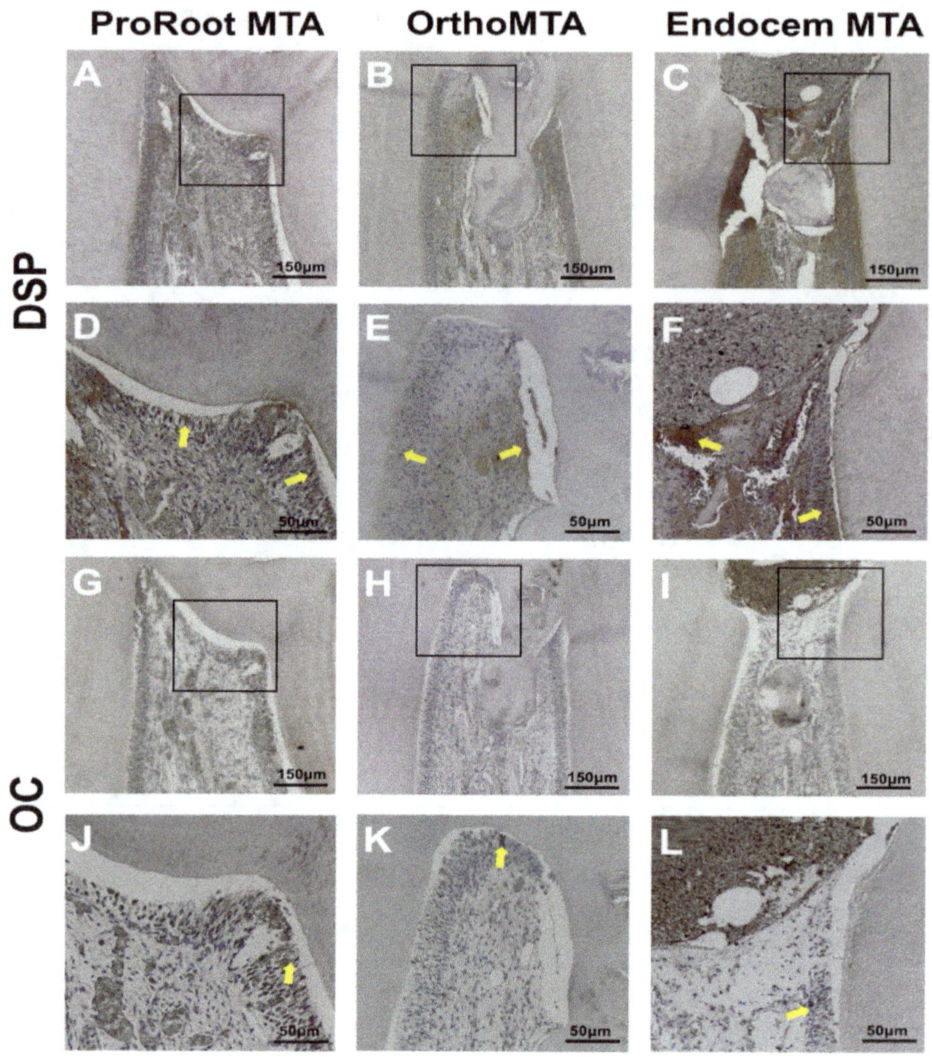

Figure 4. Immunohistochemical staining of dentin sialoprotein (DSP) and osteocalcin (OC). The DSP is highly expressed in all three groups. Although OC is expressed most clearly in odontoblast-like cells in the PMTA group, its expression was reduced in the EMTA group. Yellow arrows indicate cells with a positive signal. ((**A**–**C**,**G**–**I**): scale bars = 150 μm; (**D**–**F**,**J**–**L**): scale bars = 50 μm).

4. Discussion

Many attempts have been made to improve the clinical application of MTA by modifying chemical components or adding a setting accelerator; however, it is important to note that changes in MTA components may cause adverse effects with respect to physical and biological properties [24]. We recommend that in vivo studies explore the pulpal response when using MTA for vital pulp therapy. We recently reported the pulpal responses to pulpotomy with RetroMTA, TheraCal (Bisco Inc., Schamburg, IL, USA), and PMTA [22], and compared the biological efficacies of Endocem Zr (Maruchi, Wonju, Korea) and PMTA at 4 weeks in an in vivo study [23]. We performed this study to compare and evaluate the pulpal response associated with PMTA, OMTA, and EMTA over 8 weeks in a beagle dog pulpotomy model. To our knowledge, this is the first study to examine the biological response from OMTA compared with those from EMTA and PMTA simultaneously in an in vivo model.

Overall, both PMTA and OMTA showed favorable pulpal reactions and formed an almost complete calcific barrier. EMTA induced a slightly greater inflammatory reaction than the other two MTAs and had a lower amount of calcific barrier formation with tunnel defects. These results suggested that EMTA had relatively less biocompatibility than PMTA or OMTA. In addition, PMTA and OMTA formed favorable palisading patterns in odontoblast cells, which demonstrate that these materials had stronger odontogenic differentiation potential.

We suggest several reasons for the low biocompatibility of EMTA observed in this study. A study reported that EMTA resulted in lower cell viability than PMTA immediately after mixing because of its high pH and the heat from the cement surface [25]. This initial cytotoxic effect might contribute to denaturation of adjacent cells [26]. EMTA was also known to express a lower level of osteopontin, a specific bone mineralization marker, compared with other MTAs [27]. Reduced osteopontin production could be a result of lower hard tissue formation. However, these results were not in accordance with the results of a previous in vitro study, which reported that OMTA was significantly more cytotoxic than PMTA and EMTA [27]. The difference may result from interactions with living cells; chemical reactions in the dentin-MTA interfacial layer might have caused the differences in results between the in vivo and in vitro study models. In addition, while PMTA and OMTA exhibit similar components, EMTA contains different chemicals, such as small particles of pozzolan. A pozzolan is a siliceous and aluminous material that reacts chemically with calcium hydroxide to form calcium silicate hydrate in the presence of water [28]. Unlike the initially high pH levels after mixing, EMTA showed a significantly lower pH value than PMTA and OMTA [29]. A previous study found that an acidic environment adversely affected the physical properties and hydration behavior of MTA [30]. We recommend further study because EMTA had inferior cell viability and a low pH level after setting, but was not significantly different from the other two MTAs.

Despite the small number of reports regarding OMTA and EMTA, various in vivo and clinical studies have demonstrated successful formation of calcific barriers in vital pulp therapy with PMTA [16,17,22,23,31,32]. It is still controversial whether calcific barrier formation at the interface between the pulp and material indicates the success of the treatment. Therefore, to judge the efficacy of different MTAs, it is important to analyze the presence or absence of inflammation (the type and severity) and the continuity, structure, and tubule formation of the formed calcific barrier [33]. This study interpreted the calcific barrier as a sign of healing and a positive reaction to stimulation. In the three MTA groups, the calcific barrier interfaces had columnar cells projecting into the bridge with polarized nuclei, which indicates the formation of odontoblast cells and reparative dentin synthesis. This study also confirmed odontogenic properties with IHC by using OC and DSP. OC is a specific marker of the late odontoblastic development pathway and DSP is a marker of odontoblast regulation in reparative dentin mineralization [34]. In regards to several molecular mechanisms, in vitro studies with PMTA showed continuously increasing transcription of mRNA for DSP [35]. Further, upregulation of OC mRNA confirmed the odontoblastic pathway of cell differentiation, indicating that cells enter a quiescent phase in another calcium silicate cement, Biodentine [36]. IHC revealed that PMTA had the potential to induce greater odontoblastic differentiation than OMTA or EMTA. In the analysis of the mean calcific barrier areas, the areas of newly formed calcific barrier were significantly greater in the PMTA group than in the EMTA group. When comparing the area of newly formed calcific barrier in this study statistically, the size of the pulp would be different according to the type of tooth. Although we tried to distribute the tooth types evenly among the experimental groups, we excluded some specimens during tooth removal and specimen production, especially in the EMTA group. Further, the PMTA was regarded as a positive control, but there was no negative control group in this experiment. We recommend further study with a larger sample and the inclusion of a negative control.

In the present study, we evaluated the pulpal response in pulpotomy model for a period of 8 weeks. Other studies used the same time interval [37,38]. In one study, osteodentin matrix formation occurred during the first 2 weeks; after 3 weeks, a complete layer of reparative dentin was formed at the capping site [39]. Another study reported the presence of a calcified bridge in all specimens at 5 weeks after capping with MTA [34]. Notably, we designed the study to compare pulpal responses in a previous study with a shorter time interval (4 weeks) to determine whether there was any difference in response, compared with an 8-week interval. At 8 weeks, hard tissue formation at the exposure site was thicker with less inflammation than in our previous in vivo study at 4 weeks [22,23].

The results of the animal model may not correspond with those of human teeth. A complete hard tissue barrier appeared 1 week after pulp capping in canine teeth [33], whereas the initiation of hard tissue formation has been reported to start as early as 2 weeks after pulp capping in humans [40]. Most studies reported that it took 30 to 42 days to form a hard tissue barrier in humans [41,42]. In addition, we performed the evaluation of the pulpal response on healthy, intact teeth from dogs. Therefore, these results do not necessarily reflect the effects of newly developed MTAs on inflamed pulps. We advise clinicians to place a wet cotton pellet over the MTA in the first visit, followed by replacement with a permanent restoration at the second visit. In this experiment under G/A, the long setting time of PMTA and OMTA was a limitation. Accordingly, careful consideration is necessary when adapting these results to clinical situations.

In conclusion, the results of the present in vivo study demonstrated that PMTA and OMTA had favorable outcomes when used as pulpotomy materials. Both materials showed biocompatibility and induced high-quality calcific barrier formation at the interface with the pulp tissue. However, EMTA has appropriate characteristics and clinical advantages of a shorter setting time and no tooth discoloration. Regarding the application of these results on pulpotomy in healthy canine pulps with no inflammation, we recommend further clinical studies using human teeth for an evaluation of the biological efficacy of these materials.

Author Contributions: C.-M.K. performed data curation, formal analysis and contributed in writing original draft; J.H. contributed in formal analysis and writing original draft; J.S.S. performed conceptualization, project administration, and visualization; J.-H.L. contributed in supervision and validation. H.-J.C. contributed in project administration and supervision; Y.S. performed conceptualization, funding acquisition, and resources; C.-M.K. and J.H. contributed equally as first authors.

Acknowledgments: This study was supported by a faculty research grant of Yonsei university new faculty research fund (6-2017-0009).

References

1. Dahlkemper, P.; Dan, B.; Ang, D.; Goldberg, R.; Rubin, R.; Schultz, G.; Sheridan, B.; Slingbaum, J.; Stevens, M.; Powell, W. *Guide to Clinical Endodontics*; American Association of Endodontics: Chicago, IL, USA, 2013.
2. Zhang, W.; Yelick, P.C. Vital pulp therapy—Current progress of dental pulp regeneration and revascularization. *Inter. J. Dent.* **2010**, *2010*, 856087. [CrossRef] [PubMed]
3. Asgary, S.; Hassanizadeh, R.; Torabzadeh, H.; Eghbal, M.J. Treatment Outcomes of 4 Vital Pulp Therapies in Mature Molars. *J. Endod.* **2018**, *44*, 529–535. [CrossRef] [PubMed]
4. Parirokh, M.; Torabinejad, M.; Dummer, P. Mineral trioxide aggregate and other bioactive endodontic cements: An updated overview—Part I: Vital pulp therapy. *Inter. Endod. J.* **2018**, *51*, 177–205. [CrossRef] [PubMed]
5. Endodontology, E.S.O. Quality guidelines for endodontic treatment: Consensus report of the European Society of Endodontology. *Inter. Endod. J.* **2006**, *39*, 921–930. [CrossRef]
6. Torabinejad, M.; Parirokh, M. Mineral trioxide aggregate: A comprehensive literature review—Part II: Leakage and biocompatibility investigations. *J. Endod.* **2010**, *36*, 190–202. [CrossRef] [PubMed]
7. Barrieshi-Nusair, K.M.; Hammad, H.M. Intracoronal sealing comparison of mineral trioxide aggregate and glass ionomer. *Quintessence Int.* **2005**, *36*, 539–545. [PubMed]
8. Iwamoto, C.E.; Adachi, E.; Pameijer, C.H.; Barnes, D.; Romberg, E.E.; Jefferies, S. Clinical and histological evaluation of white ProRoot MTA in direct pulp capping. *Am. J. Dent.* **2006**, *19*, 85–90. [PubMed]
9. Parirokh, M.; Torabinejad, M. Mineral trioxide aggregate: A comprehensive literature review—Part I: Chemical, physical, and antibacterial properties. *J. Endod.* **2010**, *36*, 16–27. [CrossRef] [PubMed]
10. Schmalz, G.; Widbiller, M.; Galler, K. Material tissue interaction—From toxicity to tissue regeneration. *Oper. Dent.* **2016**, *41*, 117–131. [CrossRef] [PubMed]

11. Parirokh, M.; Torabinejad, M. Mineral trioxide aggregate: A comprehensive literature review—Part III: Clinical applications, drawbacks, and mechanism of action. *J. Endod.* **2010**, *36*, 400–413. [CrossRef] [PubMed]
12. Kum, K.Y.; Zhu, Q.; Safavi, K.; Gu, Y.; Bae, K.S.; Chang, S.W. Analysis of six heavy metals in Ortho mineral trioxide aggregate and ProRoot mineral trioxide aggregate by inductively coupled plasma-optical emission spectrometry. *Aust. Endod J.* **2013**, *39*, 126–130. [CrossRef] [PubMed]
13. Chang, S.-W.; Baek, S.-H.; Yang, H.-C.; Seo, D.-G.; Hong, S.-T.; Han, S.-H.; Lee, Y.; Gu, Y.; Kwon, H.-B.; Lee, W.; et al. Heavy Metal Analysis of Ortho MTA and ProRoot MTA. *J. Endod.* **2011**, *37*, 1673–1676. [CrossRef] [PubMed]
14. Physicochemical Analysis. Available online: www.biomta.com (accessed on 26 May 2018).
15. Yoo, J.S.; Chang, S.W.; Oh, S.R.; Perinpanayagam, H.; Lim, S.M.; Yoo, Y.J.; Oh, Y.R.; Woo, S.B.; Han, S.H.; Zhu, Q.; et al. Bacterial entombment by intratubular mineralization following orthograde mineral trioxide aggregate obturation: A scanning electron microscopy study. *Int. J. Oral Sci.* **2014**, *6*, 227–232. [CrossRef] [PubMed]
16. Kang, C.M.; Kim, S.H.; Shin, Y.; Lee, H.S.; Lee, J.H.; Kim, G.T.; Song, J.S. A randomized controlled trial of ProRoot MTA, OrthoMTA and RetroMTA for pulpotomy in primary molars. *Oral Dis.* **2015**, *21*, 785–791. [CrossRef] [PubMed]
17. Kang, C.M.; Sun, Y.; Song, J.S.; Pang, N.S.; Roh, B.D.; Lee, C.Y.; Shin, Y. A randomized controlled trial of various MTA materials for partial pulpotomy in permanent teeth. *J. Dent.* **2017**, *60*, 8–13. [CrossRef] [PubMed]
18. Lee, B.N.; Son, H.J.; Noh, H.J.; Koh, J.T.; Chang, H.S.; Hwang, I.N.; Hwang, Y.C.; Oh, W.M. Cytotoxicity of newly developed ortho MTA root-end filling materials. *J. Endod.* **2012**, *38*, 1627–1630. [CrossRef] [PubMed]
19. Park, S.J.; Heo, S.M.; Hong, S.O.; Hwang, Y.C.; Lee, K.W.; Min, K.S. Odontogenic effect of a fast-setting pozzolan-based pulp capping material. *J. Endod.* **2014**, *40*, 1124–1131. [CrossRef] [PubMed]
20. Choi, Y.; Park, S.-J.; Lee, S.-H.; Hwang, Y.-C.; Yu, M.-K.; Min, K.-S. Biological effects and washout resistance of a newly developed fast-setting pozzolan cement. *J. Endod.* **2013**, *39*, 467–472. [CrossRef] [PubMed]
21. Nowicka, A.; Lipski, M.; Parafiniuk, M.; Sporniak-Tutak, K.; Lichota, D.; Kosierkiewicz, A.; Kaczmarek, W.; Buczkowska-Radlinska, J. Response of human dental pulp capped with biodentine and mineral trioxide aggregate. *J. Endod.* **2013**, *39*, 743–747. [CrossRef] [PubMed]
22. Lee, H.; Shin, Y.; Kim, S.O.; Lee, H.S.; Choi, H.J.; Song, J.S. Comparative Study of Pulpal Responses to Pulpotomy with ProRoot MTA, RetroMTA, and TheraCal in Dogs' Teeth. *J. Endod.* **2015**, *41*, 1317–1324. [CrossRef] [PubMed]
23. Lee, M.; Kang, C.M.; Song, J.S.; Shin, Y.; Kim, S.; Kim, S.O.; Choi, H.J. Biological efficacy of two mineral trioxide aggregate (MTA)-based materials in a canine model of pulpotomy. *Dent. Mater. J.* **2017**, *36*, 41–47. [CrossRef] [PubMed]
24. Kogan, P.; He, J.; Glickman, G.N.; Watanabe, I. The effects of various additives on setting properties of MTA. *J. Endod.* **2006**, *32*, 569–572. [CrossRef] [PubMed]
25. Song, M.; Yoon, T.S.; Kim, S.Y.; Kim, E. Cytotoxicity of newly developed pozzolan cement and other root-end filling materials on human periodontal ligament cell. *Restor. Dent. Endod.* **2014**, *39*, 39–44. [CrossRef] [PubMed]
26. De Deus, G.; Ximenes, R.; Gurgel-Filho, E.D.; Plotkowski, M.C.; Coutinho-Filho, T. Cytotoxicity of MTA and Portland cement on human ECV 304 endothelial cells. *Int. Endod. J.* **2005**, *38*, 604–609. [CrossRef] [PubMed]
27. Kim, M.; Yang, W.; Kim, H.; Ko, H. Comparison of the biological properties of ProRoot MTA, OrthoMTA, and Endocem MTA cements. *J. Endod.* **2014**, *40*, 1649–1653. [CrossRef] [PubMed]
28. Koseoglu, S.; Pekbagr Yan, K.T.; Kucukyilmaz, E.; Saglam, M.; Enhos, S.; Akgun, A. Biological response of commercially available different tricalcium silicate-based cements and pozzolan cement. *Microsc. Res. Tech.* **2017**, *80*, 994–999. [CrossRef] [PubMed]
29. Che, J.-L.; Kim, J.-H.; Kim, S.-M.; Choi, N.-k.; Moon, H.-J.; Hwang, M.-J.; Song, H.-J.; Park, Y.-J. Comparison of setting time, compressive strength, solubility, and pH of four kinds of MTA. *Korean J. Dent. Mater.* **2016**, *43*, 61–71. [CrossRef]
30. Lee, Y.-L.; Lee, B.-S.; Lin, F.-H.; Lin, A.Y.; Lan, W.-H.; Lin, C.-P. Effects of physiological environments on the hydration behavior of mineral trioxide aggregate. *Biomaterials* **2004**, *25*, 787–793. [CrossRef]

31. De Rossi, A.; Silva, L.A.; Gaton-Hernandez, P.; Sousa-Neto, M.D.; Nelson-Filho, P.; Silva, R.A.; de Queiroz, A.M. Comparison of pulpal responses to pulpotomy and pulp capping with biodentine and mineral trioxide aggregate in dogs. *J. Endod.* **2014**, *40*, 1362–1369. [CrossRef] [PubMed]
32. Nair, P.N.; Duncan, H.F.; Pitt Ford, T.R.; Luder, H.U. Histological, ultrastructural and quantitative investigations on the response of healthy human pulps to experimental capping with mineral trioxide aggregate: A randomized controlled trial. *Int. Endod. J.* **2008**, *41*, 128–150. [PubMed]
33. Parirokh, M.; Asgary, S.; Eghbal, M.J.; Stowe, S.; Eslami, B.; Eskandarizade, A.; Shabahang, S. A comparative study of white and grey mineral trioxide aggregate as pulp capping agents in dog's teeth. *Dent. Traumatol.* **2005**, *21*, 150–154. [CrossRef] [PubMed]
34. Bronckers, A.L.; Farach-Carson, M.C.; Van Waveren, E.; Butler, W.T. Immunolocalization of osteopontin, osteocalcin, and dentin sialoprotein during dental root formation and early cementogenesis in the rat. *J. Bone Miner. Res.* **1994**, *9*, 833–841. [CrossRef] [PubMed]
35. Widbiller, M.; Lindner, S.; Buchalla, W.; Eidt, A.; Hiller, K.-A.; Schmalz, G.; Galler, K. Three-dimensional culture of dental pulp stem cells in direct contact to tricalcium silicate cements. *Clin. Oral Investig.* **2016**, *20*, 237–246. [CrossRef] [PubMed]
36. Zanini, M.; Sautier, J.M.; Berdal, A.; Simon, S. Biodentine induces immortalized murine pulp cell differentiation into odontoblast-like cells and stimulates biomineralization. *J. Endod.* **2012**, *38*, 1220–1226. [CrossRef] [PubMed]
37. Zarrabi, M.H.; Javidi, M.; Jafarian, A.H.; Joushan, B. Histologic Assessment of Human Pulp Response to Capping with Mineral Trioxide Aggregate and a Novel Endodontic Cement. *J. Endod.* **2010**, *36*, 1778–1781. [CrossRef] [PubMed]
38. Asgary, S.; Parirokh, M.; Eghbal, M.J.; Ghoddusi, J. SEM evaluation of pulp reaction to different pulp capping materials in dog's teeth. *Iran. Endod. J.* **2006**, *1*, 117–123. [PubMed]
39. Simon, S.; Cooper, P.; Smith, A.; Picard, B.; Naulin Ifi, C.; Berdal, A. Evaluation of a new laboratory model for pulp healing: Preliminary study. *Inter. Endod. J.* **2008**, *41*, 781–790. [CrossRef] [PubMed]
40. AlShwaimi, E.; Majeed, A.; Ali, A.A. Pulpal Responses to Direct Capping with Betamethasone/Gentamicin Cream and Mineral Trioxide Aggregate: Histologic and Micro-Computed Tomography Assessments. *J. Endod.* **2016**, *42*, 30–35. [CrossRef] [PubMed]
41. Eskandarizadeh, A.; Shahpasandzadeh, M.H.; Shahpasandzadeh, M.; Torabi, M.; Parirokh, M. A comparative study on dental pulp response to calcium hydroxide, white and grey mineral trioxide aggregate as pulp capping agents. *J. Conserv. Dent.* **2011**, *14*, 351–355. [PubMed]
42. Shahravan, A.; Jalali, S.P.; Torabi, M.; Haghdoost, A.A.; Gorjestani, H. A histological study of pulp reaction to various water/powder ratios of white mineral trioxide aggregate as pulp-capping material in human teeth: A double-blinded, randomized controlled trial. *Int. Endod. J.* **2011**, *44*, 1029–1033. [CrossRef] [PubMed]

6

Direct Pulp Capping: Which is the Most Effective Biomaterial? A Retrospective Clinical Study

Anabela Paula [1,*], Eunice Carrilho [1], Mafalda Laranjo [2], Ana M. Abrantes [2], João Casalta-Lopes [2,3], Maria Filomena Botelho [2], Carlos Miguel Marto [4] and Manuel M. Ferreira [5]

1 Institute of Integrated Clinical Practice, Institute for Clinical and Biomedical Research (iCBR), Centre for Innovative Biomedicine and Biotechnology (CIBB), Area of Environment Genetics and Oncobiology (CIMAGO), CNC.IBILI, Faculty of Medicine, University of Coimbra, 3000-075 Coimbra, Portugal; eunicecarrilho@gmail.com

2 Biophysics Institute, Institute for Clinical and Biomedical Research (iCBR), Centre for Innovative Biomedicine and Biotechnology (CIBB), Area of Environment Genetics and Oncobiology (CIMAGO), CNC.IBILI Consortium, Faculty of Medicine, University of Coimbra, 3000-548 Coimbra, Portugal; mafaldalaranjo@gmail.com (M.L.); margaridaabrantes@gmail.com (A.M.A.); joao.casalta@gmail.com (J.C.-L.); mfbotelho@fmed.uc.pt (M.F.B.)

3 Radiation Oncology Department, Coimbra University Hospital Centre, 3000-548 Coimbra, Portugal

4 Institute of Experimental Pathology, Institute for Clinical and Biomedical Research (iCBR), Centre for Innovative Biomedicine and Biotechnology (CIBB), Area of Environment Genetics and Oncobiology (CIMAGO), CNC.IBILI, Faculty of Medicine, University of Coimbra, 3000-548 Coimbra, Portugal; mig-marto@hotmail.com

5 Institute of Endodontics, Institute for Clinical and Biomedical Research (iCBR), Centre for Innovative Biomedicine and Biotechnology (CIBB), Area of Environment Genetics and Oncobiology (CIMAGO), CNC.IBILI, Faculty of Medicine, University of Coimbra, 3000-075 Coimbra, Portugal; m.mferreira@netcabo.pt

* Correspondence: anabelabppaula@sapo.pt; Tel.: +351-934-262-687

Abstract: (1) Background: Recently, tricalcium silicate cements, such as Biodentine™, have emerged. This biomaterial has a calcium hydroxide base and characteristics like mineral aggregate trioxide cements, but has tightening times that are substantially more suitable for their application and other clinical advantages. (2) Methods: A retrospective clinical study was conducted with 20 patients, which included a clinical evaluation of the presence or absence of pulp inflammation compatible symptoms, radiographic evaluation of the periapical tissues, and structural alterations of the coronary restoration that supports pulp capping therapies with Biodentine™ and WhiteProRoot®MTA. (3) Results: This clinical study revealed similar success rates between mineral trioxide cement and tricalcium silicates cements at 6 months, with 100% and 95% success rates, respectively. There were no statistically significant differences between both biomaterials and between these and the various clinical circumstances, namely the absolute isolation of the operating field, exposure size, the aetiology of exposure, and even the type of restorative material used. (4) Conclusions: Biodentine™ demonstrated a therapeutic effect on the formation of a dentin bridge accompanied by slight inflammatory signs, with a high clinical success rate, indicating the possibility of its effective and safe use in dental pulp direct capping in humans, similar to the gold standard material.

Keywords: biocompatibility; biomaterials; clinical; direct pulp capping; pulp vitality

1. Introduction

Pulp protection therapies aim to maintain the vitality of the tooth in which pulp tissue has been exposed due to trauma, carious lesions, or restorative procedures. Treatment options in this situation include direct pulp capping, pulpotomy, or pulpectomy [1,2].

Traditionally, direct pulp capping therapies were performed on young permanent teeth with iatrogenic pulp exposures or trauma. When pulpal exposures occurred after carious tissue removal, in most situations, the recommendation was to perform pulpotomies or even pulpetomies. Direct pulp capping was restricted to very specific cases with very narrow indications. Many materials have been used for this type of therapy, as Pereira Paula et al. described [3]. Although calcium hydroxide-based cements have been the material of choice for many years, it presents some disadvantages, as has been widely reported: poor adherence to dentin, dissolution over time, and multiple tunnel defects in the formed dentin bridges [1]. Further, its success rates ranged from 30% to 85% [4–6]. With the development of other biomaterials, aggregate-based cements of mineral trioxides have emerged, which present higher success rates, form structurally more consistent dentin bridges, and with high antibacterial effects, they are now considered the gold standard materials for this type of therapy [1,7–10]. Mineral trioxide aggregate-based cements are bioactive materials that can create an environment that enhances tissue regeneration and healing. When applied in direct contact with tissues, it forms calcium hydroxide, which releases calcium ions, of which are fundamental for cell adhesion and proliferation. Additionally, it creates an antibacterial environment by increasing the pH (alkalizing the medium), modulates cytokine production, induces differentiation and migration of cells that are capable of producing dentin or bone tissue, and forms hydroxyapatite or carbonate apatite on its surface, inducing a biological sealing [11]. Hydroxyapatite can release calcium and phosphorus ions continuously, contributing to hard tissue metabolism, marginal sealing with dentine tissue, and hard tissue regeneration and remineralization [12–14]. MTA (mineral trioxide aggregate) also has the lowest cytotoxicity values [15]. However, MTA-based cements present great difficulties regarding clinical manipulation, high costs, and long setting times [1,16].

The emergence of new bioceramic materials, with properties similar to MTA-based cements and with improved handling characteristics, suggests the possibility of a clinical alternative [9,16–19]. Tricalcium silicate is bioactive and, when hydrated, turns into hydrated calcium silicate and calcium hydroxide. These react in the presence of physiological fluids, producing hydroxyapatite, which is biocompatible and induces pulp cell differentiation in the same way as calcium hydroxide [20].

The present retrospective preliminary clinical study aims to address clinical success/failure factors following the treatment of direct pulpal exposure with WhiteProRoot®MTA or Biodentine™. The evaluation of these factors included the clinical evaluation of the absence or presence of symptomatology that are compatible with inflammatory pulp states and radiographic evaluation of the structural alterations of coronary restoration that support pulp tissue repair and changes in the pulp tissue itself. Overall, we sought to evaluate the advantage of the clinical use of Biodentine™ compared to other similar materials, such as WhiteProRoot®MTA, by searching for clinical signs of pulp tissue vitality preservation in patients who were treated with this material.

2. Materials and Methods

The retrospective clinical study was approved by the FMUC/CHUC Ethics Committee with number 005-CE-2014.

2.1. Sample Selection

The medical files of patients who underwent direct pulp capping therapies at the Operative Dentistry appointment of the Faculty of Medicine, University of Coimbra and Coimbra University' Hospital Centre, Portugal between 2012 and 2016 were evaluated. Only patients with direct pulp cappings with two dentinogenesis-inducing materials, a mineral trioxide aggregate, WhiteProRoot®MTA (Dentsply,

Maillefer, Tulsa Dental Specialties, Switzerland), and a tricalcium silicate, Biodentine™ (Septodont, Saint-Maur-des-Fosses, France), were included. The goal was to standardize the sample, with a similar number of clinical cases for each of the biomaterials.

2.2. Inclusion Criteria

The included patients met certain criteria which were reported in the clinical chart, namely: thermal sensitivity response compatible with vital tooth diagnosis and corroboration by radiographic examination; patients aged 18 to 55; and a reasonable state of health and oral hygiene, without periodontal pathology. The included treatments were made on absolute isolation with a rubber dam or with a relative isolation of the operative field with cotton rolls. Cavity disinfection was performed with 2% chlorhexidine. Teeth in which restorations were performed using either total-etch adhesive or self-etching adhesive systems were included. The restorative materials that were used in all the therapies were light-cured composite resins.

2.3. Evaluation of the Clinical Procedures of Direct Pulp Capping Therapies

Twenty-one direct pulp capping therapies performed on 20 patients were included, divided into two groups—one with 11 teeth that were treated with WhiteProRoot® MTA and the other with 10 teeth that were treated with Biodentine™. The aetiologies of the pulp exposures were different, namely due to extensive carious lesion and iatrogenic causes and, therefore, different dimensions of the exposure sites were reported. Some clinical files also referred to the need for pulp cappings before the complete removal of the active caries lesion. In all of the selected patients, the therapies were performed with one of the biomaterials, followed by the placement of a resin-modified glass ionomer cement. The definitive restorations were performed at the appointment in which the direct pulp capping was performed or, in some cases due to various constraints, within 15 days after. At the end of each therapy, the radiographic evaluation was reported. All these clinical procedures were performed following the standards of good clinical practice [21].

2.4. Evaluation of the Teeth after Therapy

Clinical controls were performed at one week, one month, three months, and six months after treatment. Broader follow-ups could not be obtained because no clinical record of further evaluations was found after 6 months. In these controls, qualitative tests had been performed such as the pulp sensitivity test, which included the ethyl chloride cold test and the vertical and horizontal percussion test. The criteria that were used in the qualitative assessment have already been established as good practice procedures and are described in Table 1. Clinical controls over time assessed the restoration success, including the search for fractures and/or marginal infiltration, through clinical examination and complementary exams with periapical radiography. This radiographic examination also allowed the evaluation of secondary signs of treatment failure, namely the formation of apical root injury and the appearance of secondary caries. Therapies on teeth that remained asymptomatic, with normal ethyl chloride sensitivity tests and no radiographic signs of periapical pathology, were considered as clinical successes.

2.5. Statistical Analysis

The age factor was evaluated through descriptive analysis and the application of normality tests, namely the Kolmogorov-Smirnov and Shapiro-Wilk tests. For comparisons of the biomaterials that were used in the therapies and pulp exposure characteristics, namely aetiology and size, the chi-square test or Fisher's exact test according to Cochrane rules were used. To evaluate the variables that characterize the symptoms over time, a frequency analysis was performed.

Table 1. Qualitative evaluation criteria for the pulp sensitivity tests.

Test	Normal State of the Pulp Tissue	Pathological State of Pulp Tissue		
		Reversible Pulpitis	Irreversible Pulpitis	Necrosis
Test with ethyl chloride	positive (no change in intensity or duration after stimulation)	positive (with change in intensity and/or duration after lower stimulus 5 s)	positive (with change in intensity and/or duration after upper stimulus 5 s)	negative
Horizontal Percussion Test	negative	negative	positive	positive
Vertical Percussion Test	negative	negative	positive	positive

3. Results

The distribution of the clinical parameters that were considered can be seen in Figure 1. The present clinical study included patients aged 18 to 55 years, most of which were aged 18 to 25 years, with a percentage of 45%. The age group of 46 to 55 years was the second-highest group to be represented, with a percentage of 30% of the total patients. The mean age was 32.2 ± 13.85 years, with a non-normal distribution, a median of 26, and an interquartile range (AiQ) of 28.

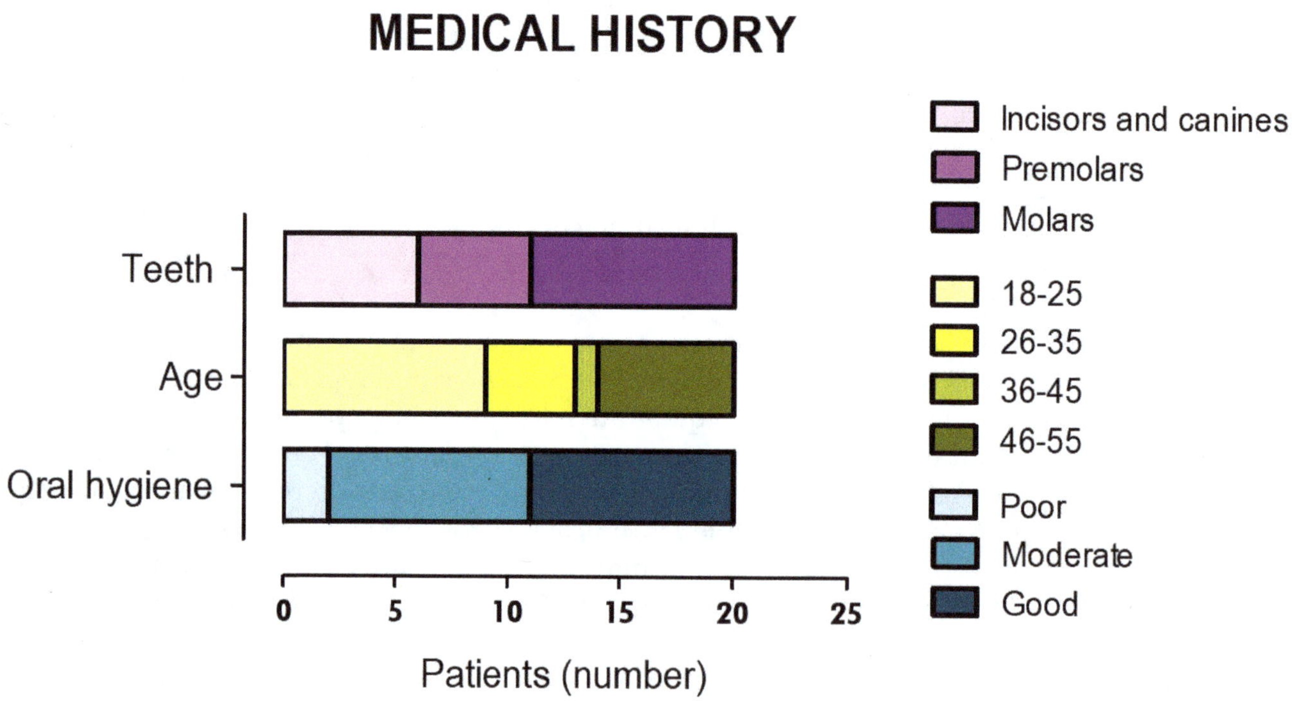

Figure 1. Relevant aspects of the clinical history of patients who were included in the clinical study, namely age, hygiene habits, and type of teeth intervened. Results corresponded to 20 patients in whom pulp capping therapies were performed on 21 teeth.

Regarding the type of teeth with pulp capping therapy, the distribution was uniform with a higher percentage of molars, 42.9%, followed by the group of incisors and canines with 33.3% and, finally, premolars with 23.8%. Hygiene habits were mostly moderate and good, with a percentage of 42.9% in both groups. Only a small percentage of 14.3% was referred to as having poor hygiene habits.

The biomaterials that were used to protect the pulp tissue and the adhesive and restorative materials that were used in the restorative phase can be seen in Figure 2.

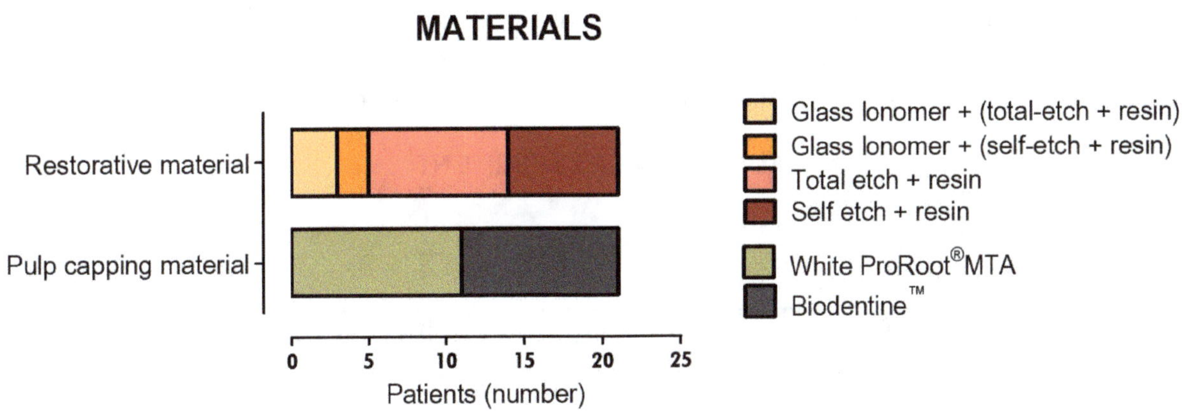

Figure 2. Types of material used for the direct pulp capping and restoration of the dental structure. The results are for 21 teeth, in which pulp capping therapies were performed.

WhiteProRoot®MTA was used in 52.4% of the teeth and Biodentine™ in 47.6%. Regarding restorative materials, about 23.8% of the teeth were initially restored provisionally with a glass ionomer cement and about 76.2% were permanently restored. In the permanent restoration of all the teeth that were submitted to pulp capping therapy, a total-etch dentin bonding system was used in 57.2% and a self-etch dentin bonding system was used in 42.8%. The definitive restorations were made with composite resins, as already mentioned.

Relevant pre-therapeutic diagnostic factors and those that occurred during therapy and were relevant for prognosis were also recorded, as shown in Figure 3.

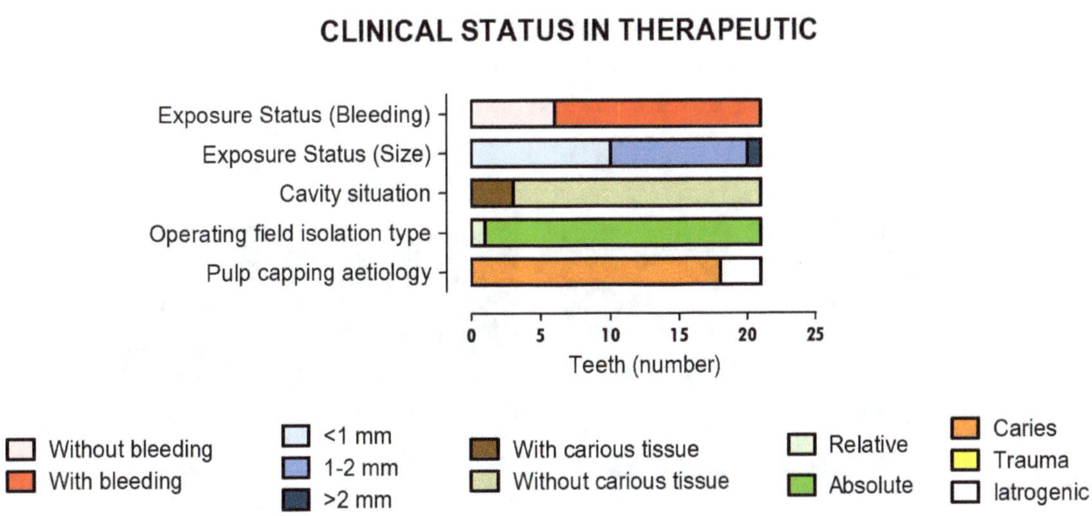

Figure 3. Diagnostic factors of pre-therapeutic clinical status, such as the cause of pulp capping and the type of isolation performed; and relevant clinical factors for prognosis, such as cavity status and pulp exposure status (size and bleeding). The results correspond to 21 teeth in which pulp capping therapies were performed.

Regarding pre-therapeutic diagnosis factors, pulp exposure in about 85.7% of the intervened teeth was caused by dental caries. On the other hand, about 14.3% of pulp exposure was iatrogenic. No pulp exposure due to dental trauma was reported. For the therapies that were applied to the 21 teeth, about 95.2% were performed under rubber dam isolation and in the others, relative insulation with cotton rolls was used. In 14.3% of the therapies that were reported, there was decayed dentin at the time of pulp exposure. Regarding pulp exposure, its size was less than 1 mm in 47.6% of the treated teeth and an average size of 1 to 2 mm was reported in 47.6% of the teeth. Exposures that were larger than 2 mm were reported in 4.8% of the teeth. There were reports of bleeding in 71.4% of clinical situations and no bleeding was reported in 28.6% of pulp exposures.

As mentioned, data from the initial clinical evaluation were extracted from all the intervention teeth to confirm the diagnosis of vital or reversible pulpitis, compatible with the direct pulp capping therapy that was instituted as the treatment. These initial assessment data are described in Figure 4.

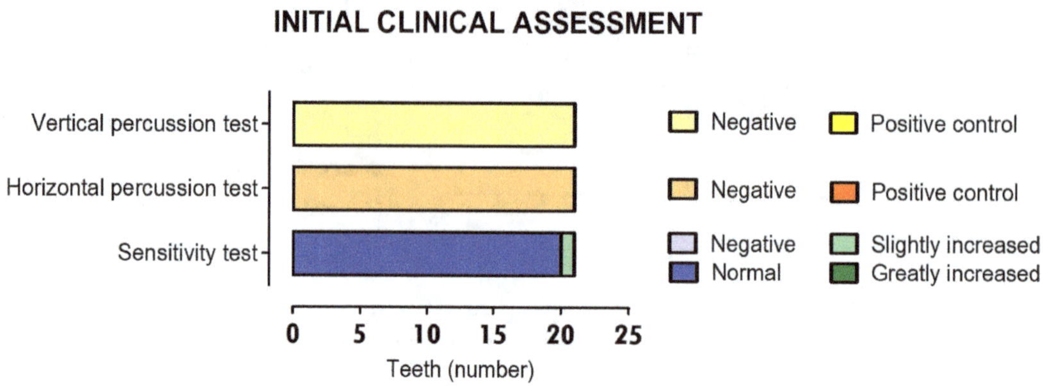

Figure 4. Pre-therapeutic clinical assessment, assessment of changes in cold and horizontal and vertical percussion sensitivity tests. The results correspond to 21 teeth in which pulp capping therapies were performed.

Thus, in all teeth undergoing therapy, the reported horizontal and vertical percussion tests were negative. Sensitivity testing with ethyl chloride revealed a normal response in 95.2% of the teeth and slightly increased, i.e., was compatible with reversible pulpit tooth, in 4.8% of the teeth.

Evaluations were performed at 1 week, 1 month, 3 months, and 6 months after treatments, considering the various parameters to measure the pulp state of the teeth that were intervened. In all the controls, a radiographic evaluation was performed, which contributed to the evaluation of some of these parameters. Figure 5 shows periapical radiographs, by way of example, from two clinical cases in which pulp capping with different biomaterials was made.

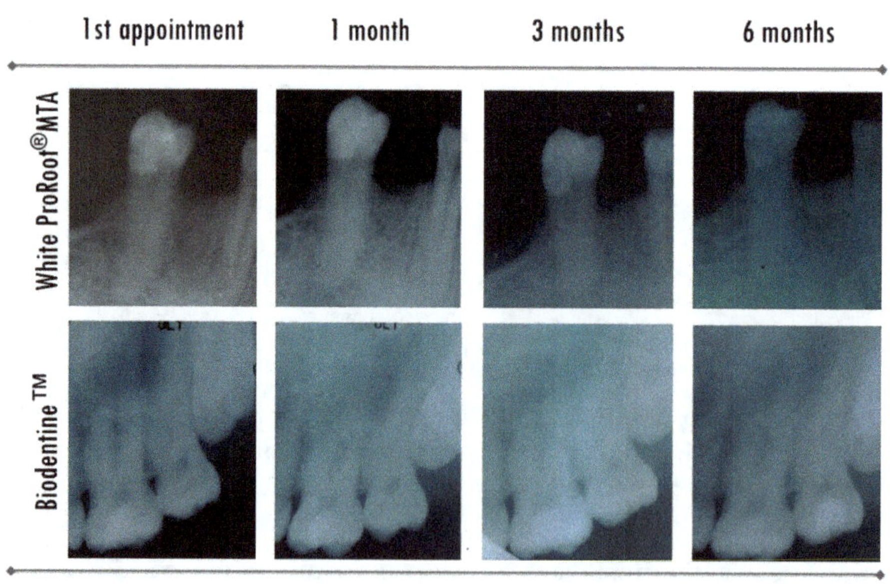

Figure 5. Radiographic images corresponding to direct pulp capping therapies with WhiteProRoot®MTA and Biodentine™ biomaterials. Therapy with WhiteProRoot®MTA was performed on tooth 35, with iatrogenic pulp exposure <2 mm, with haemorrhage and under absolute isolation. The definitive restoration was performed after therapy at the same appointment with a total-etch adhesive Scotchbond 1® (3M/ESPE, Burgdorf, Schweiz) and composite resin Synergy D6® (Coltène/Whaledent AG, Altstätten, Switzerland). Biodentine™ therapy was performed on tooth 26, with pulpal exposure due to carious lesion between 1 and 2 mm, without bleeding and under absolute isolation, and was definitively restored after therapy with a total-etch adhesive Scotchbond 1® and resin composite Synergy D6®.

The post-treatment evaluations considered five parameters and the results can be seen in Figure 6. In evaluations that were performed in the first-week control, the sensitivity test was normal in 71.4% of teeth and slightly increased in 28.6% of teeth. In the horizontal percussion test, it was reported that 95.2% of the teeth responded negatively and 4.8% responded positively (reported for the Biodentine® group). Regarding the vertical percussion test, it was reported that 90.5% of the teeth presented negative answers and 9.5% reported positive answers (reported to the Biodentine® group and the WhiteProRoot®MTA group by an equal percentage). Radiographic evaluation revealed that 100% of the intervened teeth showed no signs of secondary caries, nor any signs of apical tissue injury.

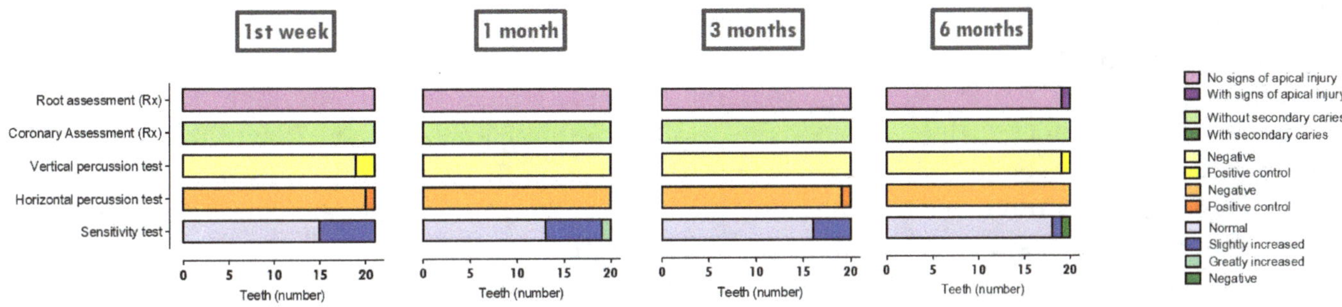

Figure 6. Therapeutic control times. Five parameters were analyzed: cold sensitivity tests (negative, normal, slightly increased, and greatly increased); horizontal and vertical percussion tests (negative and positive); coronary radiography (with or without secondary caries); root radiography (with or without apical lesion). The results express the evaluation of 21 teeth at 1 week and the evaluation of 20 teeth at 1 month, 3 months, and 6 months.

At 1 month, evaluation sensitivity testing was normal in 65% of teeth, slightly increased in 30% of teeth, and greatly increased in 5% of teeth. On the other hand, in all subjects undergoing therapy, the horizontal and vertical percussion tests were negative. Radiographic evaluation revealed that 100% of the intervened teeth showed no signs of secondary caries, nor any signs of apical tissue injury.

In the 3 months assessment, the percentage of teeth with a normal sensitivity test increased to 80%. A slight increase in sensitivity was revealed in about 20% of the teeth. The reported vertical percussion tests were negative in 100% of the teeth, as opposed to the horizontal percussion test, which was positive in 5%. As in the 1 week and 1 month controls, complementary radiographic examinations revealed that 100% of the intervened teeth showed no signs of secondary caries or injury to the apical tissues.

The post-therapeutic evaluation at 6 months revealed some changes from the other control times. Thus, pulp necrosis was diagnosed in one tooth (5%) and a marked increase in sensitivity was diagnosed in another (5%), both of which reported to the Biodentine® group. Sensitivity testing was normal for 90% of the teeth that were evaluated. Corroborating the evaluation of the sensitivity tests, the vertical percussion test was positive in one tooth (5%) and negative for the remaining 95% of the teeth. The horizontal percussion test was negative in 100% of the teeth. Radiographic evaluation, both at the coronary level and at the root level, retained negative results regarding the appearance of secondary caries and only had signs of periapical tissue damage in one tooth (5%), which was reported to the Biodentine® group as referred.

In addition to this descriptive analysis, comparisons were also made between the results that were obtained. Thus, comparisons were made between the clinical situations that were presented before therapy and the results that were obtained after therapy. Some patient data, including age, were compared with the results of the sensitivity tests over time, and hygiene habits were compared with the results of the radiographic assessment of coronary restoration over time. These comparisons showed no statistically significant differences. Comparisons were also made between the circumstances of pulp tissue exposure (caries or iatrogenic), the cavity situation at the time of exposure (with or without caries), and the size of the exposure, with the results of sensitivity tests over time. From these comparisons, it was concluded that there were no significant differences between the various circumstances and the results of these tests.

Finally, comparisons were also made between the two biomaterials that were studied and the results of the sensitivity tests with ethyl chloride and the horizontal and vertical percussion and the radiographic evaluation radicular. It was concluded that there were no statistically significant differences between the biomaterials and the results that were obtained after therapy.

Both biomaterials had similar success rates at 6 months, i.e., 100% for WhiteProRoot®MTA and 95% for Biodentine™. In this last group, there was a clinical situation of necrosis.

4. Discussion

Whenever possible, this study sought to rigorously apply the methodological items for non-randomized studies, MINORS version, to increase its reproducibility and quality. Since this is a retrospective study, the inclusion criteria were applied in the search and selection of the clinical files. Retrospective data were collected from each clinical process, at the endpoints that were determined in the study's objective, without biased evaluation. No prospective sample size calculation was performed as this is a preliminary study. Considering published meta-analysis studies, which revealed very similar clinical performances between MTA-based cement and tricalcium silicate-based cement, and in order to clinically evaluate the efficacy of these therapies, only two biomaterials were chosen [3,22,23]. Thus, with such restrictive criteria in the choice of biomaterial, it was not possible to obtain a large sample. Additional criteria for comparative studies were applied, with the choice of the gold standard biomaterial as the control group, the contemporaneity of the biomaterials, the base equivalence in both groups, and appropriate statistical analysis.

The results that were observed in the present study are comparable with others, showing success rates of 92.5% for Biodentine™ and 84.6% for WhiteProRoot®MTA [2]. Other studies mention success rates of 85%, 91.7%, and 97.1% for MTA-based cements after 3, 1, and 9 years of follow up, respectively; and 83.3% and 85.37% for 1-year follow-up with tricalcium silicate cements [1,10,24–28]. Some authors report similar success rates between the two types of biomaterials in immature permanent teeth [29–31].

The treatment failure is referred to in some studies as occurring in the first weeks after therapy, mainly due to previous impairment of the pulp state [2]. This is difficult to diagnose through sensitivity tests as these tests do not assess pulp vitality, but only measure sensitivity through subjective symptomatic assessment of the patient. In the present study, the only treatment failure occurred after 6 months, which was evaluated with the positive vertical percussion test and negative ethyl chloride test, inferring that pre-therapeutic diagnoses were correctly made. An individual cause is likely to be related to this loss of vitality since throughout the other assessment times, the tooth never changed in sensitivity testing and radiographic assessment. However, the small sample size of the present study may have contributed to the absence of statistically significant differences in the success rates of the different groups. In fact, over the various post-therapy periods, only the time and intensity of the positive response to the ethyl chloride test increased in some cases. Nevertheless, it was found that this change in response gradually decreased from week 1 to 6 months, either in the percentage of clinical cases or in response intensity. Percussion tests were positive in some cases, but sporadically and without recurrence in the various subsequent control times.

It is recognized that the direct pulp capping therapies' success depends on the rigorous selection of cases and the appropriate application of the treatment protocol [32]. Thus, the inclusion criteria for this clinical study took this premise into account. Many of the cases that were included in the present study had the aetiology of dental caries exposure. In this case, it is difficult clinically to assess the true pulp state, which is of extreme importance for prognosis. Some authors suggest that the degree of haemorrhage after exposure is a good indicator to measure the inflammatory state of the pulp tissue [32]. The occurrence of intense bleeding, which is difficult to control, is suggestive of pulp with a moderate to severe inflammatory stage and, therefore, without indication for direct pulp capping therapy [33]. Control of this pulp haemorrhage and cavity disinfection during direct pulp capping therapies are decisive steps that can affect pulp tissue regeneration. Bleeding should be controlled by exerting pressure at the exposure site for 3 to 5 min with a sterile cotton ball soaked in the haemostatic/disinfection solution. Several authors have studied the efficacy and influence of these solutions on pulp tissue regeneration [34–37]. Although saline has limited effects, it is traditionally the most widely used. Some authors report that 0.9% of saline has acceptable results, but is inferior to other solutions such as chlorhexidine and sodium hypochlorite [35–37]. The established protocol recommends the use of chlorhexidine at a concentration of 2% and with a 3 min application time to achieve maximum efficacy with minimal cytotoxicity, according to the literature [35,38,39]. In all clinical processes that were consulted, chlorhexidine was the cavity disinfectant that was chosen in the direct pulp capping therapies, and the procedure was made according to the protocol.

The radiographic technique of long cone parallelism is not a practice that is established in outpatient dentistry appointments and there are no standardized radiographic records of the therapies that were performed in the clinical processes. Thus, it was not possible to perform a radiographic comparison study. This would have been useful in gauging the formation and quality of the dental bridge, as was done in other studies [31,40]. The results of those report very similar values between biomaterials, between 85% and 95%, when the evaluation refers to the existence of dentin bridge, although incomplete [24,30]. However, it is also described in the literature that the relatively low radiopacity of tricalcium silicate-based cement, when compared with MTA-based cements, can make this type of assessment difficult [2,41–43].

In extracting data from clinical files, it was found that the use of glass ionomer cement liner had always been performed after biomaterials were applied to the exposure sites. However, according to some authors and the manufacturer of the tricalcium silicate-based biomaterial, the setting time is very short and definitive restoration can be performed in the same appointment without the need to place a base between the biomaterial and the restorative materials. Some authors also report the use of tricalcium silicate cement as an integral substitute for all dentine tissue using a sandwich restorative technique [1,16,18,19].

The adhesive techniques that were performed in this study, whether using total-etch or self-etch adhesive systems with selective enamel etching, are recommended by many authors as having the best adhesion values and, consequently, the best performance [44–49]. It was also observed that the definitive restorations were performed by direct or indirect technique with the composite resins, as recommended by the literature [39,50–54]. The results of the radiographic evaluations that were performed on the restorations throughout the study that reveal the absence of signs of secondary caries corroborate this recommendation.

Histologically, it is established that mineral trioxide aggregates induce the formation of a thicker hard tissue barrier than calcium hydroxide-based materials, accompanied by less tissue inflammation. In addition, pulp tissue has progenitor cells that are capable of differentiating into odontoblast cells type, with the capacity to mineralize tissue deposition. This mechanism is facilitated by mineral trioxide aggregates by inducing the secretion of morphogenetic proteins and growth factors such as BMP-2 and TGF-β1 [55,56]. The technology behind the biosilicate manufacturing process, the main constituent of Biodentine™, removes metallic impurities that are present in other cements. The main reaction involves the hydration of tricalcium silicate and the production of a calcium silicate and calcium hydroxide based gel which in contact with phosphate ions, has the ability to precipitate a hydroxyapatite-like compound [57]. Some studies even report that due to its low cytotoxicity and high bioinductive capacity, Biodentine™ can be considered the ideal material for the treatment of pulp exposures [55]. The repair mechanism by deposition of mineralized tissue depends on the pH and the ability of tricalcium silicate cement to release various ions. Extracellular calcium ions represent a potent factor that affects cell function and has significant effects on cell proliferation and differentiation. Calcium ions are known to be involved in a number of proliferation signaling pathways and represent a key point for the investigation of the action mechanisms of these biomaterials and the eventual development of others.

The main limitations of this retrospective clinical study are the small sample size and the short evaluation period, so it was considered preliminary. Longer evaluation times and larger samples would be important to assess intrapulpar changes resulting from these therapies and the effective formation of a dentin bridge at the site of exposure [58]. It would also be advisable to histologically evaluate pulp capping therapies over time if possible. This evaluation would only be feasible in randomized clinical studies involving teeth with an indication for extraction.

5. Conclusions

As the use of tricalcium silicate cement is relatively new, there are few studies regarding its clinical performance in permanent teeth. In the present study, success rates of tricalcium silicate cement were 95%, which are high and similar to the 100% success rate of MTA-based cement. Comparisons showed that the success rates obtained are not dependent on age or tooth type or on the cavity or aetiology of pulp exposure. Tricalcium silicate cement could be an alternative to pulp capping with low costs, more clinically friendly setting times, and the same therapeutic performance as the gold-standard, MTA-based cement.

Author Contributions: Conceptualization, A.P., E.C. and M.F.B.; Data curation, M.L. and C.M.M.; Formal analysis, A.P., E.C., A.M.A., J.C.-L. and M.M.F.; Funding acquisition, E.C. and M.F.B.; Investigation, A.P., E.C., M.L. and C.M.M.; Methodology, A.P., E.C. and C.M.M.; Project administration, A.M.A. and M.M.F.; Resources, M.L., J.C.-L., M.F.B. and C.M.M.; Software, A.M.A. and J.C.-L.; Supervision, M.F.B. and M.M.F.; Validation, A.P., J.C.-L., C.M.M. and M.M.F.; Visualization, A.P., M.L. and A.M.A.; Writing—original draft, A.P., E.C. and J.C.-L.; Writing—review and editing, M.L., M.F.B. and C.M.M. The second author had an equivalent contribution to the first author in the conduct of the work and preparation of the article.

References

1. Hegde, S.; Sowmya, B.; Mathew, S.; Bhandi, S.H.; Nagaraja, S.; Dinesh, K. Clinical evaluation of mineral trioxide aggregate and biodentine as direct pulp capping agents in carious teeth. *J. Conserv. Dent.* **2017**, *20*, 91–95.
2. Linu, S.; Lekshmi, M.S.; Varunkumar, V.S.; Sam Joseph, V.G. Treatment Outcome Following Direct Pulp Capping Using Bioceramic Materials in Mature Permanent Teeth with Carious Exposure: A Pilot Retrospective Study. *J. Endod.* **2017**, *43*, 1635–1639. [CrossRef]
3. Pereira Paula, A.B.; Laranjo, M.; Marto, C.-M.; Paulo, S.; Abrantes, A.; Casalta-Lopes, J.; Marques-Ferreira, M.; Botelho, M.F.; Carrilho, E. Direct pulp capping: What is the most effective therapy?—Systematic review and meta-analysis. *J. Evid. Based Dent. Pract.* **2018**, *18*, 298–314. [CrossRef]
4. Auschill, T.M.; Arweiler, N.B.; Hellwig, E.; Zamani-Alaei, A.; Sculean, A. Success rate of direct pulp capping with calcium hydroxide. *Schweizer Monatsschrift fur.* **2003**, *113*, 946–952.
5. Barthel, C.R.; Rosenkranz, B.; Leuenberg, A.; Roulet, J.F. Pulp capping of carious exposures: Treatment outcome after 5 and 10 years: A retrospective study. *J. Endod.* **2000**, *26*, 525–528. [CrossRef]
6. Hörsted-Bindslev, P.; Vilkinis, V.; Sidlauskas, A. Direct capping of human pulps with a dentin bonding system or with calcium hydroxide cement. *Oral Surg. Oral Med. Oral Pathol. Oral Radiol. Endod.* **2003**, *96*, 591–600. [CrossRef]
7. Accorinte, M.L.R.; Loguercio, A.D.; Reis, A.; Bauer, J.R.O.; Grande, R.H.M.; Murata, S.S.; Souza, V.; Holland, R. Evaluation of two mineral trioxide aggregate compounds as pulp-capping agents in human teeth. *Int. Endod. J.* **2009**, *42*, 122–128. [CrossRef] [PubMed]
8. De Accorinte, M.L.R.; Holland, R.; Reis, A.; Bortoluzzi, M.C.; Murata, S.S.; Dezan, E.; Souza, V.; Alessandro, L.D. Evaluation of mineral trioxide aggregate and calcium hydroxide cement as pulp-capping agents in human teeth. *J. Endod.* **2008**, *34*, 1–6. [CrossRef] [PubMed]
9. Kim, J.; Song, Y.-S.; Min, K.; Kim, S.; Koh, J.-T.; Lee, B.; Chang, H.; Hwang, I.-N.; Oh, W.-M.; Hwang, Y.-C. Evaluation of reparative dentin formation of ProRoot MTA, Biodentine and BioAggregate using micro-CT and immunohistochemistry. *Restor. Dent. Endod.* **2016**, *41*, 29–36. [CrossRef]

10. Kundzina, R.; Stangvaltaite, L.; Eriksen, H.M.; Kerosuo, E. Capping carious exposures in adults: A randomized controlled trial investigating mineral trioxide aggregate versus calcium hydroxide. *Int. Endod. J.* **2017**, *50*, 924–932. [CrossRef]
11. Camilleri, J.; Pitt Ford, T.R. Mineral trioxide aggregate: A review of the constituents and biological properties of the material. *Int. Endod. J.* **2006**, *39*, 747–754. [CrossRef] [PubMed]
12. Asgary, S.; Eghbal, M.J.; Parirokh, M.; Ghanavati, F.; Rahimi, H. A comparative study of histologic response to different pulp capping materials and a novel endodontic cement. *Oral Surg. Oral Med. Oral Pathol. Oral Radiol. Endod.* **2008**, *106*, 609–614. [CrossRef] [PubMed]
13. Asgary, S.; Shahabi, S.; Jafarzadeh, T.; Amini, S.; Kheirieh, S. The Properties of a New Endodontic Material. *J. Endod.* **2008**, *34*, 990–993. [CrossRef] [PubMed]
14. Parirokh, M.; Torabinejad, M. Mineral Trioxide Aggregate: A Comprehensive Literature Review—Part I: Chemical, Physical, and Antibacterial Properties. *J. Endod.* **2010**, *36*, 16–27. [CrossRef] [PubMed]
15. Okiji, T.; Yoshiba, K. Reparative Dentinogenesis Induced by Mineral Trioxide Aggregate: A Review from the Biological and Physicochemical Points of View. *Int. J. Dent.* **2009**, *2009*, 464280. [CrossRef]
16. Martens, L.; Rajasekharan, S.; Cauwels, R. Pulp management after traumatic injuries with a tricalcium silicate-based cement (Biodentine™): A report of two cases, up to 48 months follow-up. *Eur. Arch. Paediatr. Dent.* **2015**, *16*, 491–496. [CrossRef]
17. Nikfarjam, F.; Beyer, K.; König, A.; Hofmann, M.; Butting, M.; Valesky, E.; Kippenberger, S.; Kaufmann, R.; Heidemann, D.; Bernd, A.; et al. Influence of Biodentine®—A Dentine Substitute—On Collagen Type I Synthesis in Pulp Fibroblasts In Vitro. *PLoS ONE* **2016**, *11*, e0167633. [CrossRef]
18. Koubi, G.; Colon, P.; Franquin, J.-C.; Hartmann, A.; Richard, G.; Faure, M.-O.; Lambert, G. Clinical evaluation of the performance and safety of a new dentine substitute, Biodentine, in the restoration of posterior teeth—A prospective study. *Clin. Oral Investig.* **2013**, *17*, 243–249. [CrossRef]
19. Rajasekharan, S.; Martens, L.C.; Cauwels, R.G.E.C.; Verbeeck, R.M.H. Biodentine™ material characteristics and clinical applications: A review of the literature. *Eur. Arch. Paediatr. Dent.* **2014**, *15*, 147–158. [CrossRef]
20. Camilleri, J.; Sorrentino, F.; Damidot, D. Investigation of the hydration and bioactivity of radiopacified tricalcium silicate cement, Biodentine and MTA Angelus. *Dent. Mater.* **2013**, *29*, 580–593. [CrossRef]
21. Kravitz, A.; Bullock, A.; Cowpe, J. *Manual of Dental Practice 2015*; The Council of European Dentists, Ed.; 5.1.; Cardiff University: Wales, UK, 2015.
22. Deng, Y.; Zhu, X.; Zheng, D.; Yan, P.; Jiang, H. Laser use in direct pulp capping: A meta-analysis. *J. Am. Dent. Assoc.* **2016**, *147*, 935–942. [CrossRef] [PubMed]
23. Luiz de Oliveira da Rosa, W.; Machado da Silva, T.; Fernando Demarco, F.; Piva, E.; Fernandes da Silva, A. Could the application of bioactive molecules improve vital pulp therapy success? A systematic review. *J. Biomed. Mater. Res. A* **2017**, *105*, 941–956. [CrossRef] [PubMed]
24. Bogen, G.; Kim, J.S.; Bakland, L.K. Direct pulp capping with mineral trioxide aggregate: An observational study. *J. Am. Dent. Assoc.* **2008**, *139*, 305–315. [CrossRef] [PubMed]
25. Jang, Y.; Song, M.; Yoo, I.-S.; Song, Y.; Roh, B.-D.; Kim, E. A Randomized Controlled Study of the Use of ProRoot Mineral Trioxide Aggregate and Endocem as Direct Pulp Capping Materials: 3-month versus 1-year Outcomes. *J. Endod.* **2015**, *41*, 1201–1206. [CrossRef]
26. Awawdeh, L.; Al-Qudah, A.; Hamouri, H.; Chakra, R.J. Outcomes of Vital Pulp Therapy Using Mineral Trioxide Aggregate or Biodentine: A Prospective Randomized Clinical Trial. *J. Endod.* **2018**, *44*, 1603–1609. [CrossRef]
27. Parinyaprom, N.; Nirunsittirat, A.; Chuveera, P.; Na Lampang, S.; Srisuwan, T.; Sastraruji, T.; Bua-on, P.; Simprasert, S.; Khoipanich, I.; Sutharaphan, T.; et al. Outcomes of Direct Pulp Capping by Using Either ProRoot Mineral Trioxide Aggregate or Biodentine in Permanent Teeth with Carious Pulp Exposure in 6- to 18-Year-Old Patients: A Randomized Controlled Trial. *J. Endod.* **2018**, *44*, 341–348. [CrossRef]
28. Brizuela, C.; Ormeño, A.; Cabrera, C.; Cabezas, R.; Silva, C.I.; Ramírez, V.; Mercade, M. Direct Pulp Capping with Calcium Hydroxide, Mineral Trioxide Aggregate, and Biodentine in Permanent Young Teeth with Caries: A Randomized Clinical Trial. *J. Endod.* **2017**, *43*, 1776–1780. [CrossRef]
29. Bhat, S.S.; Hegde, S.K.; Adhikari, F.; Bhat, V.S. Direct pulp capping in an immature incisor using a new bioactive material. *Contemp. Clin. Dent.* **2014**, *5*, 393–396. [CrossRef]

30. Katge, F.A.; Patil, D.P. Comparative Analysis of 2 Calcium Silicate-based Cements (Biodentine and Mineral Trioxide Aggregate) as Direct Pulp-capping Agent in Young Permanent Molars: A Split Mouth Study. *J. Endod.* **2017**, *43*, 507–513. [CrossRef]
31. Nowicka, A.; Lipski, M.; Parafiniuk, M.; Sporniak-Tutak, K.; Lichota, D.; Kosierkiewicz, A.; Kaczmarek, W.; Buczkowska-Radlińska, J. Response of Human Dental Pulp Capped with Biodentine and Mineral Trioxide Aggregate. *J. Endod.* **2013**, *39*, 743–747. [CrossRef]
32. Aguilar, P.; Linsuwanont, P. Vital pulp therapy in vital permanent teeth with cariously exposed pulp: A systematic review. *J. Endod.* **2011**, *37*, 581–587. [CrossRef] [PubMed]
33. Andreasen, J.O. Pulp and periodontal tissue repair—Regeneration or tissue metaplasia after dental trauma. A review. *Dent. Traumatol.* **2012**, *28*, 19–24. [CrossRef] [PubMed]
34. Accorinte, M.; Loguercio, A.; Reis, A.; Holland, R. Effects of hemostatic agents on the histomorphologic response of human dental pulp capped with calcium hydroxide. *Quintessence Int.* **2007**, *38*, 843–852.
35. Bal, C.; Alacam, A.; Tuzuner, T.; Tirali, R.E.; Baris, E. Effects of Antiseptics on Pulpal Healing under Calcium Hydroxide Pulp Capping: A Pilot Study. *Eur. J. Dent.* **2011**, *5*, 265–272. [CrossRef]
36. Gomes, B.P.; Ferraz, C.C.; Vianna, M.E.; Berber, V.B.; Teixeira, F.B.; Souza-Filho, F.J. In vitro antimicrobial activity of several concentrations of sodium hypochlorite and chlorhexidine gluconate in the elimination of Enterococcus faecalis. *Int. Endod. J.* **2001**, *34*, 424–428. [CrossRef]
37. Rôças, I.N.; Siqueira, J.F. Comparison of the in vivo antimicrobial effectiveness of sodium hypochlorite and chlorhexidine used as root canal irrigants: A molecular microbiology study. *J. Endod.* **2011**, *37*, 143–150. [CrossRef]
38. Silva, A.F.; Tarquinio, S.B.C.; Demarco, F.F.; Piva, E.; Rivero, E.R.C. The influence of haemostatic agents on healing of healthy human dental pulp tissue capped with calcium hydroxide. *Int. Endod. J.* **2006**, *39*, 309–316. [CrossRef]
39. Baldissera, R.; Corrêa, M.B.; Schuch, H.S.; Collares, K.; Nascimento, G.G.; Jardim, P.S.; Moraes, R.R.; Opdam, N.J.M.; Demarco, F.F. Are there universal restorative composites for anterior and posterior teeth? *J. Dent.* **2013**, *41*, 1027–1035. [CrossRef]
40. Zarrabi, M.H.; Javidi, M.; Jafarian, A.H.; Joushan, B. Histologic assessment of human pulp response to capping with mineral trioxide aggregate and a novel endodontic cement. *J. Endod.* **2010**, *36*, 1778–1781. [CrossRef]
41. Tanalp, J.; Karapınar-Kazandağ, M.; Dölekoğlu, S.; Kayahan, M.B. Comparison of the radiopacities of different root-end filling and repair materials. *Sci. World J.* **2013**, *2013*, 594950. [CrossRef]
42. Kaup, M.; Schäfer, E.; Dammaschke, T. An in vitro study of different material properties of Biodentine compared to ProRoot MTA. *Head Face Med.* **2015**, *11*, 16. [CrossRef] [PubMed]
43. Saghiri, M.A.; Gutmann, J.L.; Orangi, J.; Asatourian, A.; Sheibani, N. Radiopacifier particle size impacts the physical properties of tricalcium silicate-based cements. *J. Endod.* **2015**, *41*, 225–230. [CrossRef] [PubMed]
44. Abdalla, A.I.; El Zohairy, A.A.; Abdel Mohsen, M.M.; Feilzer, A.J. Bond efficacy and interface morphology of self-etching adhesives to ground enamel. *J. Adhes. Dent.* **2010**, *12*, 19–25. [PubMed]
45. Nawareg, M.M.A.; Zidan, A.Z.; Zhou, J.; Chiba, A.; Tagami, J.; Pashley, D.H. Adhesive sealing of dentin surfaces in vitro: A review. *Am. J. Dent.* **2015**, *28*, 321–332. [PubMed]
46. Peumans, M.; De Munck, J.; Mine, A.; Van Meerbeek, B. Clinical effectiveness of contemporary adhesives for the restoration of non-carious cervical lesions. A systematic review. *Dent. Mater.* **2014**, *30*, 1089–1103. [CrossRef] [PubMed]
47. Reis, A.; Dourado Loguercio, A.; Schroeder, M.; Luque-Martinez, I.; Masterson, D.; Cople Maia, L. Does the adhesive strategy influence the post-operative sensitivity in adult patients with posterior resin composite restorations?: A systematic review and meta-analysis. *Dent. Mater.* **2015**, *31*, 1052–1067. [CrossRef] [PubMed]
48. Zhang, Y.; Wang, Y. Distinct photopolymerization efficacy on dentin of self-etch adhesives. *J. Dent. Res.* **2012**, *91*, 795–799. [CrossRef]
49. Zhang, Y.; Wang, Y. Effect of application mode on interfacial morphology and chemistry between dentine and self-etch adhesives. *J. Dent.* **2013**, *41*, 231–240. [CrossRef]
50. Baroudi, K.; Rodrigues, J.C. Flowable Resin Composites: A Systematic Review and Clinical Considerations. *J. Clin. Diagn. Res.* **2015**, *9*, ZE18–ZE24. [CrossRef]
51. Ferracane, J.L. Resin composite—State of the art. *Dent. Mater.* **2011**, *27*, 29–38. [CrossRef]

52. Opdam, N.J.M.; van de Sande, F.H.; Bronkhorst, E.; Cenci, M.S.; Bottenberg, P.; Pallesen, U.; Gaengler, P.; Lindberg, A.; Huysmans, M.C.; van Dijken, J.W. Longevity of posterior composite restorations: A systematic review and meta-analysis. *J. Dent. Res.* **2014**, *93*, 943–949. [CrossRef]
53. Van de Sande, F.H.; Opdam, N.J.; Rodolpho, P.A.D.R.; Correa, M.B.; Demarco, F.F.; Cenci, M.S. Patient risk factors' influence on survival of posterior composites. *J. Dent. Res.* **2013**, *92*, 78S–83S. [CrossRef] [PubMed]
54. Syed, M.; Chopra, R.; Sachdev, V. Allergic Reactions to Dental Materials—A Systematic Review. *J. Clin. Diagn. Res.* **2015**, *9*, ZE04–ZE09. [CrossRef] [PubMed]
55. Poggio, C.; Ceci, M.; Beltrami, R.; Dagna, A.; Colombo, M.; Chiesa, M. Biocompatibility of a new pulp capping cement. *Ann. Stomatol.* **2014**, *5*, 69–76. [CrossRef]
56. Poggio, C.; Arciola, C.R.; Beltrami, R.; Monaco, A.; Dagna, A.; Lombardini, M.; Visai, L. Cytocompatibility and Antibacterial Properties of Capping Materials. *Sci. World J.* **2014**, *2014*, 1–10. [CrossRef] [PubMed]
57. Nuñez, C.M.; Bosomworth, H.J.; Field, C.; Whitworth, J.M.; Valentine, R.A. Biodentine and mineral trioxide aggregate induce similar cellular responses in a fibroblast cell line. *J. Endod.* **2014**, *40*, 406–411. [CrossRef] [PubMed]
58. Olsson, H.; Petersson, K.; Rohlin, M. Formation of a hard tissue barrier after pulp cappings in humans. A systematic review. *Int. Endod. J.* **2006**, *39*, 429–442. [CrossRef] [PubMed]

7

Microstructures and Mechanical Properties of Laser-Sintered Commercially Pure Ti and Ti-6Al-4V Alloy for Dental Applications

Yoshimitsu Okazaki [1,*] and **Akira Ishino** [2]

1 Department of Life Science and Biotechnology, National Institute of Advanced Industrial Science and Technology, 1-1 Higashi 1-chome, Tsukuba, Ibaraki 305-8566, Japan
2 IDS Co. Ltd., 3-5-4 Hongo, Bunkyo-ku, Tokyo 113-0033, Japan; a-isino@idscoltd.jp
* Correspondence: y-okazaki@aist.go.jp; Tel.: +81-29-861-7179

Abstract: To apply laser-sintered titanium (Ti) materials to dental prostheses with a three-dimensional structure such as partial dentures, we examined the microstructures and mechanical properties of commercially pure (CP) Ti grade (G) 2 annealed after laser sintering and laser-sintered (as-built) Ti-6Al-4V alloy. The tensile and fatigue properties of CP Ti G 2 annealed at 700 °C for 2 h after laser sintering were close to those of wrought CP Ti G 2 annealed at the same temperature after hot forging. The ultimate tensile strengths (σ_{UTS}) of 90°- and 0°-direction-built CP Ti G 2 rods after laser sintering 10 times were 553 and 576 MPa and the total elongations (TE) of these rods were 26% and 28%, respectively. The fatigue strengths (σ_{FS}) at 10^7 cycles of the 90°- and 0°-direction-built CP Ti G 2 rods after laser sintering 10 times were ~320 and ~365 MPa, respectively. The ratio σ_{FS}/σ_{UTS} was in the range of 0.5–0.7. The changes in the chemical composition and mechanical properties after laser sintering 10 times were negligible. The fatigue strength of the laser-sintered Ti-6Al-4V alloy was ~600 MPa, which was close to that of wrought Ti-6Al-4V alloy. These findings indicate that the laser-sintered CP Ti and Ti-6Al-4V alloy can also be applied in dental prostheses similarly to laser-sintered Co–Cr–Mo alloy. In particular, it was clarified that laser sintering using CP Ti G 4 powder is useful for dental prostheses.

Keywords: titanium materials; laser sintering; microstructure; tensile property; fatigue property; physical property; dental prostheses

---

1. Introduction

Metallic materials such as titanium (Ti) materials and cobalt–chromium–molybdenum (Co–Cr–Mo) alloys with excellent mechanical properties and structural stability have been widely used for dental prostheses (especially metal frames for partial dentures, complete dentures, and implant superstructures) [1–3]. Ti materials (commercially pure (CP) Ti and Ti alloys) with high biocompatibility have been widely used for orthopedic implants and dental prostheses. CP Ti for orthopedic implants is classified into grades (G) G 1 (O ≤ 0.18 mass %), G 2 (O ≤ 0.25 mass %), G 3 (O ≤ 0.35 mass %), and G 4 (O ≤ 0.4 mass %) in International Organization for Standardization (ISO) 5832-2 [4]. As the grade of CP Ti increases, the amount of trace elements such as oxygen (O) increases.

Ti-6%Al-4%V alloy (here and hereafter values of alloy compositions indicate mass %) is also widely used in the medical field and is standardized in ISO 5832-3 [5]. Since the O concentration in laser-sintered Ti-6Al-4V alloy increases upon laser sintering [6], high-purity Ti-6Al-4V G 5 powder for additive manufacturing (AM) has been standardized in ASTM F 2924 [7]. The O concentration in this standard is defined according to the particle size of the Ti-6Al-4V alloy powder. In the Ti alloys containing Al, the O concentration is limited to ≤0.2% [5]. On the other hand, since CP Ti does not contain Al, it is expected that the O concentration can be increased to 0.4% as standardized in ISO 5832-2 [4]. Ti materials have the advantage of being lower in density and lighter than Co–Cr–Mo alloys. Dental prostheses (metal frames for partial dentures, complete dentures, and implant superstructures) fabricated using Ti materials are also suitable for patients sensitive to Co ions released from Co–Cr–Mo alloys [2].

The mechanical properties of dental-cast CP Ti and Ti alloys have been reported [8–10]. In conventional dental casts with Ti materials, a brittle (hard) surface oxide (alpha-case) layer and blow holes in the central part of casts are formed owing to the reaction of Ti materials with the mold material during the casting process. These casting defects cause problems such as the breakage of partial dentures and clasps. This hard alpha-case layer has also made it difficult to adapt Ti materials to crowns, bridges, and so forth [11,12]. In the case of using a computer-aided machining (CAM) milling system, it is difficult to manufacture complicated shapes, and long processing times are required [2]. Therefore, AM is expected to be a new technology for manufacturing Ti dental prostheses. In the AM of Ti materials, since no investment mold material is used, no reaction occurs between the mold material and the Ti material. Thus, as Ti has a strong affinity to O, for the AM of Ti materials, it is important to examine the change in the O concentration of Ti materials after laser sintering. However, there have been few studies on the mechanical and microstructural properties of laser-sintered CP Ti and Ti-6Al-4V alloys for dental prostheses. In particular, there are few reports on the fatigue properties of laser-sintered Ti materials.

To obtain regulatory approval for dental prostheses and orthopedic devices produced by 3-D layer manufacturing in Japan, evaluation of the chemical composition, powder recycling, melting point, microstructure, tensile property, immersion property, and fatigue property is desirable [1]. We acquired experimental data according to these requirements for regulatory approval in dental prostheses.

The microstructures and mechanical properties of laser-sintered Co–Cr–Mo alloys for dental prostheses have been investigated [1–3]. These days, the tensile and fatigue properties of Co-25Cr-5Mo-5W (SP2) and W-free Co-28Cr-6Mo alloys are extremely superior to those of conventional dental-cast Co–Cr–Mo alloys [1]. The ultimate tensile strength (σ_{UTS}) and total elongation (TE) of Co-28Cr-6Mo alloys are close to those of hot-forged Co-28Cr-6Mo alloys. The fatigue strengths (σ_{FS}) at 10^7 cycles of the 90°- and 0°-direction-built Co-28Cr-6Mo alloys are ~500 and ~600 MPa, respectively [1]. These superior mechanical properties result from the precipitation of fine intermetallic compound π-phase (lattice parameter a = b = c = 0.633 nm) particles in the grains and grain boundaries of the fine face-centered-cubic (fcc) matrix formed owing to rapid solidification [1]. The changes in the chemical composition and mechanical properties of Co-25Cr-5Mo-5W and Co-28Cr-6Mo alloys after laser sintering 20 times are also negligible.

In this study, we investigated the chemical composition, immersion property, microstructure, tensile property, and fatigue strength of CP Ti G 2 annealed at 700 °C for 2 h after laser sintering for dental application with 3-D structures (metal frames for partial dentures, complete dentures, and implant superstructures). The purpose of this study was to compare the mechanical properties of laser-sintered Ti materials with those of laser-sintered Co–Cr–Mo alloy. To develop dental prostheses with high strength, these properties were also compared with those of laser-sintered (as-built) Ti-6Al-4V alloy.

Moreover, to obtain similar two-phase equiaxed grains of the alpha (α)-phase [hexagonal-close-packed (hcp) structure] and beta (β)-phase [body-centered-cubic (bcc) structure] as the wrought Ti-6Al-4V alloy [13], the effect of the heat treatment temperature on as-built Ti-6Al-4V alloy rods was also investigated.

In particular, we focused on the fatigue properties of laser-sintered and wrought Ti materials. The results obtained in this study are expected to be useful for the development of Ti dental prostheses by 3-D layer manufacturing.

2. Experimental Procedure

2.1. Test Specimens

2.1.1. Laser Sintering and Dental Casting

CP Ti G 2 (EOS (EOS GmbH Electro Optical System, Krailling, Germany) and TILOP (Osaka Titanium Technologies Co., Ltd., Osaka, Japan) powders were prepared by plasma and Ar gas atomization processes, respectively. The CP Ti G 2 powder was laser-sintered using a system comprising an EOS M290 or EOS M270 machine ((EOS GmbH Electro Optical System, Krailling, Germany), EOSPRINT v. 1.3 (EOS GmbH Electro Optical System, Krailling, Germany) and HCS v. 2.3.29 software (EOS GmbH Electro Optical System, Krailling, Germany), and the TiCP 30 μm FlexLine parameter set. Ti-6Al-4V (EOS) alloy powder and a CP Ti G 2 ingot for preparing conventional dental casts were used for comparison. The Ti-6Al-4V alloy powder was laser-sintered in an Ar atmosphere using a system comprising an EOS M290 machine, EOSPRINT v. 1.5 and HCS v. 2.4.14 software, and the Ti64 Performance M291 1.10 parameter set.

The laser beam power (P) and the hatch spacing between scan passes (H) were 150–300 W (mainly 280–300 W) and 0.1–0.15 mm (mainly 0.13–0.14 mm), respectively. The laser scan speed (V) and powder stacking (deposited layer) thickness (T) were fixed from 1000 to 1300 mm/s (mainly 1200–1300 mm/s) and 0.02–0.04 mm (mainly 0.03 mm), respectively. The laser spot focus diameter was from 0.1 to 0.3 mm (mainly 0.1 mm). The volumetric energy density (E) = P/(H·T·V) was 50–120 J/mm^3 (mainly 60 J/mm^3). Cylindrical specimens built by laser sintering were cut from the support materials.

Cylindrical specimens with a diameter of 9 mm and a height of 50 mm were fabricated by laser sintering under the above conditions using EOSINT M 290 and EOSINT M 270 machines on support materials using the CP Ti G 2 powders. As shown in Figure 1, to investigate the effect of the building direction of laser sintering, the building direction was set to 0° (hereafter, 0° direction), 45° (45° direction), and 90° (90° direction) for the base plate using the CP Ti G 2 powders [1]. CP Ti G 2 cylindrical specimens after laser sintering were heat-treated at 700 °C for 2 h followed by air cooling. This heat treatment (annealing) at 700 °C (±10 °C) for 2 h is recommended by the FlexLine EOS material data. These conditions are also widely used for wrought Ti materials [14]. In the actual laser sintering of dental prostheses, a certain percentage of virgin powder is added. The number of repeated uses of the same powder of up to 10 times in this work was decided considering the effect of a small amount of residual powder. In the case of laser sintering from two to nine times, two cylindical specimens with a diameter of 9 mm and a height of 50 mm were laser-sintered in the 90° direction in each sintering.

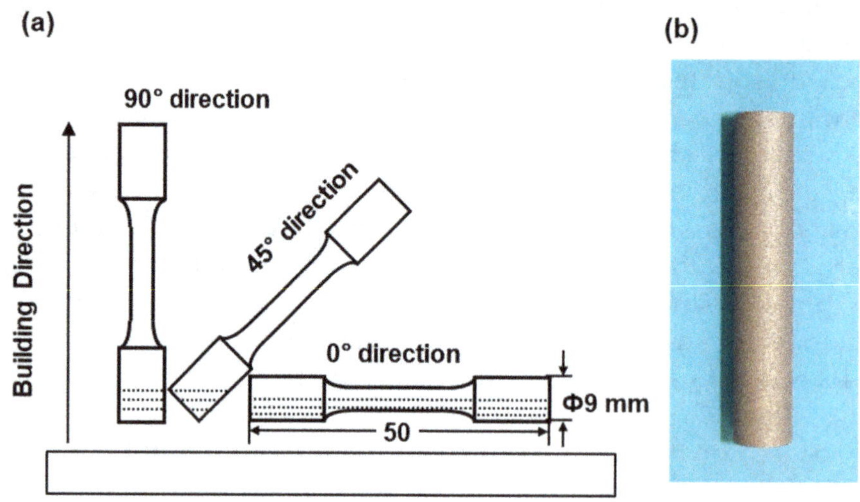

Figure 1. (**a**) Building directions of cylindrical specimens in laser sintering; (**b**) laser-sintered cylindrical specimens.

For comparison, Ti-6Al-4V alloy was laser-sintered in the 90° direction with the EOSINT M 290 machine (as-built Ti-6Al-4V alloy). To obtain two-phase grains with the α (hcp) and β (bcc) phases, as seen in wrought Ti-6Al-4V alloy, the test specimens subjected to heat treatment were prepared from the laser-sintered Ti-6Al-4V alloy. The test specimens were heat-treated at 840, 860, 880, 900, 920, 940, 960, and 980 °C for 2 h followed by air cooling [14]. The microstructure after annealing was observed by optical microscopy and scanning electron microscopy (SEM, Talos Thermo Fisher Scientific, Tokyo, Japan, Quanta 200FEG; acceleration voltage, 15 kV). The phases were also identified by X-ray diffraction with Cu Kα radiation (Rigaku, SmartLab, Tokyo, Japan; tube voltage, 45 kV; tube current, 200 mA; 2°/min; scan range (2θ) of 30°–80°).

An Ar gas pressure dental casting machine manufactured by Wada Precision Dental Laboratories (EZ Titan, Osaka, Japan) and an alumina phosphate investment mold (SUPER-VEST-D, Okazaki Minerals and Refining Co. Ltd., Osaka, Japan) were used to manufacture the cylindrical dental casts. CP Ti G 2 ingots of 40 g (30 mm diameter and 13 mm height; GC Corporation, Tokyo, Japan) used for conventional dental casts were employed as reference materials.

2.1.2. Laser-Sintered Powders and Ti Material Rods

Figure 2 shows (a) the particle size distribution and (b) SEM images of the CP Ti G 2 powders. Figure 2a also shows the D_{10}, D_{50}, and D_{90} particle sizes corresponding to 10%, 50%, and 90% of the cumulative distribution, respectively. The particle size distributions of the powders were measured using an LA-750 particle size analyzer (Horiba, Ltd., Tokyo, Japan) in accordance with ISO 133320 [15]. EOS CP Ti G 2 particles were larger than TILOP CP Ti G 2 particles. The particle size distributions of the virgin TILOP powders and 10-times-sintered CP Ti powders showed the same tendency.

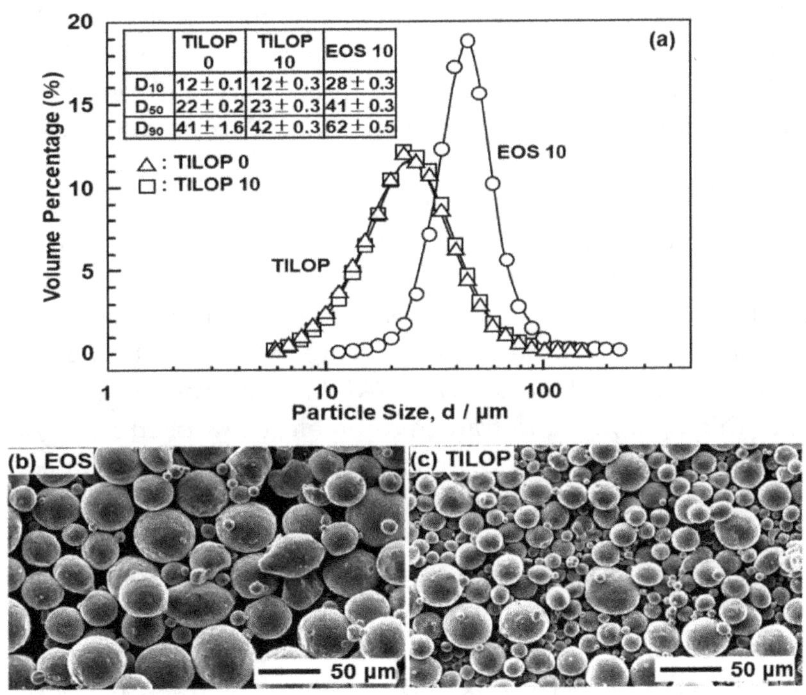

Figure 2. (**a**) Particle size distributions of 10-times-sintered EOS (EOS 10) and once-sintered (TILOP 0) and 10-times-sintered TILOP (TILOP 10) commercially pure (CP) Ti G 2 powders; SEM images of (**b**) 10-times-sintered EOS and (**c**) TILOP CP Ti G 2 powders.

The changes in the D_{10}, D_{50}, and D_{90} particle sizes of Ti-6Al-4V powders when the number of repetitions in AM is incresaed from once to five times are small according to the literature [6].

The chemical compositions of these powders and laser-sintered (as-built) CP Ti G 2 and Ti-6Al-4V alloy, and dental-cast CP Ti G 2 rods are shown in Table 1. The H, N, O, Fe, C, Al, and V concentrations in the laser-sintered and dental-cast CP Ti G 2 rods and laser-sintered Ti-6Al-4V alloy rods were measured in accordance with Japanese Industrial Standard (JIS) H 1619 [16], JIS H 1612 [17], JIS H 1620 [18], JIS H 1614 [19], JIS H 1617 [20], JIS H 1622 [21], and JIS H 1624 [22], respectively. These chemical analyses were performed at Kobelco Research Institute, Inc. (Hyogo, Japan). Even when the number of repetitions in AM was increased from once to 10 times, the changes in metal concentrations (impurities) of the laser-sintered CP Ti G 2 rods were very small.

Table 1. Chemical compositions (mass %) of CP Ti G 2 virgin powders, laser-sintered CP Ti G 2 and Ti-6Al-4V alloy, and dental-cast CP Ti G 2 rods.

Alloy	Al	V	Fe	O	N	H	C	Ti
EOS CP Ti G 2 virgin powder			0.16	0.15	0.01	0.002	0.01	Bal.
10-times-sintered powder			0.17	0.15	0.008	0.0013	0.009	Bal.
10-times-sintered CP Ti G 2 rod			0.17	0.16	0.017	0.0014	0.008	Bal.
TILOP CP Ti G 2 virgin powder			0.015	0.11	<0.005	0.0037	0.005	Bal.
10-times-sintered CP Ti powder			0.015	0.12	0.006	0.0035	0.005	Bal.
Once-sintered CP Ti G 2 rod			0.02	0.12	0.009	0.0032	0.002	Bal.
10-times-sintered CP Ti G 2 rod			0.02	0.12	0.007	0.0037	0.004	Bal.
Dental-cast CP Ti G 2 rod			0.103	0.17	0.007	0.0022	0.007	Bal.
Ti-6Al-4V powder	6.05	3.89	0.21	0.11	0.003	0.002	0.006	Bal.
Laser-sintered Ti-6Al-4V rod	5.93	3.91	0.20	0.14	0.022	0.002	0.007	Bal.

2.2. *Evaluation of Physical Properties*

The liquidus temperature of the laser-sintered CP Ti was measured by differential thermal analysis (DTA, TG-DTA 2200SA, Bruker Corp., Kanagawa, Japan) [14]. Test specimens of 3 mm diameter and 1.5 mm height were cut from the laser-sintered CP Ti G 2. Heat flows in DTA were measured at a heating rate of 10 °C/min in Ar at a flow rate of 200 mL/min. The densities (ρ) of powder and laser-sintered CP Ti G 2 were measured using an Ultrapycnometer 1000 M-UPYC (Quantachrome Instruments, Kanagawa, Japan) by gas pycnometry in accordance with JIS R1620 [23]. The Vickers hardness (Hv) of each laser-sintered CP Ti G 2 rod at room temperature was measured with a Vickers hardness tester (FV-310, Future-Tech Corp., Kanagawa, Japan) at three to five points at a load of 10 kg.

2.3. *Microstructural Observation*

The CP Ti G 2 annealed after laser sintering and laser-sintered (as-built) Ti-6Al-4V alloy were embedded in resin and polished to a mirrorlike finish with 200–4200 grit waterproof emery paper and an oxide polishing (OP-S) suspension. Then, each specimen was etched with nitric acid solution containing 3 vol% hydrogen fluoride. The microstructures of the CP Ti G 2 annealed at 700 °C for 2 h after laser sintering and laser-sintered (as-built) Ti-6Al-4V alloy were analyzed by optical microscopy (Nikon ECLIPSE LV150, Tokyo, Japan) and transmission electron spectroscopy (TEM, Hitachi HF-2000, Tokyo, Japan; acceleration voltage, 200 kV) with energy dispersive X-ray spectroscopy (EDS 2008 ver. 1.2 RevE, IXRF Systems, Tokyo, Japan). After etching, the surfaces of the annealed CP Ti G 2 and as-built Ti-6Al-4V alloy were observed by optical microscopy at magnifications of 50× and 400×. TEM was performed using disc-shaped specimens of 3 mm diameter, which were prepared by electrolytic polishing with 5 vol% perchloric acid +60 vol% methanol +35 vol% butanol solution under conditions of 30 V and 75 mA at −30 °C. After electrolytic polishing, the transverse cross-sectional structure was observed by TEM at magnifications of 15,000× and 60,000×. The fracture surfaces after the tensile and fatigue tests were observed by SEM.

2.4. *Static Immersion Test*

The specimens (n = 2), each with dimensions of 15 mm × 32 mm × 1 mm, were laser-sintered (as-built) and dental-cast CP Ti G 2 plates. Immersion tests were conducted at 37 ± 1 °C in an incubator using 0.1 mol/L lactic acid +0.1 mol/L NaCl solution (pH = 2.3) [1] in accordance with ISO 10271 [24] and JIS T 6115 [25]. The concentration of Ti released into the solution over 7 d was determined (ng/mL) by inductively coupled plasma mass spectrometry (ICP-MS, NexION 300D, PerkinElmer, Kanagawa, Japan; isotopic mass number of Ti, 48). An internal standard solution of Y (isotopic mass number, 89) was used for correction of the Ti concentration. The mean amount of Ti released ($\mu g/cm^2$/week) and the standard deviation were calculated for two specimens.

2.5. Room-Temperature Tensile Tests

Uniform rod specimens (rod diameter, 3 mm; gauge length, 15 mm) were cut from cylindrical specimens with a diameter of 9 mm and a height of 50 mm [1,26,27]. Tensile test specimens for dental-cast CP Ti G 2 were also cut from cylindrical specimens without defects as determined by X-ray inspection. The tensile test specimens were pulled with an Instron 5567 testing machine at a crosshead speed of 0.5% of the gauge length (GL)/min until the proof stress reached 0.2%. The crosshead speed was then changed to 3 mm/min and maintained at this speed until the specimen fractured. The 0.2% proof stress ($\sigma_{0.2\%PS}$), σ_{UTS}, total elongation (TE) at breaking, reduction in area (RA), and elastic modulus (E) were measured in tensile tests. The mean and standard deviation were calculated from the results of at least four specimens.

2.6. Fatigue Tests

Miniature hourglass-shaped rod specimens (3 mm minimum diameter and 50 mm total length) cut from cylindrical specimens were used for fatigue tests [1,28]. The fatigue tests were carried out with a sine wave at a stress ratio R(minimum cyclic stress (σ_{min})/(maximum cyclic stress (σ_{max})) of 0.1 and a frequency of 15 Hz in air. To obtain profiles of the relationship between σ_{max} and the number of cycles to failure N (S–N curves), the specimens were subjected to cycling at various constant maximum cyclic loads up to N = 10^7 cycles, at which the specimens remained intact. The fatigue strength at 10^7 cycles (fatigue limit, σ_{FS}) was measured from the S–N curves.

3. Results and Discussion

3.1. Chemical Compositions and Physical Properties

Table 1 shows the chemical compositions of laser-sintered (as-built) CP Ti G 2 and Ti-6Al-4V alloy rods with virgin powders (hereafter, once-sintered CP Ti G 2 rod), and the compositions after laser sintering 10 times (10-times-sintered CP Ti G 2 rod) with the same CP Ti G 2 powders without the virgin powder added. The changes in the chemical composition of the 10-times-sintered CP Ti G 2 rod were negligible. The results shown in Table 1 were in good agreement with the FlexLine EOS material data sheet and the Ti-6Al-4V material mill test certificate.

Figure 3 shows the oxygen (O) concentration in laser-sintered EOS CP Ti G 2 rods, laser-sintered TILOP CP Ti G 2 rods, and TILOP CP Ti G 2 powders as a function of the number of times of repeated laser sintering. The bars in Figure 3 indicate the standard deviation. In Figure 3, the results for the Ti-6Al-4V alloy were taken from the literature [6]. The increase in the O concentration of the laser-sintered CP Ti G 2 rods was found to be negligible. The O concentration in the laser-sintered Ti-6Al-4V alloy slightly increased from 0.11% in the virgin powder to 0.14% in the once-sintered alloy. On the other hand, in a previous report, the O concentration of the laser-sintered Ti-6Al-4V alloys was increased to up to 0.21% by laser sintering [6]. In particular, almost no increase in O concentration was observed after sintering 10 times. Thus, it was found that CP Ti powder can be recycled up to 10 times in the laser sintering of CP Ti. These tendencies were similar to those obtained with laser-sintered Co–Cr–Mo alloys [1].

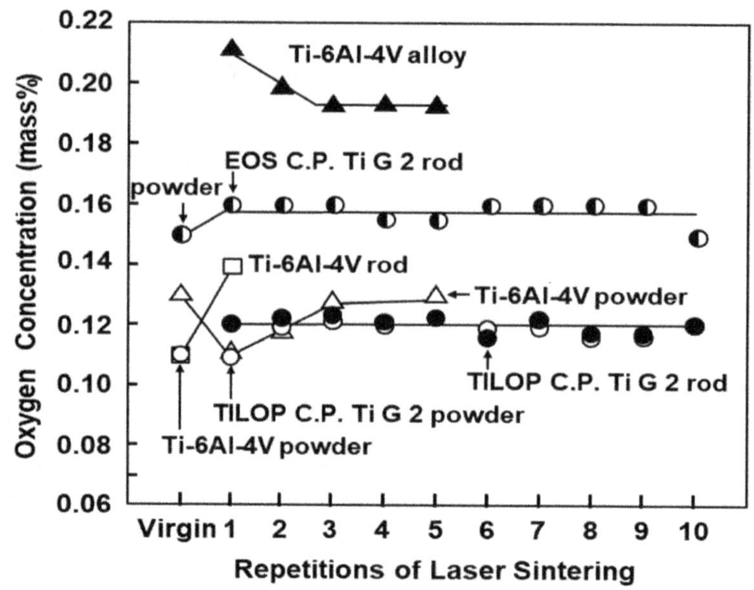

Figure 3. Effect of repeated laser sintering on oxygen concentration in Ti powders and laser-sintered Ti materials.

The densities of EOS virgin powder and once-sintered and 10-times-sintered (as-built) CP Ti G 2 rods were 4.49, 4.50, and 4.50 g/cm^3, respectively. The densities of TILOP virgin CP Ti G 2 powder and 10-times-sintered CP Ti G 2 rod were the same. These values are also consistent with the value (4.50 g/cm^3) shown in the FlexLine EOS material data sheet. Moreover, these densities of laser-sintered CP Ti G 2 were close to that (4.5 g/cm^3) of the wrought CP Ti G 2 ([29], p. 126). These values are much lower than the densities (8.4–8.8 g/cm^3) of the laser-sintered Co–Cr–Mo alloys [1].

The liquidus temperatures of once-sintered and 10-times-sintered TILOP CP Ti G 2 rods measured by DTA were 1659 and 1662 °C, respectively. These liquidus temperatures were close to those (1663 ± 1 °C) of wrought CP Ti G 2 reported in the literature [14]. The liquidus temperature of CP Ti G 2 was much higher than those (1458–1463 °C) of laser-sintered Co–Cr–Mo alloys [1].

The amounts of Ti ions released from the once-sintered TILOP and dental-cast CP Ti G 2 plates were 1.90 ± 0.10 and 1.10 ± 0.05 μg/cm^2/week, respectively. These values were close to the amount (1.2 μg/cm^2/week) of Ti ions released from wrought Ti-6Al-4V alloy at pH = 2.3 reported in the literature [30].

The Hv values (n = 5) of transverse sections of the 10-times-sintered 90° EOS and once-sintered 90° TILOP CP Ti G 2 rods, and dental-cast CP Ti G 2 were 187 ± 4, 207 ± 6, and 169 ± 6, respectively. These values were close to the Hv (approximately 200–210) of dental-cast CP Ti G 2 in the literature [8,12].

3.2. Microstructure of Laser-Sintered Ti Materials

Figure 4 shows optical microscopy images of transverse (T) and longitudinal (L) sections of annealed CP Ti G 2 rods after laser sintering (90° and 0° directions). Similar microstructures were observed in the transverse and longitudinal sections of 0°- and 45°-direction-built specimens. As clearly shown in Figure 4e, the structure of CP Ti G 2 annealed at 700 °C for 2 h after laser sintering was similar to that of CP Ti G 2 annealed under the same conditions after hot forging. On the other hand, as shown in Figure 4f, the center part of the dental-cast CP Ti G 2 rod had an α phase with an hcp crystal structure [8]. Figure 5 shows TEM images of transverse sections of annealed CP Ti G 2 after 90°-direction-built laser sintering. The bcc structure (lattice parameters a = b = c = 0.331 nm) precipitated in the grain boundaries of the hcp structure (a = b = 0.295, c = 0.468 nm) matrix. The values of these lattice parameters were consistent with those in a handbook of Ti material properties ([29], p. 125).

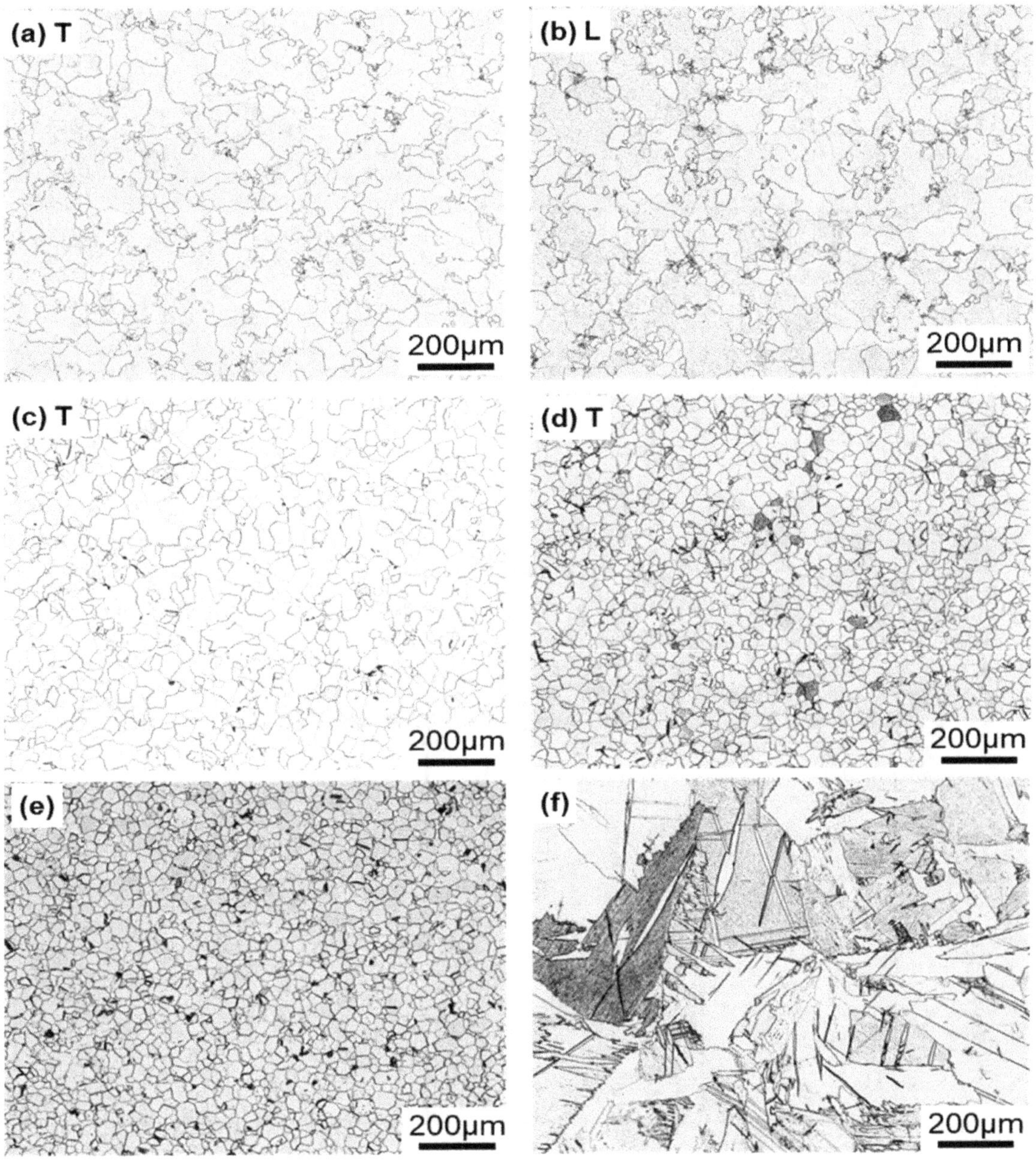

Figure 4. Optical microscopy images of (**a**,**b**) 10-times-laser-sintered EOS CP Ti G 2 and (**c**,**d**) once-sintered TILOP CP Ti G 2 built in (**a**–**c**) 90° and (**d**) 0° directions; (**a**,**c**,**d**) transverse (T) sections to the building direction and (**b**) longitudinal (L) section perpendicular to the building direction; (**e**,**f**) optical microscopy images of wrought and dental-cast (center part) CP Ti G 2 rods, respectively.

For comparison, optical microscopy and SEM images of laser-sintered Ti-6Al-4V alloy are shown in Figure 6a–d. The laser-sintered Ti-6Al-4V alloy had an acicular structure. Figure 6e,f show TEM images of transverse sections of 90°-direction-built laser-sintered Ti-6Al-4V alloy. TEM images of the laser-sintered (as-built) Ti-6Al-4V alloy show that it consisted of a fine martensitic (α') needle-like microstructure (hcp, a = b = 0.295, c = 0.468 nm) formed owing to rapid solidification [31–38].

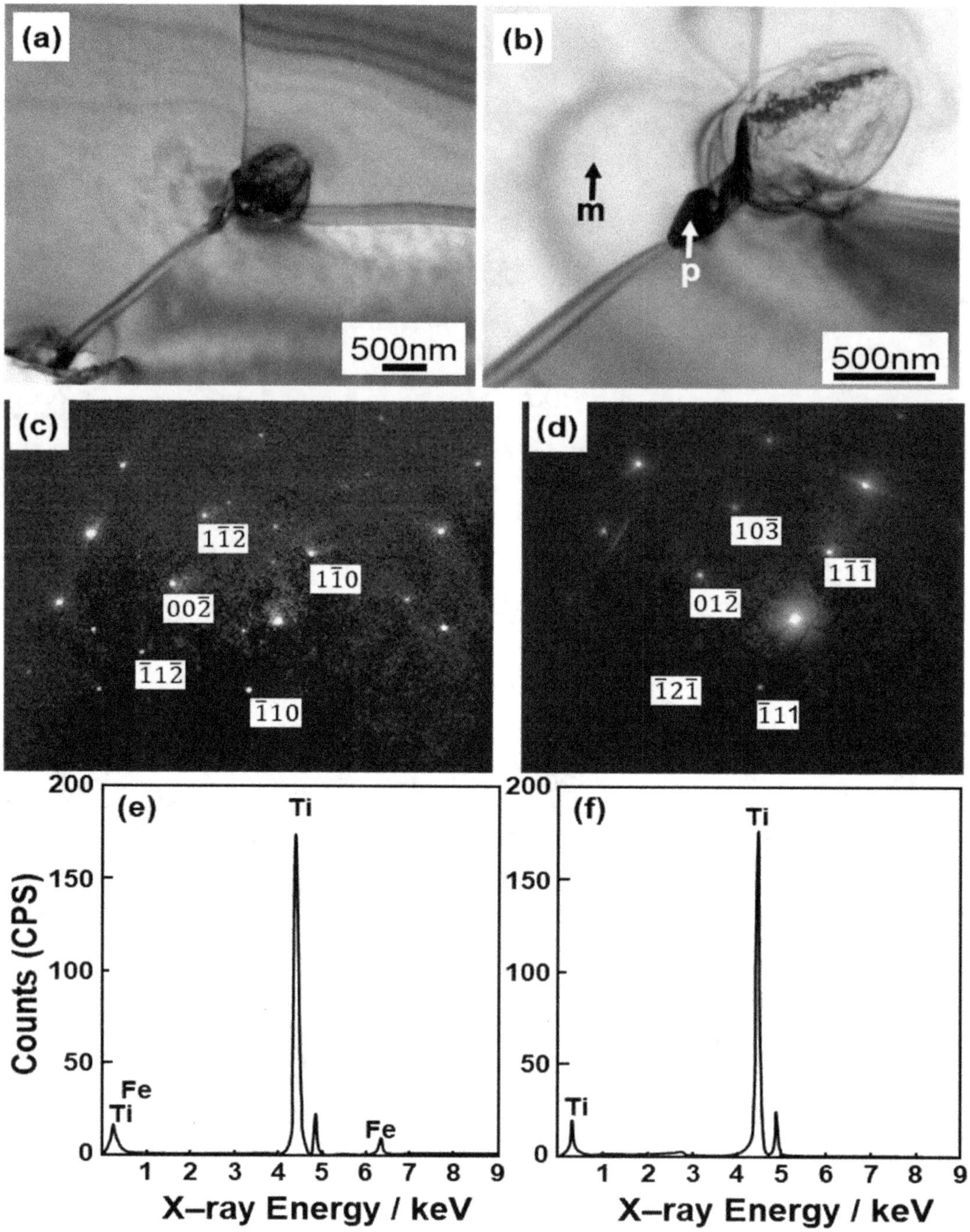

Figure 5. TEM images of transverse sections of (**a**,**b**) once-sintered TILOP CP Ti G 2 built in 90° direction; (**c**,**d**) electron beam diffraction patterns obtained at the location indicated by p (precipitation) and m (matrix) in (**b**), respectively; (**e**,**f**) EDS patterns of precipitate indicated by p and m in (**b**).

Figure 7 shows optical microscopy and SEM images of the Ti-6Al-4V alloy annealed at 840, 900, and 920 °C for 2 h after laser sintering of the alloy built in the 90° direction. In X-ray diffraction, most of the α-phase (hcp) contained a very small amount of the β-phase (bcc). Similar microstructures were observed in the optical images of specimens annealed at 860, 880, 940, 960, and 980 °C. The α-phase tended to become coarse with increasing annealing temperature. The annealed alloy retained its needle-like structure and did not change to a two-phase structure of α (hcp)–β (bcc), in contrast to the wrought Ti-6Al-4 V alloy [13,39]. Hv (n = 5) of each transverse section in the heat treatment range decreased from 342 to 316 and tended to decrease slowly with increasing annealing temperature.

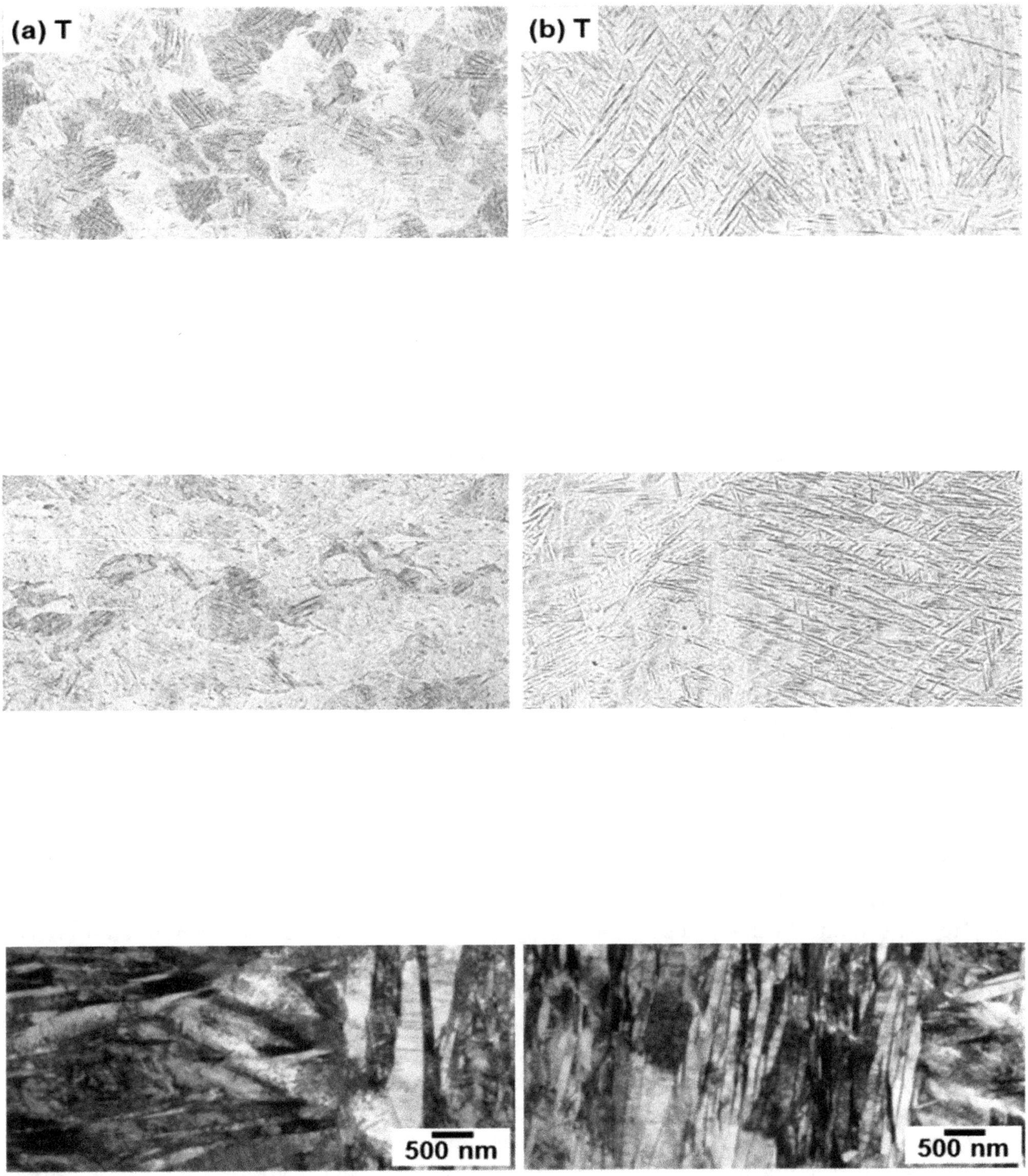

Figure 6. Optical microscopy images of once-sintered Ti-6Al-4V alloys built in 90° direction; (**a**,**b**) transverse (T) sections to the building direction and (**c**,**d**) longitudinal (L) sections perpendicular to the building direction; (**e**,**f**) TEM images of transverse section of once-sintered Ti-6Al-4V alloys built in 90° direction.

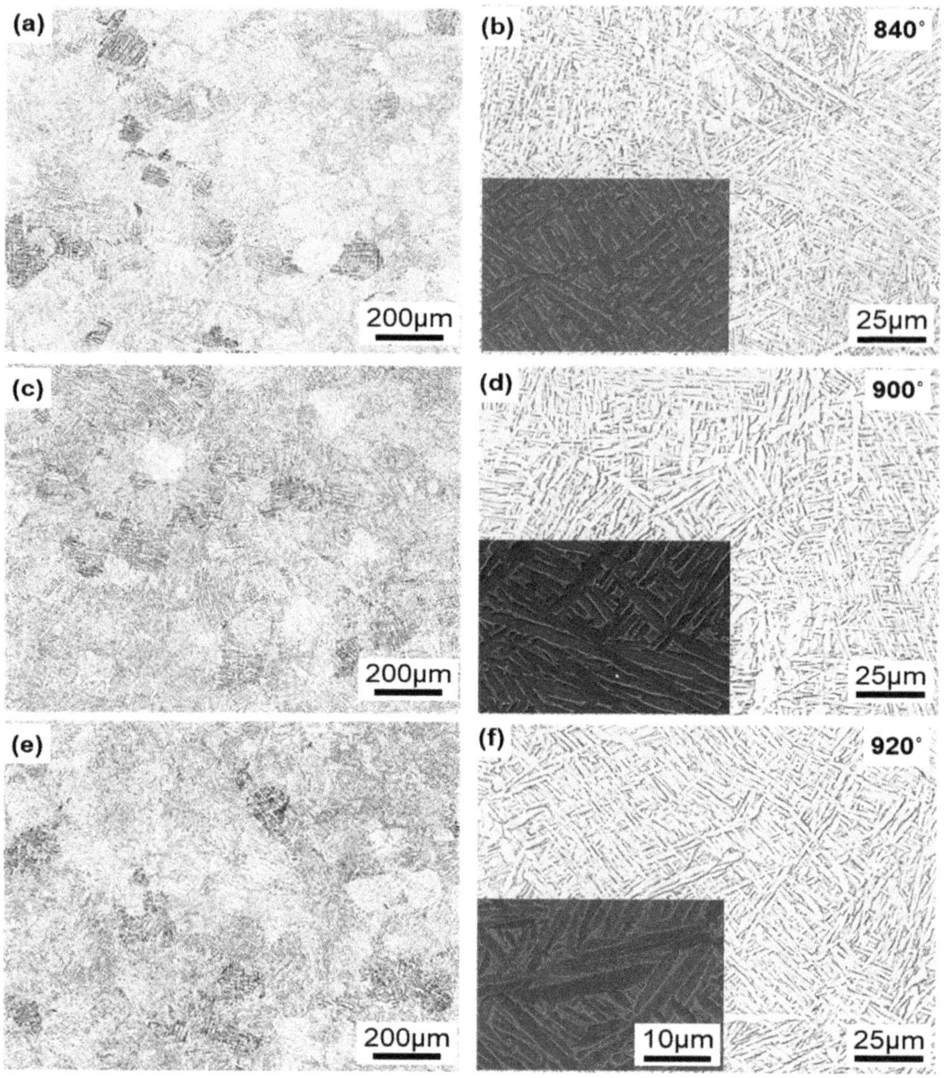

Figure 7. Optical microscopy and SEM images of Ti-6Al-4V alloy annealed at (**a**,**b**) 840, (**c**,**d**) 900, and (**e**,**f**) 920 °C for 2 h after laser sintering.

3.3. Mechanical Properties of Laser-Sintered Ti Materials

Figure 8 shows the mechanical properties ($\sigma_{0.2\%PS}$, σ_{UTS}, TE, and RA) of laser-sintered EOS CP Ti G 2 rods as a function of number of the repetitions of laser sintering. Hardly any effect of the number of repetitions on $\sigma_{0.2\%PS}$, σ_{UTS}, TE, and RA was observed up to 10 repetitions.

Table 2 summarizes the tensile properties (mean ± standard deviation) of the CP Ti G 2 annealed after laser sintering, the laser-sintered (as-built) Ti-6Al-4V alloy, and the dental-cast CP Ti G 2. The tensile properties of annealed (wrought) CP Ti G 2 and Ti-6Al-4V alloy after hot forging shown in Table 2 are taken from the literature [39]. The strengths of the 10-times-sintered CP Ti were similar to those of the once-sintered CP Ti. In particular, it was found that the tensile strengths of the annealed CP Ti G 2 after laser sintering were close to those of the annealed (wrought) CP Ti G 2 after hot forging. Table 2 also shows the tensile properties of wrought CP Ti G 2 specified in ISO 5832-3 [4]. The mechanical properties of the CP Ti G 2 annealed after laser sintering obtained in this study satisfied these standard values. However, $\sigma_{0.2\%PS} \geq 500$ MPa specified in the dental standard ISO 22674 was not satisfied [26]. These characteristics of the laser-sintered CP Ti G 4 materials (O ≤ 0.4%) with CP Ti G 4 powder were expected because the same annealed microstructure as the wrought CP Ti G 4 material was obtained. The elastic moduli of the laser-sintered and dental-cast CP Ti G 2 rods were 113 ± 2 and 115 ± 4 GPa, respectively. These values were lower than the value in ISO 22674 (≥150 GPa) [26].

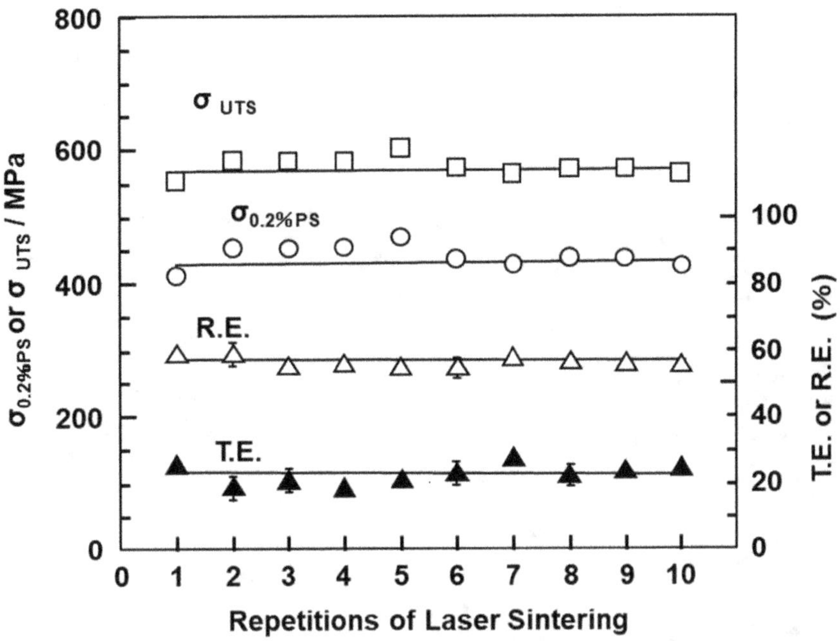

Figure 8. Effects of repeated laser sintering on mechanical properties ($\sigma_{0.2\%\ PS}$, $\sigma_{\ UTS}$, TE, and RA) of laser-sintered EOS CP Ti G 2 rods.

Table 2. Tensile properties ($\sigma_{0.2\%PS}$, σ_{UTS}, TE, and RA), fatigue strength (σ_{FS}), and fatigue ratio (σ_{FS}/σ_{UTS}) of CP Ti G 2 and Ti-6Al-4V alloys manufactured under various conditions.

Specimen	$\sigma_{0.2\%PS}$ /MPa	σ_{UTS} /MPa	TE (%)	RA (%)	σ_{FS} /MPa	σ_{FS} /σ_{UTS}
EOS CP Ti G 2						
Once-sintered 90°	412 ± 2	553 ± 3	26 ± 1	59 ± 1	320	0.58
10-times-sintered 0°	437 ± 2	576 ± 1	28 ± 2	55 ± 1	365	0.63
10-times-sintered 90°	426 ± 1	565 ± 1	25 ± 1	56 ± 1	320	0.57
TILOP CP Ti G 2						
Once-sintered 90°	445 ± 2	578 ± 3	27 ± 5	36 ± 10	330	0.57
Once-sintered 0°	432 ± 6	576 ± 5	26 ± 3	50 ± 1	380	0.66
Once-sintered 45°	419 ± 4	557 ± 3	22 ± 5	47 ± 6	290	0.52
10-times-sintered 90°	371 ± 4	481 ± 6	22 ± 8	41 ± 14	340	0.71
Dental-cast CP Ti G 2	351 ± 2.2	466 ± 3	30 ± 6	68 ± 5	290	0.62
Wrought CP Ti G 2	276 ± 6	410 ± 4	40 ± 2	60 ± 6	280	0.68
Laser-sintered Ti-6Al-4V	1171 ± 3	1305 ± 2	13 ± 1	31 ± 3	600	0.46
Wrought Ti-6Al-4V	849 ± 1	934 ± 1	16 ± 1	42 ± 3	680	0.73
ISO 5832-4	≥275	≥345	≥20			

Considering the dental application of high-strength Ti alloy, the mechanical properties of laser-sintered Ti-6Al-4V alloy are compared in Table 2. The tensile properties of the laser-sintered Ti-6Al-4V alloy were higher than those of the dental-cast Ti alloys [8,10]. The mechanical strength of laser-sintered Ti-6Al-4V alloy was also higher than that of wrought Ti-6Al-4V alloy [39]. On the other hand, the ductility of laser-sintered Ti-6Al-4V alloy was close to that of wrought Ti-6Al-4V alloy. The tensile properties of laser-sintered Ti-6Al-4V alloy fully satisfied the tensile properties ($\sigma_{0.2\%PS} \geq 780$, $\sigma_{UTS} \geq 860$ MPa, TE ≥ 10%) specified in ISO 5832-3 [5]. The tensile properties obtained in this study were also similar to those reported in the literature [32–37]. The tensile strength of Ti-6Al-4V alloy annealed after laser sintering tended to be lower than that of the as-built Ti-6Al-4V alloy [36,38]. To increase the ductility of alloys, it is effective to improve the morphology of the needle-like microstructure by heat treatment [33–35].

The Ti-6Al-4V alloy has much lower fracture toughness (Charpy V-notch impact toughness) than CP Ti G 2 ([29], p. 238). The fracture toughness of laser-sintered Ti-6Al-4V alloy should be evaluated in the future.

Figure 9 shows SEM images of the fracture surfaces of laser-sintered CP Ti G 2 after the tensile test. Magnified images of the rectangular areas in Figure 9a,b are shown in Figure 9b,c, respectively. Dimples were observed on the fracture surfaces, as shown in Figure 9c. Similar fracture surfaces were observed on all the other laser-sintered CP Ti G 2 specimens.

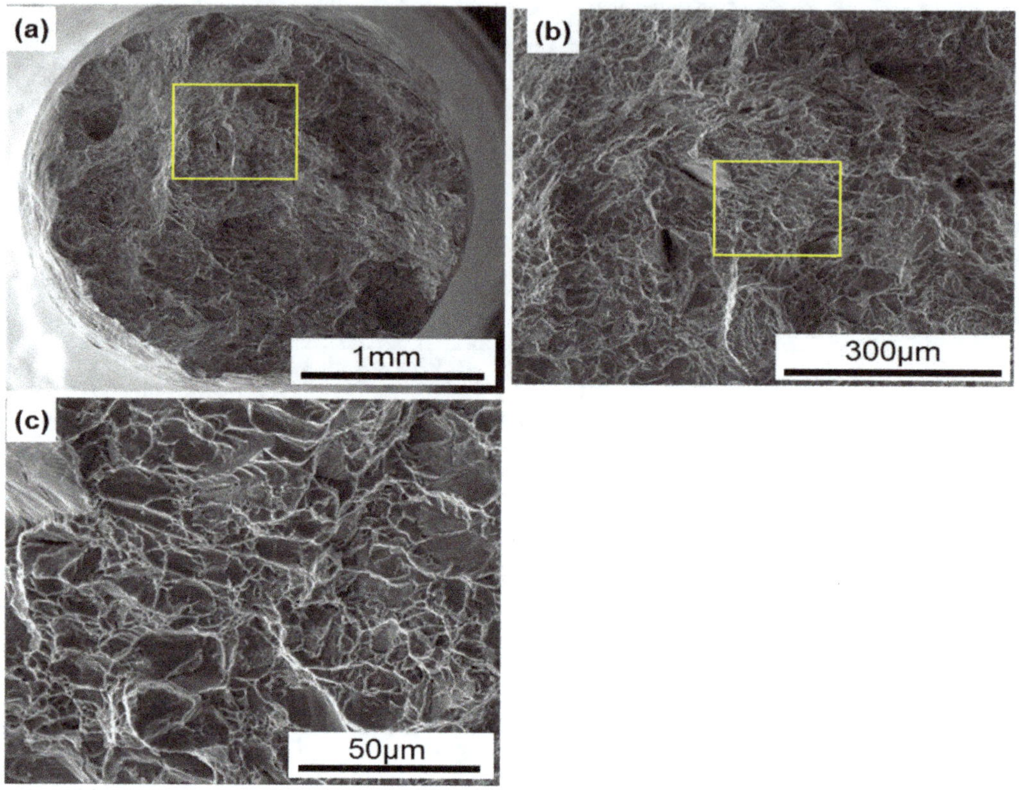

Figure 9. SEM images of fracture surfaces of the tensile-tested TILOP CP Ti G 2 (10-times-sintered); (**b**) magnification of rectangular area in (**a**), and (**c**) magnification of rectangular area in (**b**).

3.4. Fatigue Strengths of Laser-Sintered Ti Materials

Figure 10a,b shows S–N curves of annealed CP Ti G 2 rods ((a) EOS and (b) TIROP powders) after laser sintering and dental-cast CP T G 2 (shown in Figure 10a). Figure 10b also shows S–N curves of CP Ti G 2 annealed after hot forging taken from the literature for comparison [39]. The fatigue strengths of the 90°-, 45°-, and 0°-direction-built CP Ti G 2 rods were ~330, ~290, and ~380 MPa, respectively. The effects of the laser sintering direction on σ_{FS} of CP Ti G 2 were considered to be small because the anisotropy factor of the fatigue strength was 0.87 ((fatigue strength in 90° direction)/(fatigue strength in 0° direction)). This value was similar to those obtained for the laser-sintered Co–Cr–Mo alloy (0.83–1.0) [1] and the anisotropy of $\sigma_{0.2\%PS}$ caused by forging of Ti-15Zr-4Nb-4Ta alloys (0.83–0.94) [40]. Thus, it was considered that the effect of the laser sintering direction is negligible for CP Ti G 2. The fatigue strength of the 90°-direction-built 10-times-sintered CP Ti G 2 was ~340 MPa.

Figure 11 shows S–N curves of laser-sintered (as-built) Ti-6Al-4V alloy and wrought Ti-6Al-4V alloy annealed at 700 °C for 2 h after hot forging; the curve for wrought Ti-6Al-4V alloy is taken from the literature for comparison [39]. The fatigue strength of the 90°-direction-built Ti-6Al-4V alloy was ~600 MPa, which is close to that of wrought Ti-6Al-4V alloy. The improvements in the fatigue strength and durability of dental prostheses (such as partial dentures and clasps) are effective in improving the needle-like structure and reducing the thermal stress caused by laser sintering. We would like to investigate in detail the other orthopedic applications of laser-sintered Ti-6Al-4V alloy in future studies.

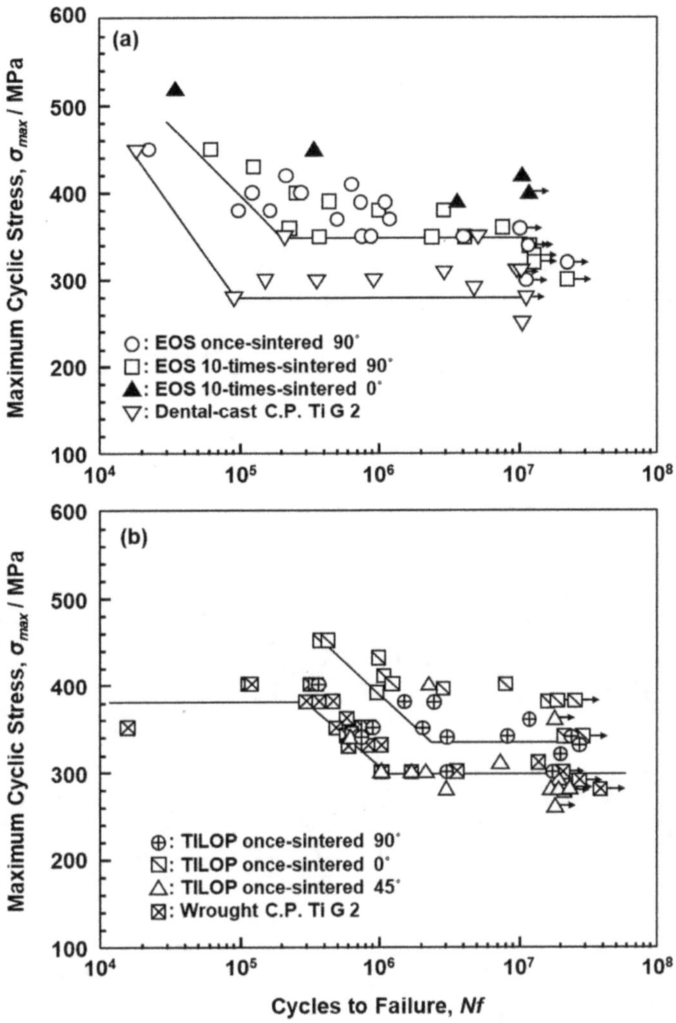

Figure 10. S–N curves of laser-sintered (**a**) EOS (once- and 10-times-sintered) and (**b**) TILOP (once-sintered) CP Ti G 2 rods; dental-cast CP Ti G 2 in (**a**) and wrought CP Ti G 2 in (**b**).

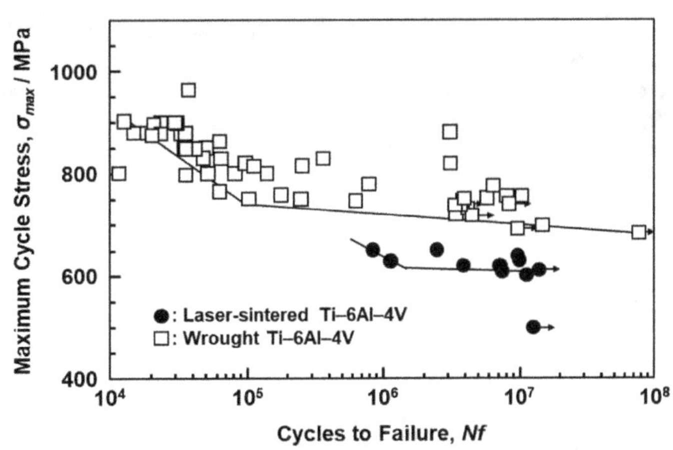

Figure 11. S–N curves of once-sintered Ti-6Al-4V alloy built in 90° direction and wrought Ti-6Al-4V alloy.

Figure 12 shows SEM images of the surface of 0°-direction-built CP Ti G 2. A fatigue crack developed with a fatigue fracture from the periphery of the specimen, and river-like patterns and striations were observed, as shown in Figure 12e,f [38].

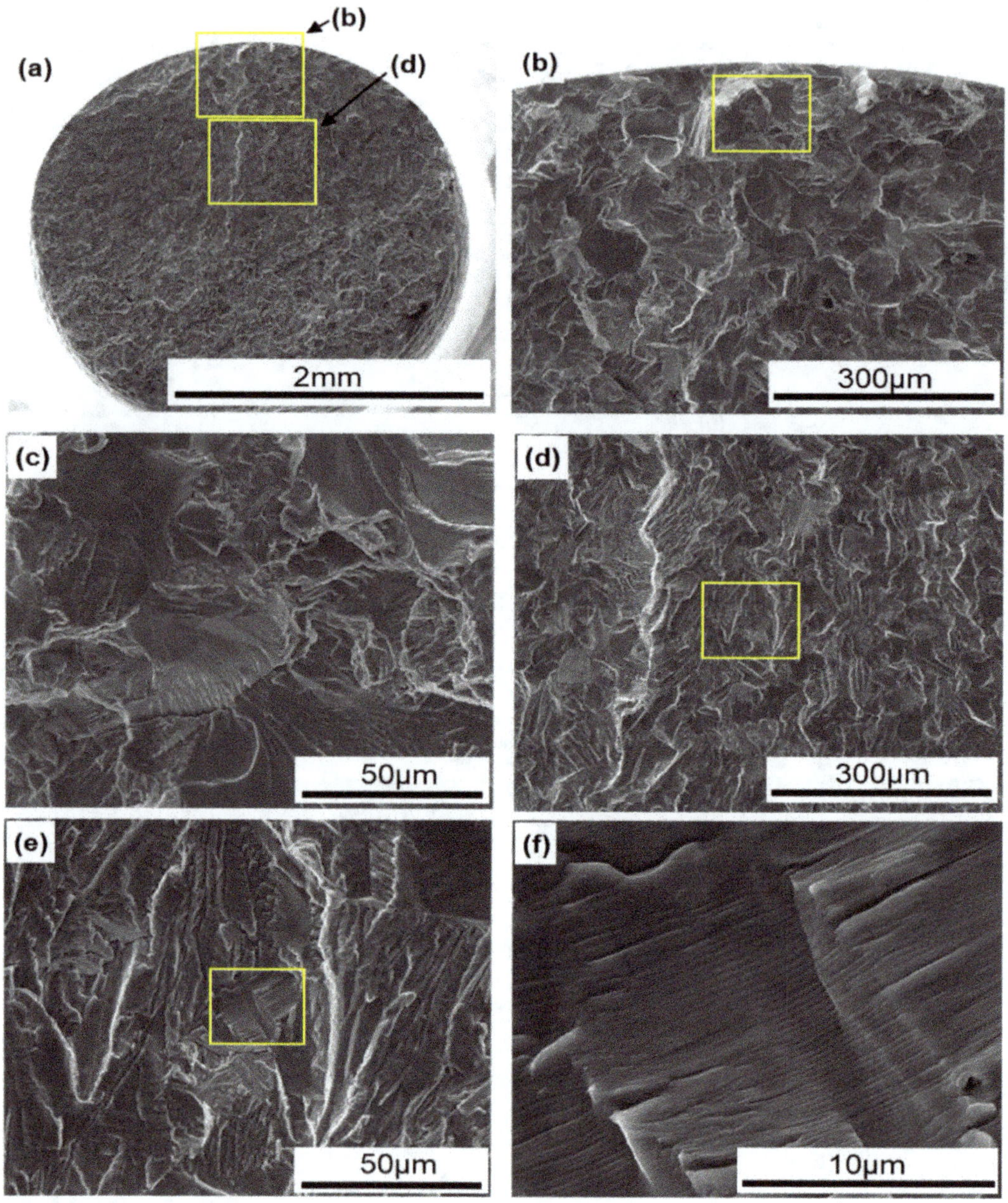

Figure 12. SEM images of fracture surfaces of fatigue-tested TILOP CP Ti G 2 (once-sintered 0°); (**b**) magnification of upper rectangular area in (**a**), (**c**) magnification of rectangular area in (**b**), (**d**) magnification of lower rectangular area in (**a**), (**e**) magnification of rectangular area in (**d**), and (**f**) magnification of rectangular area in (**e**).

It was found that the strength and ductility of CP Ti G 2 annealed at 700 °C for 2 h after laser sintering were excellent owing to the dispersion of fine hcp and bcc particles. AM of CP Ti materials may be a promising new manufacturing technology to replace dental Ti casting as shown in Figure 13. The fatigue strength of the laser-sintered Ti-6Al-4V alloy was ~600 MPa, which is close to that of wrought Ti-6Al-4V alloy. Therefore, laser-sintered Ti-6Al-4V alloy can also be applied in dental prostheses such as high-durability partial dentures and clasps.

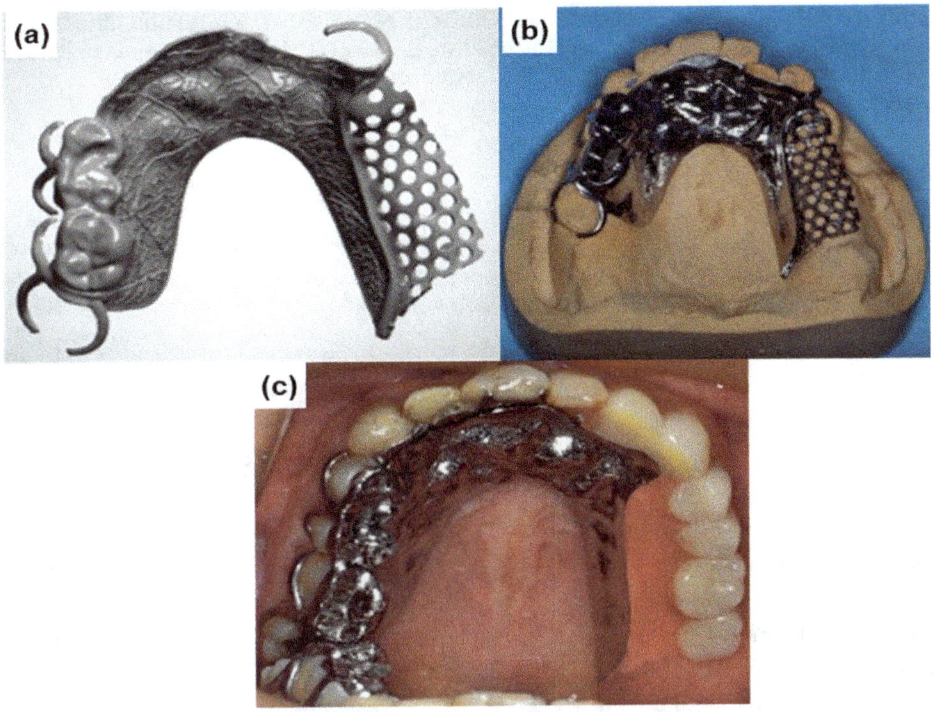

Figure 13. Partial dentures manufactured by laser sintering with CP Ti G 2 powder. (**a**) laser-sintered metal frame; (**b**) polished metal frame; (**c**) partial denture.

4. Conclusions

We evaluated the chemical composition, physical properties, microstructure, immersion property, tensile property, and fatigue strength of CP Ti G 2 annealed at 700 °C for 2 h after laser sintering and laser-sintered (as-built) Ti-6Al-4V alloy for dental applications.

The changes in the chemical composition and mechanical properties of CP Ti G 2 after laser sintering up to 10 times were negligible. The rates of Ti ion release were low, with CP Ti and dental-cast CP Ti showing release rates of 1.90 ± 0.05 and 1.10 ± 0.05 μg/cm^2/week, respectively.

The fatigue strengths of the 90°-, 45°-, and 0°-direction-built CP Ti were ~330, ~290, and 380 MPa, respectively. The fatigue strength of the 90°-direction-built alloys after laser sintering 10 times was also ~340 MPa. The ratios of the fatigue strength at 10^7 cycles to the ultimate tensile strength (σ_{FS}/σ_{UTS}) were 0.5–0.7.

Precipitates identified to be bcc particles (a = b = c = 0.322 nm) were found in the grain boundaries of the hcp matrix. The structure of the annealed CP Ti G 2 after laser sintering was similar to that of the annealed CP Ti G 2 after hot forging.

It was found that the strength and ductility of annealed CP Ti G 2 after laser sintering are excellent owing to the dispersion of the fine bcc particles. AM of CP Ti materials (G 2 and G 4) may be a promising new manufacturing technology to replace dental Ti casting. In particular, it was clarified that laser sintering with CP Ti G 4 powder (O ≤ 0.4 mass %) is useful for dental prostheses.

The fatigue strength of the laser-sintered Ti-6Al-4V alloy was ~600 MPa, which is close to that of wrought Ti-6Al-4V alloy. Therefore, laser-sintered Ti-6Al-4V alloy can also be applied in dental prostheses such as high-durability partial dentures and clasps, and orthopedic implants such as artificial hip-joint stems.

Author Contributions: Mechanical tests, microstructural analysis, chemical and physical analysis, data curation, conceptualization, writing and editing of paper, Y.O.; selection of test items, regulatory approval for dental prostheses, A.I. All authors have read and agreed to the published version of the manuscript.

Acknowledgments: TEM analysis was supported by Kazushi Nakamura, Materials Characterization Division, Nippon Steel Technology Co., Ltd. (Chiba, Japan). Laser sintering of CP Ti G 2 rods was conducted by EOS Japan (Osaka, Japan) or Osaka Titanium Technologies Co., Ltd. (Osaka, Japan). Dental-cast CP Ti G 2 rods were cast by Wada Precision Dental Laboratories (Osaka, Japan).

References

1. Okazaki, Y.; Ishino, A.; Higuchi, S. Chemical, physical, and mechanical properties and microstructures of laser-sintered Co–25Cr–5Mo–5W (SP2) and W-free Co–28Cr–6Mo alloys for dental application. *Materials* **2019**, *12*, 4039. [CrossRef] [PubMed]
2. Nakata, T.; Shimpo, H.; Ohkubo, C. Clasp fabrication using one-process molding by repeated laser sintering and high-speed milling. *J. Prosthodont. Res.* **2017**, *61*, 276–282. [CrossRef] [PubMed]
3. Takaichi, A.; Suyalatu; Nakamoto, T.; Joko, N.; Nomura, N.; Tsutumi, Y.; Migita, S.; Doi, H.; Kurosu, S.; Chiba, A.; et al. Microstructures and mechanical properties of Co–29Cr–6Mo alloy fabricated by selective laser melting process for dental applications. *J. Mech. Behav. Biomed. Mater.* **2013**, *21*, 67–76. [CrossRef] [PubMed]
4. *Implants for Surgery–Metallic Materials–Part 2: Unalloyed Titanium, ISO 5832–2*; International Organization for Standardization: Geneva, Switzerland, 2018.
5. *Implants for Surgery–Metallic Materials–Part 3: Wrought Titanium 6–Aluminum 4–Vanadium Alloy, ISO 5832–3*; International Organization for Standardization: Geneva, Switzerland, 2016.
6. O'Leary, R.; Setchi, R.; Prickett, P.; Hankins, G.; Jones, N. An investigation into the recycling of Ti–6Al–4V powder used within SLM to improve sustainability. In Proceedings of the 2nd International Conference on Sustainable Design and Manufacturing, Seville, Spain, 12–14 April 2015; pp. 377–388. Available online: http://orca.cf.ac.uk/id/eprint/81260 (accessed on 10 January 2020).
7. *Standard Specification for Additive Manufacturing Titanium–6 Aluminum–4 Vanadium with Powder Bed Fusion, ASTM F 2924*; American Society for Testing and Materials: West Conshohocken, PA, USA, 2014.
8. Lin, C.W.; Ju, C.P.; Lin, J.H.C. Comparison among mechanical properties of investment-cast C.P. Ti, Ti-6Al-7Nb and Ti-15Mo-1Bi alloys. *Mater. Trans.* **2004**, *45*, 3028–3032. [CrossRef]
9. Takahashi, M.; Kikuchi, M.; Takada, Y.; Okuno, O. Mechanical properties and microstructures of dental cast Ti-Ag and Ti-Cu alloys. *Dent. Mater. J.* **2002**, *21*, 270–280. [CrossRef] [PubMed]
10. Koizumi, H.; Ishii, T.; Okazaki, T.; Kaketani, M.; Matumura, H.; Yoneyama, T. Castability and mechanical properties of Ti-15Zr-5Zr-3Al alloy in dental casting. *J. Oral Sci.* **2018**, *60*, 285–292. [CrossRef] [PubMed]
11. Tamaki, Y.; Miyazaki, T. Problems on titanium castings for clinical use. *J. Jpn. Prosthodont. Soc.* **1998**, *42*, 528–539. [CrossRef]
12. Ida, K.; Togaya, T.; Tsutsumi, S.; Takeuchi, M. Effect of magnesia investments in the dental casting of pure titanium or titanium alloys. *Dent. Mater. J.* **1982**, *1*, 8–21. [CrossRef] [PubMed]
13. Collings, E.W.; Boyer, R.; Welsch, G.; Collings, E.W. (Eds.) *ASM Materials Properties Handbook: Classification of Titanium Alloys*; The Materials Information Society: Materials Park, OH, USA, 1994; p. 5.
14. Okazaki, Y. Development of low-cost manufacturing process and effects of adding small amounts of Ta, O, and N on the physical and mechanical properties of highly biocompatible Ti alloys. *Mater. Trans.* **2019**, *60*, 1769–1778. [CrossRef]
15. *Particle Size Analysis–Laser Diffraction Methods, ISO 13332*; International Organization for Standardization: Geneva, Switzerland, 2009.
16. *Titanium and Titanium Alloys–Determination of Hydrogen Content, JIS H 1619*; Japanese Standards Association: Tokyo, Japan, 2012.
17. *Methods for Determination of Nitrogen in Titanium and Titanium Alloys, JIS H 1612*; Japanese Standards Association: Tokyo, Japan, 1993.
18. *Methods for Determination of Oxygen in Titanium and Titanium Alloys, JIS H 1620*; Japanese Standards Association: Tokyo, Japan, 1995.
19. *Methods for Determination of Iron in Titanium and Titanium Alloys, JIS H 1614*; Japanese Standards Association: Tokyo, Japan, 1995.

20. *Methods for Determination of Carbon in Titanium and Titanium Alloys, JIS H 1617*; Japanese Standards Association: Tokyo, Japan, 1995.
21. *Titanium Alloys–Methods for Determination of Aluminium, JIS H 1622*; Japanese Standards Association: Tokyo, Japan, 1998.
22. *Titanium Alloys–Method for Determination of Vanadium, JIS H 1624*; Japanese Standards Association: Tokyo, Japan, 2005.
23. *Testing Methods for Particle Density of Fine Ceramic Powder, JIS R 1620*; Japanese Standards Association: Tokyo, Japan, 1995.
24. *Dentistry–Corrosion Test Methods for Metallic Materials, ISO 10271*; International Organization for Standardization: Geneva, Switzerland, 2011.
25. *Dental Casting Cobalt Chromium Alloys, JIS T 6115*; Japanese Standards Association: Tokyo, Japan, 2013.
26. *Dentistry–Metallic Materials for Fixed and Removable Restorations and Appliances, ISO 22674*; International Organization for Standardization: Geneva, Switzerland, 2016.
27. *Metallic Materials–Tensile Testing–Method of Test at Room Temperature, JIS Z 2241*; Japanese Standards Association: Tokyo, Japan, 2011.
28. *Test Method for Fatigue Properties of Metallic Biomaterials, JIS T 0309*; Japanese Standards Association: Tokyo, Japan, 2009.
29. Boyer, R.; Welsch, G.; Collings, E.W. (Eds.) *ASM Materials Properties Handbook: Titanium Data Sheets*; The Materials Information Society: Materials Park, OH, USA, 1994.
30. Okazaki, Y.; Nagata, H. Comparisons of immersion and electrochemical properties of highly biocompatible Ti–15Zr–4Nb–4Ta alloy and other implantable metals for orthopedic implants. *Sci. Technol. Adv. Mater.* **2012**, *13*, 064216. [CrossRef] [PubMed]
31. Simonell, M.; Tse, Y.Y.; Tuck, C. Microstructure of Ti–6Al–4V produced by selective laser melting. *J. Phys. Conf. Ser.* **2012**, *371*, 012084. [CrossRef]
32. Rafi, H.K.; Karthik, N.V.; Gong, H.; Starr, T.L.; Stucker, B.E. Microstructures and mechanical properties of Ti6Al4V parts fabricated by selective laser melting and electron beam melting. *J. Mater. Eng. Perform.* **2013**, *22*, 3872–3883. [CrossRef]
33. Haar, G.M.T.; Becker, T.H. Selective laser melting produced Ti–6Al–4V: Post-process heat treatment to achieve superior tensile properties. *Materials* **2018**, *11*, 146. [CrossRef] [PubMed]
34. Facchini, L.; Molinari, A.; öges, S.H.; Wissenbach, K. Ductility of a Ti–6Al–4V alloy produced by selective laser melting of prealloyed powders. *Rapid Prototyp. J.* **2010**, *16*, 450–459. [CrossRef]
35. Qiu, C.; Adkins, N.J.E.; Attallah, M.M. Microstructure and tensile properties of selectively laser-melted and HIPed laser-melted Ti–6Al–4V. *Mater. Sci. Eng. A* **2013**, *578*, 230–239. [CrossRef]
36. Vrancken, B.; Thijs, L.; Kruth, J.P.; Humbeeck, J.V. Heat treatment of Ti6Al4V produced by selective laser melting: Microstructure and mechanical properties. *J. Alloys Compd.* **2012**, *541*, 177–185. [CrossRef]
37. Gong, H.; Rafi, K.; Gu, H.; Ram, G.D.J.; Starr, T.; Stucker, B. Influence of defects on mechanical properties of Ti–6Al–4V components produced by selective laser melting and electron beam melting. *Mater. Des.* **2015**, *86*, 545–554. [CrossRef]
38. Leuders, S.; Thöne, M.; Riemer, A.; Niendorf, T.; Tröster, T.; Richard, H.A.; Maier, H.J. On the mechanical behaviour of titanium alloy TiAl6V4 manufactured by selective laser melting: Fatigue resistance and crack growth performance. *Int. J. Fatigue* **2013**, *48*, 300–307. [CrossRef]
39. Okazaki, Y.; Gotoh, E. Comparison of fatigue strengths of biocompatible Ti–15Zr–4Nb–4Ta alloy and other titanium materials. *Mater. Sci. Eng. C* **2011**, *33*, 325–333. [CrossRef]
40. Okazaki, Y. On the effects of hot forging and hot rolling on the microstructural development and mechanical response of a biocompatible Ti alloy. *Materials* **2012**, *5*, 1439–1461. [CrossRef]

8

Dental Resin Cements—The Influence of Water Sorption on Contraction Stress Changes and Hydroscopic Expansion

Grzegorz Sokolowski [1], Agata Szczesio [2], Kinga Bociong [2], Karolina Kaluzinska [2], Barbara Lapinska [3], Jerzy Sokolowski [3], Monika Domarecka [3] and Monika Lukomska-Szymanska [3,*]

1 Department of Prosthetic Dentistry, Medical University of Lodz, 251 Pomorska St., 92-213 Lodz, Poland; grzegorz.sokolowski@umed.lodz.pl

2 University Laboratory of Materials Research, Medical University of Lodz, 251 Pomorska St., 92-213 Lodz, Poland; agata.szczesio@umed.lodz.pl (A.S.); kinga.bociong@umed.lodz.pl (K.B.); karolina.kaluzinska@umed.lodz.pl (K.K.)

3 Department of General Dentistry, Medical University of Lodz, 251 Pomorska St., 92-213 Lodz, Poland; barbara.lapinska@umed.lodz.pl (B.L.); jerzy.sokolowski@umed.lodz.pl (J.S.); monika.domarecka@umed.lodz.pl (M.D.)

* Correspondence: monika.lukomska-szymanska@umed.lodz.pl

Abstract: Resin matrix dental materials undergo contraction and expansion changes due to polymerization and water absorption. Both phenomena deform resin-dentin bonding and influence the stress state in restored tooth structure in two opposite directions. The study tested three composite resin cements (Cement-It, NX3, Variolink Esthetic DC), three adhesive resin cements (Estecem, Multilink Automix, Panavia 2.0), and seven self-adhesive resin cements (Breeze, Calibra Universal, MaxCem Elite Chroma, Panavia SA Cement Plus, RelyX U200, SmartCem 2, and SpeedCEM Plus). The stress generated at the restoration-tooth interface during water immersion was evaluated. The shrinkage stress was measured immediately after curing and after 0.5 h, 24 h, 72 h, 96 h, 168 h, 240 h, 336 h, 504 h, 672 h, and 1344 h by means of photoelastic study. Water sorption and solubility were also studied. All tested materials during polymerization generated shrinkage stress ranging from 4.8 MPa up to 15.1 MPa. The decrease in shrinkage strain (not less than 57%) was observed after water storage (56 days). Self-adhesive cements, i.e., MaxCem Elite Chroma, SpeedCem Plus, Panavia SA Plus, and Breeze exhibited high values of water expansion stress (from 0 up to almost 7 MPa). Among other tested materials only composite resin cement Cement It and adhesive resin cement Panavia 2.0 showed water expansion stress (1.6 and 4.8, respectively). The changes in stress value (decrease in contraction stress or built up of hydroscopic expansion) in time were material-dependent.

Keywords: resin cements; shrinkage stress; water sorption; hydroscopic expansion; photoelastic investigation

---

1. Introduction

Resin composite cements have been widely used with ceramic, resin, or metal alloy-based prosthodontic restorations [1]. The cementation technique used in adhesive dentistry is one of the major factors, which exerts influence on the clinical success of indirect restorative procedures. Cement is used to bond tooth and restoration simultaneously creating a barrier against microbial leakage [2]. The universal cement that can be applied in all indirect restorative procedures has not been introduced into the market yet. Therefore, clinicians should understand the influence of applied material properties and preparation design on the clinical performance of the restoration [3].

The composition of resin composite cements is almost the same as of resin composites [4]. Resin cements mainly consist of various methacrylate resins and inorganic fillers which are often coated with organic silanes to provide adhesion between the filler and the matrix. These materials often include bonding agents to promote the adhesion between resin cement and tooth structure. Main monomers are, i.e., hydroxyethyl methacrylate (HEMA), 4-methacryloyloxyethy trimellitate anhydride (4-MET), carboxylic acid, and organophospate 10-methacryloxydecyl dihydrogen phosphate (10-MDP) (Figure 1). The acidic group bonds calcium ions in the tooth structure [5,6].

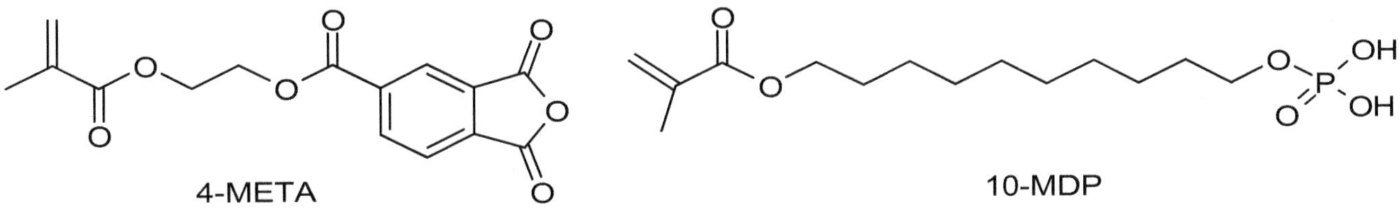

Figure 1. Monomers used as bonding agents in resin cements.

Resin composite cements are used in combination with adhesive systems. This procedure aims at creating micro-mechanical retention to both enamel and dentin. The material may also form a strong adhesion to an adequately-treated surface of the composite, ceramic, and metallic restorations [7]. Taking into account the surface preparation before the cementation process, resin cements can be divided into: (1) composite resin cement (used with total-etch adhesive systems); (2) adhesive resin cement (used with separate self-etching adhesive systems); and (3) self-adhesive resin cement (containing a self-adhesive system) [1].

The application of resin matrix-based cements is time-consuming and susceptible to manipulation errors [8]. The self-adhesive resin cements are proposed to simplify the restoration procedure. These materials bond dentin in one step without any surface conditioning or pre-treatment (priming) [9,10].

All currently available resin-based materials exhibit polymerization shrinkage. Moreover, resin cements are generally applied as a thin layer, particularly when used to lute posts, inlays, and crowns. In the aforementioned clinical cases, the cavity design has a high C-factor (high number of bonded surfaces and a low number of un-bonded surfaces) [11]. Additionally, low-viscosity composites exhibit a relatively high shrinkage amounting up to 6% (comparable to resin cements) [12,13]. These factors may generate sufficient stress resulting in debonding of the luting material, thereby increasing microleakage [14]. Nevertheless, there is little data on the stress generated by these materials. The sorption characteristic of resin-based dental cements has been extensively evaluated [15–17]. However, the analysis of the influence of water sorption on the change in contraction stress is inadequate. The purpose of this study was to evaluate the development of the stress state, i.e., the contraction stress generated during photopolymerization and hydroscopic expansion within different types of resin cements which undergo water ageing by means of photoelastic analysis.

2. Materials and Methods

The composition of investigated resin cements and bonding systems is presented in Tables 1 and 2.

Table 1. The composition of resin cements.

Material	Type	Composition	Curing Time (s)	Manufacturer
Cement-It	Composite resin cement	bis-GMA, UDMA, HDDMA, PEGDMA, barium-boro-silicate glass (65 wt %)	20	Jeneric Pentron (Wallingford, CT, USA)
NX3	Composite resin cement	TEGDMA, bis-GMA, fluoro-aluminosilicate glass (67.5 wt %/47 vol %), activators, stabilizers, radiopaque agent	20	Kerr (Orange, CA, USA)
Variolink Esthetic DC	Composite resin cement	UMDA and further methacrylate monomers, ytterbium trifluoride, spheroid mixed oxide (67 wt %/38 vol %), initiators, stabilizers and pigments	10	Ivoclar Vivadent (Ellwangen, Germany)
Estecem	Adhesive resin cement	bis-GMA, TEGDMA, bis-MPEPP, silica-zirconia filler (74 wt %), camphorquinone	20	Tokuyama Dental (Taitou, Japan)
Multilink Automix	Adhesive resin cement	dimethacrylate and HEMA, barium glass and silica filler, ytterbiumtrifluoride (68 wt %), catalysts, stabilizers, pigments	10	Ivoclar Vivadent (Ellwangen, Germany)
Panavia 2.0	Adhesive resin cement	10-MDP, BPEDMA, hydrophobic aliphatic metahrylates, hydrophilic aliphatic metahrylate, silanated silica filler, silanated barium glass filler, sodium fluoride (70.8 wt %)	20	Kuraray (Osaka, Japan)
Breeze	Self-adhesive resin cement	bis-GMA, UDMA, TEGDMA, HEMA, 4-MET, silane treated barium glass, silica, BiOCl, Ca-Al-F-silicate, curing system	20	Jeneric Pentron (Wallingford, CT, USA)
Calibra Universal	Self-adhesive resin cement	UDMA, trimethylolpropane trimethacrylate TMPTMA, bis-EMA—Bisphenol A ethoxylate dimethacrylate, TEGDMA, HEMA, 3-(acryloyloxy)-2-hydroxypropyl methacrylate, urethane modified bis-GMA, PENTA, silanated barium glass, fumed silica (48 vol %)	10	Dentsply Sirona (York, PA, USA)
MaxCem Elite Chroma	Self-adhesive resin cement	HEMA, GDM, UDMA, 1,1,3,3-tetramethylbutyl hydroperoxide TEGDMA, fluoroaluminosilicate glass, GPDM, barium glass filler, fumed silica (69 wt %)	10	Kerr (Orange, CA, USA)
Panavia SA Cement Plus	Self-adhesive resin cement	bis-GMA, TEGDMA, HEMA, 10-MDP, hydrophobic aromatic dimethacrylate, hydrophobic aliphatic dimethacrylate, sodium fluoride, silanated barium glass filler, silanated colloidal silica (70 wt %/40 vol %)	10	Kuraray (Osaka, Japan)
RelyX U200	Self-adhesive resin cement	methacrylate monomers containing phosphoric acid groups, methacrylate monomers, silanated fillers (70 wt %/43 vol %), initiator components, stabilizers, rheological additives, alkaline(basic) initiator components, stabilizers, pigments	20	3M ESPE (St. Paul, MN, USA)
SmartCem 2	Self-adhesive resin cement	UDMA, urethane modified bis-GMA, TEGDMA, PENTA, dimethacrylate resins, barium boron fluoroaluminosilicate glass amorphous silica (69 wt %/46 vol %)	10	Dentsply Sirona (York, PA, USA)
SpeedCEM Plus	Self-adhesive resin cement	UDMA, TEGDMA, PEGDMA, methacrylated phosphoric acid ester, 1,10-decandiol dimethacrylate, copolymers, dibenzoyl peroxide, ytterbium trifluoride, barium glass, silicon dioxide (75 wt %/45 vol %)	20	Ivoclar Vivadent (Ellwangen, Germany)

bis-GMA—bisphenol A glycol dimethacrylate, UDMA—urethane dimethacrylate , TEGDMA—triethylene glycol dimethacrylate, GDM—glycerol 1,3-dimethacrylate, GPDM—glycerol phosphate dimethacryalte, bis-MPEPP—bisphenol A polyethoxy methacrylate, HEMA—hydroxyethyl methacrylate, PEGDMA—polyethylene glycol dimethacrylate, NPGDMA—neopentyldimethacrylate, 10-MDP—10-methacryloxydecyl dihydrogen phosphate, BPEDMA—bisphenol-A-polyethoxy dimethacrylate, PENTA—dipentaerythritol penttacrylate monophosphate, HDDMA—1,6-hexanediol dimethacrylate, 4-MET—4-methacryloyloxyethy trimellitate anhydride, MAC-10—11-methacryloyloxy-1,1-undecanedicarboxylic acid, TMPTMA—trimethylolpropane trimethacrylate.

Table 2. The curing time of bonding systems.

Bonding system	Manufacturer	Curing Time (s)	Bonding System Dedicated to
Bond-1 C&B Primer/Adhesive	Jeneric Pentrton (Wallingford, CT, USA)	10	Cement It, Breeze
Clearfil SE bond	Kuraray (Osaka, Japan)	10	Panavia 2.0, Panavia SA Cement Plus
Easy Bond	3M ESPE (St. Paul, MN, USA)	10	RelyX U200
Estelink	Tokuyam Dental (Taitou, Japan)	10	Estecem
Monobond Plus	Ivoclar Vivadent (Ellwangen, Germany)	10	Variolink Esthetic DC, Multilink Automix, SpeedCEM Plus
OptiBond XRT	Kerr (Orange, CA, USA)	10	NX3, MaxCem Elite Chroma
Prime&Bond Elect Universal	Dentsply Sirona (York, PA, USA)	10	SmartCem 2, Calibra Universal

2.1. Absorbency Dynamic Study

Absorbency dynamic was determined by means of procedure as described by Bociong et al. [18]. The samples were prepared according to ISO 4049 [19]. Curing time was consistent with the manufacturer's instructions (Table 2).

In order to characterize absorbency dynamic, the cylindrical samples with dimensions of 15 mm in diameter and of 1 mm in width were prepared. The tested materials were applied in one layer and cured with LED light lamp (Mini L.E.D., Acteon, Mérignac Cedex, France) in nine zones partially overlapping each other with direct contact of optical fiber with the material surface. Exposure time was applied according to the manufacturer's instructions (Table 1).

Five samples were prepared for each tested cement. The samples' weight was determined (RADWAG AS 160/C/2, Poland) immediately after preparation and then for 30 consecutive days, and after 1344 h (56 days) and 2016 h (84 days). The absorbency was calculated according to the Equation (1) [20]:

$$A = \frac{m_i - m_0}{m_0} \cdot 100\% \tag{1}$$

where A is the absorbency of water, m_0 is the mass of the sample in dry condition, and m_i is the mass of the sample after storage in water for a specified (i) period of time.

2.2. Water Sorption and Solubility

Water sorption and solubility were investigated according to ISO 4049 [19]. The detailed procedure of tests has been described extensively in the previously published literature [18,21]. Curing time was consistent with the manufacturer's instructions (Table 1).

Water sorption and solubility were calculated according to following equations:

$$W_{sp} = \frac{m_2 - m_3}{V} \tag{2}$$

$$W_{sl} = \frac{m_1 - m_3}{V} \tag{3}$$

where: W_{sp} is the water sorption, W_{sl} is the water solubility, m_1 is the initial constant mass (μg), m_2 is the mass after seven days of water immersion (μg), m_3 is the final constant mass (μg), V is the specimen volume (mm^3).

2.3. Photoelastic Study

Photoelastic analysis allows for quantitative measurement and visualization of stress concentration that develops during photopolymerization or water sorption of resin composites [22,23]. The modified method enables analysis of the relationship between water sorption and the change of stress state (contraction or expansion) of resin materials. This test was described extensively in our previous articles [18,24]. Photoelastically-sensitive plates of epoxy resin (Epidian 53, Organika-Sarzyna SA, Nowa Sarzyna, Poland) were used in this study. Calibrated orifices of 3 mm in diameter and of 4 mm in depth were prepared in resin plates in order to mimic an average tooth cavity. The generated strains in the plates were visualized in circular transmission polariscope FL200 (Gunt, Barsbüttel, Germany) and photoelastic strain calculations were based on the Timoshenko equation [25].

3. Results

3.1. Absorbency Dynamic Study

Water absorbency and contraction stress mean values were presented in Figures 2–14. The water immersion resulted in an increase in weight of all tested materials. The water sorption (wt%) increased for Breeze up to three times. The lowest value of absorbency after 2016 h (84 days) was observed for Variolink Esthetic DC.

3.2. Water Sorption and Solubility

Mean values of water sorption and solubility were presented in Table 3. Maxcem Elite Chroma and Breeze exhibited the highest, while Estecem showed the lowest values of water sorption.

Table 3. Stress state before and after 2016 h (84 days) of water immersion, contraction stress drop, absorbency, and solubility of tested materials.

Material	Stress State (MPa)		Contraction Stress Drop (%)	Sorption (μg/mm³)	Solubility (μg/mm³)
	0.5 h	2016 h			
Cement It	10.9 ± 2.2	−1.6 ± 0.4	115 *	27.8 ± 0.8	1.9 ± 0.4
NX3	6.3 ± 0.1	1.6 ± 0.1	79	23.8 ± 0.6	3.7 ± 1.2
Variolink Esthetic	10.9 ± 0.4	4.7 ± 0.1	57	22.4 ± 0.8	10.0 ± 2.0
Estecem	6.8 ± 0.9	1.6 ± 0.2	76	12.5 ± 2.2	4.6 ± 1.9
Multilink Automix	12.5 ± 0.4	2.1 ± 0.9	83	25.3 ± 1.5	2.2 ± 0.8
Panavia 2.0	5.3 ± 1.8	−4.8 ± 0.4	191 *	33,9 ± 1.7	11.1 ± 1.0
Breeze	7.8 ± 1.6	−6.3 ± 1.6	180 *	47.7 ± 3.1	3.1 ± 0.5
Calibra Universal	11.1 ± 0.7	0.0 ± 0.8	100	30.9 ± 1.5	5.0 ± 2.6
MaxCem Elite Chroma	10.4 ± 0.9	−6.3 ± 0.3	160 *	50.4 ± 1.3	8.5 ± 1.3
Panavia SA Plus	4.8 ± 0.4	−1.6 ± 0.2	133 *	26.4 ± 1.3	1.7 ± 0.4
RelyX U200	13.5 ± 0.8	2.6 ± 0.9	81	29.6 ± 1.3	0.4 ± 0.2
SmartCem 2	15.1 ± 0.9	1.6 ± 0.9	89	33.0 ± 0.9	4.9 ± 1.2
SpeedCEM Plus	11.9 ± 1.1	−1.6 ± 0.4	113 *	28.2 ± 0.5	2.5 ± 0.4

* represents materials with over-compensated polymerization stress due to water expansion.

3.3. Photoelastic Study

All materials exhibited shrinkage and the associated contraction stress during hardening process. The significant reduction in contraction stress was observed due to hygroscopic expansion of cements (Figures 2–16). Water ageing of six cements resulted in additional stress characterized by the opposite direction of forces. The investigated materials exhibited various contraction stress values.

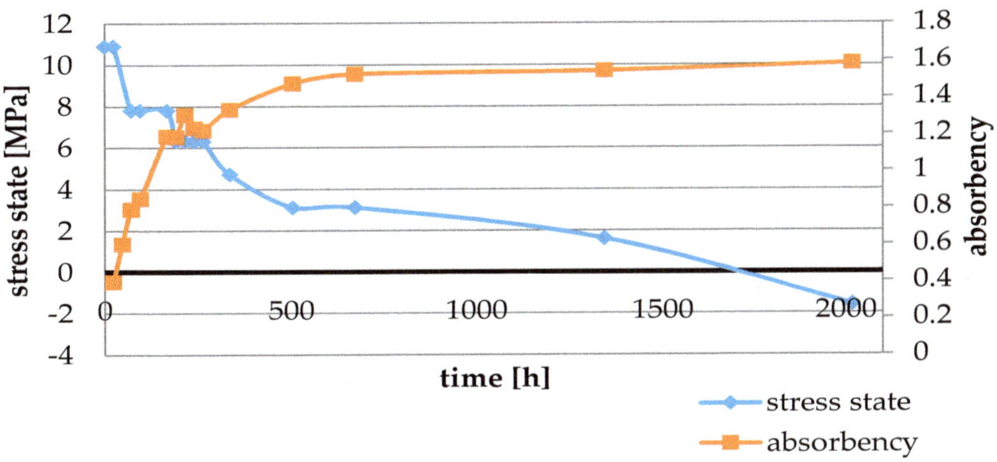

Figure 2. The influence of water sorption (2016 h water ageing) on the absorbency and contraction stress generated during the photopolymerization of Cement It.

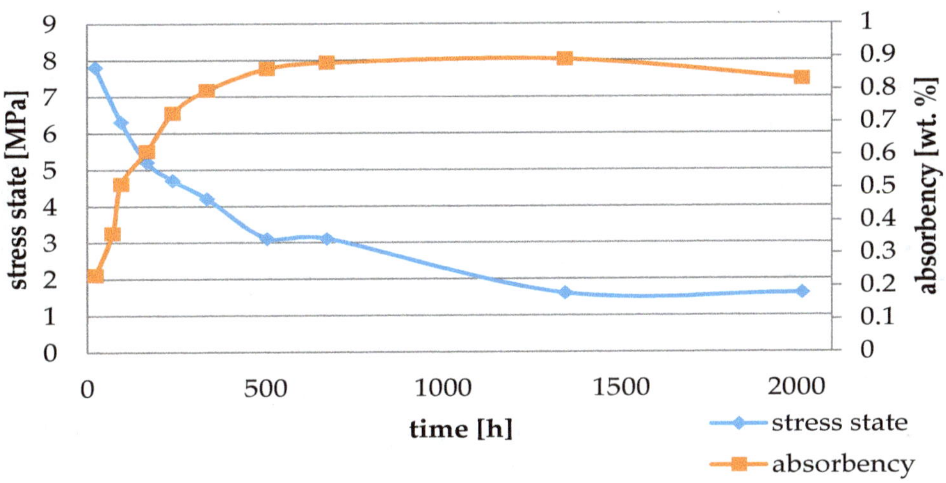

Figure 3. The influence of water sorption (2016 h water ageing) on the absorbency and contraction stress generated during the photopolymerization of NX3.

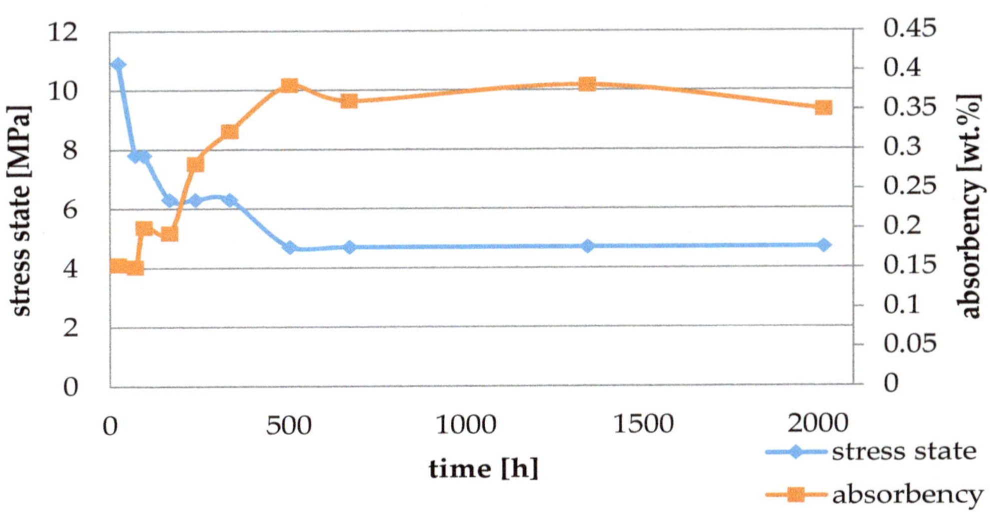

Figure 4. The influence of water sorption (2016 h water ageing) on the absorbency and contraction stress generated during the photopolymerization of Variolink Esthetic DC.

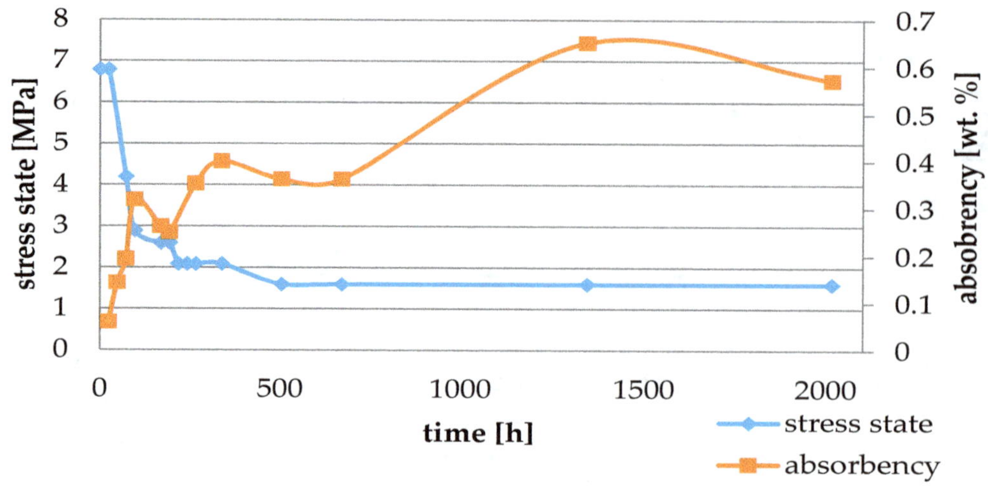

Figure 5. The influence of water sorption (2016 h water ageing) on the absorbency and contraction stress generated during the photopolymerization of Estecem.

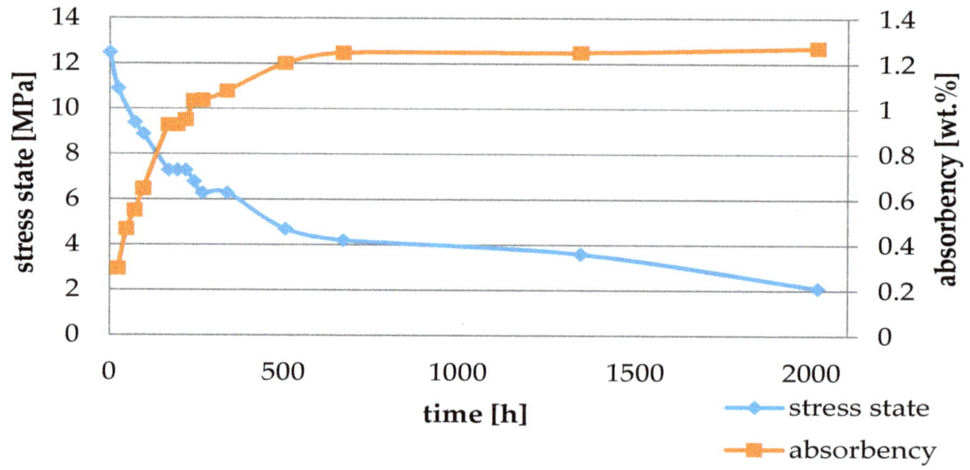

Figure 6. The influence of water sorption (2016 h water ageing) on the absorbency and contraction stress generated during the photopolymerization of Multilink Automix.

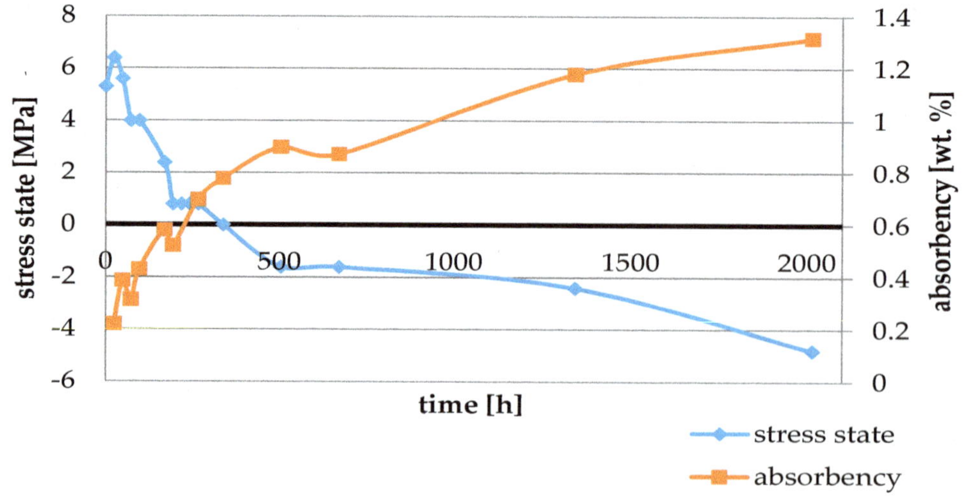

Figure 7. The influence of water sorption (2016 h water ageing) on the absorbency and contraction stress generated during the photopolymerization of Panavia 2.0.

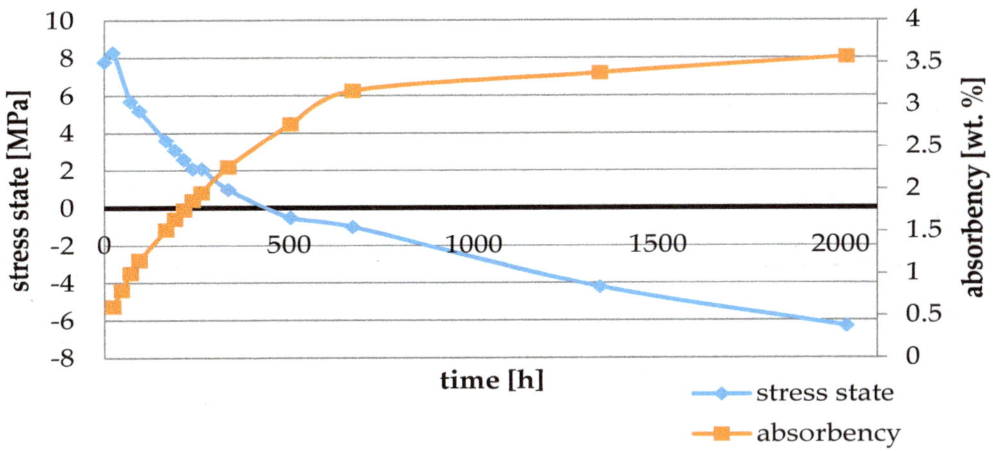

Figure 8. The influence of water sorption (2016 h water ageing) on the absorbency and contraction stress generated during the photopolymerization of Breeze.

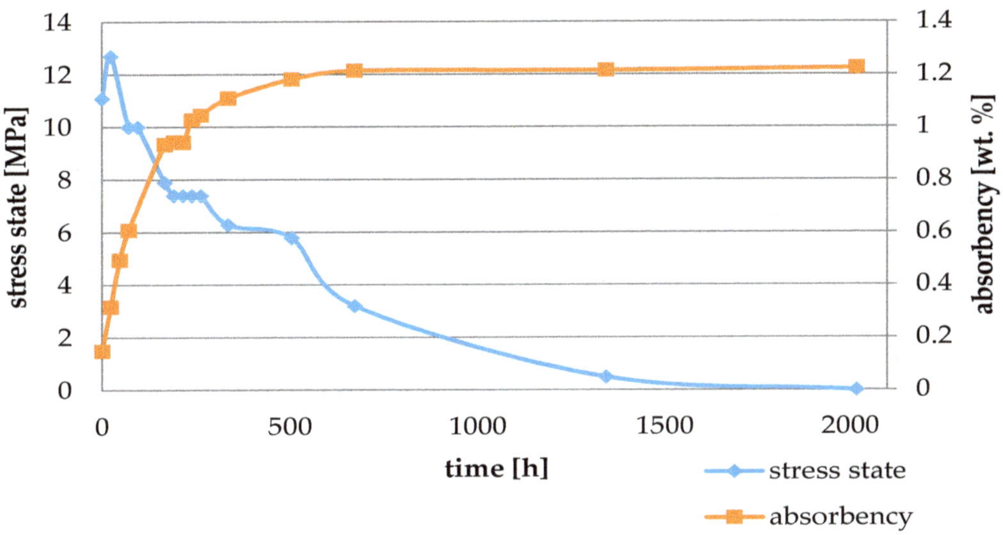

Figure 9. The influence of water sorption (2016 h water ageing) on the absorbency and contraction stress generated during the photopolymerization of Calibra Universal.

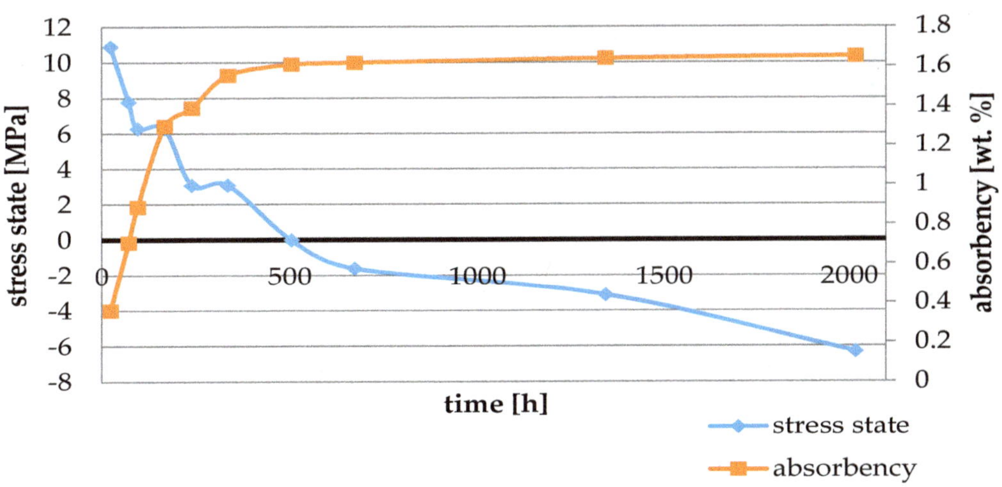

Figure 10. The influence of water sorption (2016 h water ageing) on the absorbency and contraction stress generated during the photopolymerization of Maxcem Elite Chroma.

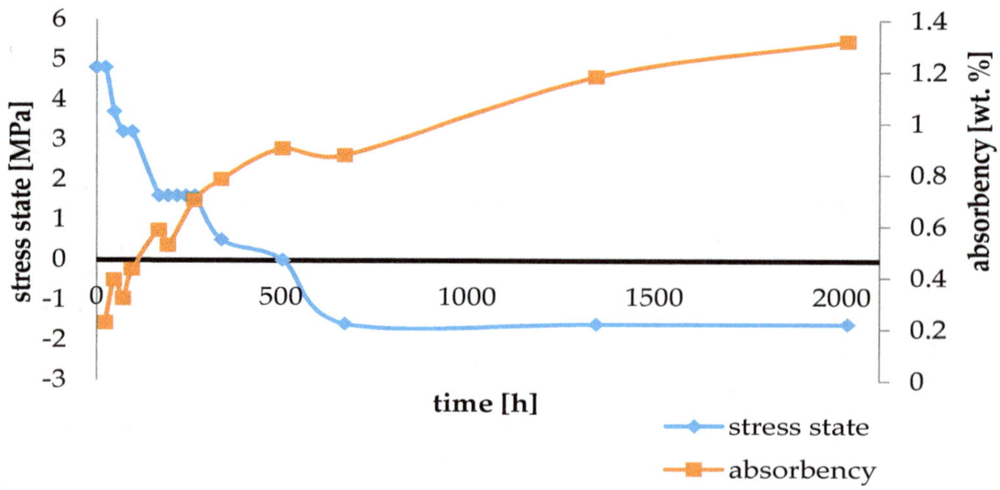

Figure 11. The influence of water sorption (2016 h water ageing) on the absorbency and contraction stress generated during the photopolymerization of Panavia SA Plus.

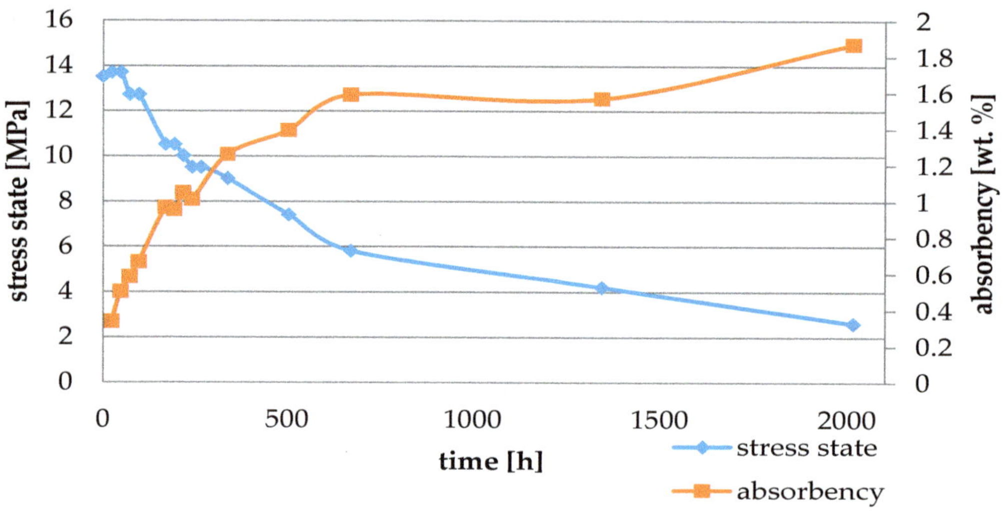

Figure 12. The influence of water sorption (2016 h water ageing) on the absorbency and contraction stress generated during the photopolymerization of Rely U200.

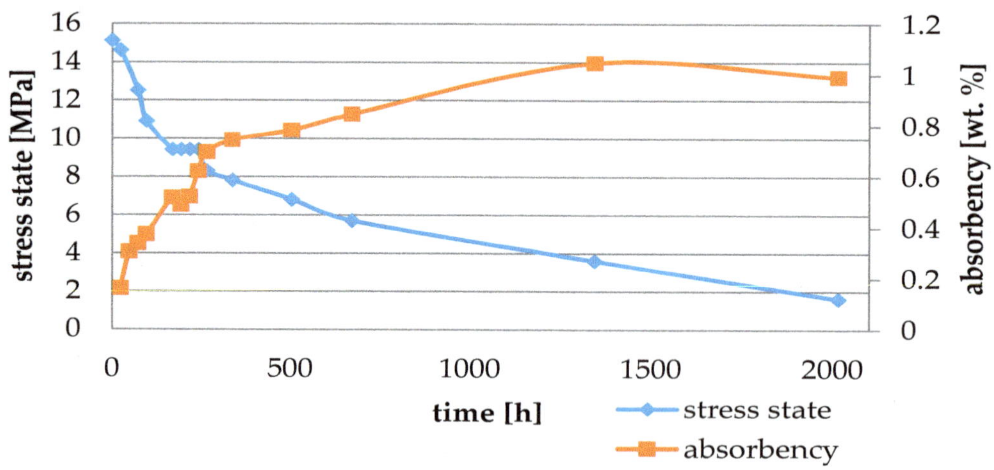

Figure 13. The influence of water sorption (2016 h water ageing) on the absorbency and contraction stress generated during the photopolymerization of SmartCem 2.

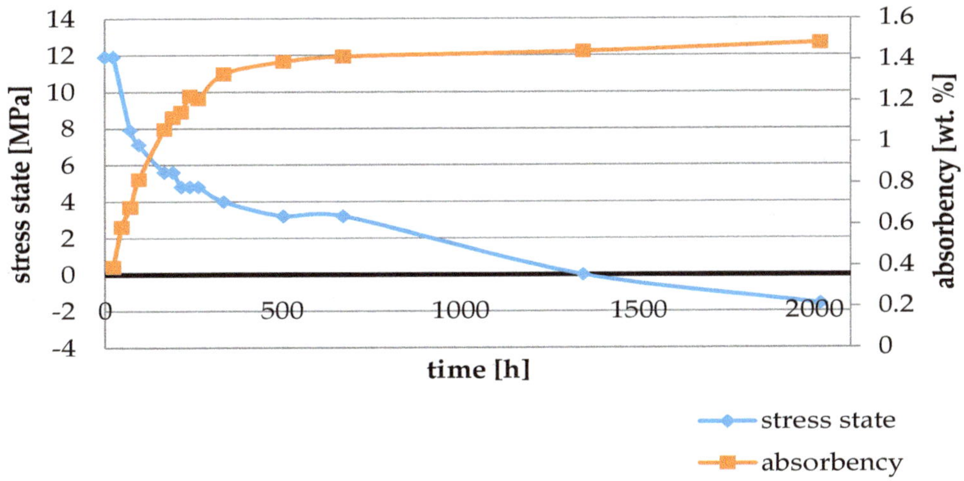

Figure 14. The influence of water sorption (2016 h water ageing) on the absorbency and contraction stress generated during the photopolymerization of SpeedCEM Plus.

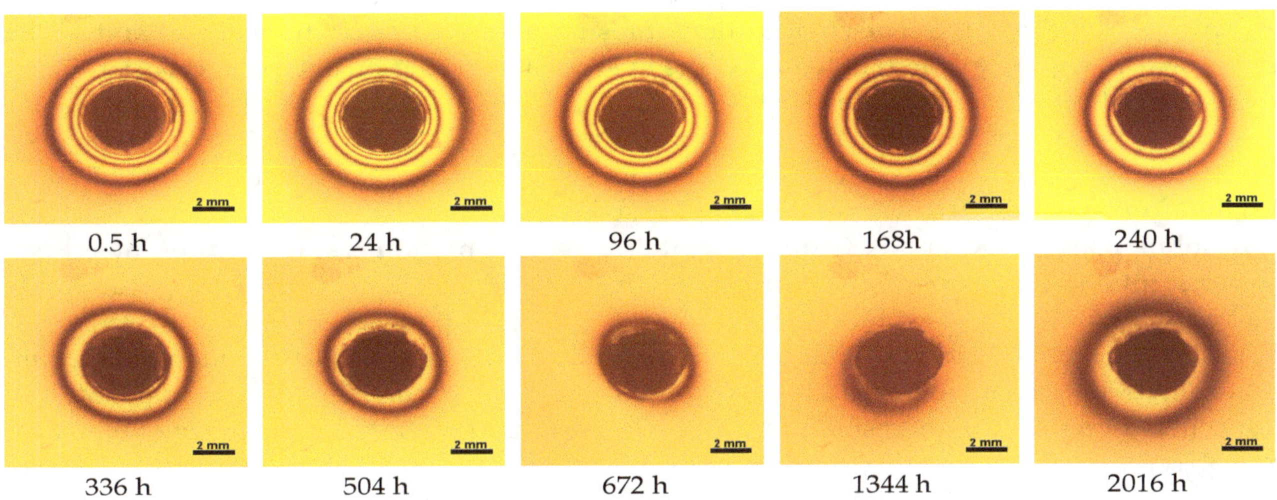

Figure 15. Isochromes in an epoxy plate around Maxcem Elite Chroma restoration before and after water storage; 0.5–2016 h.

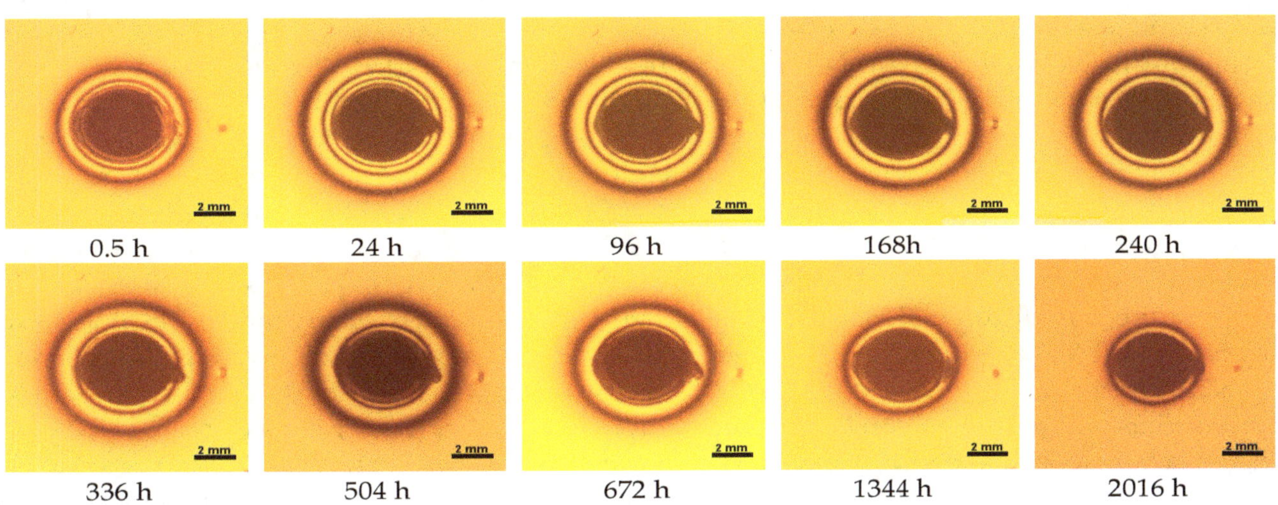

Figure 16. Isochromes in an epoxy plate around NX3 restoration before and after water storage; 0.5–2016 h.

The lowest contraction stress from tested materials exhibited Panavia SA Plus. The contraction stress decreased from 4.8 up to 0.0 MPa after 504 h (21 days) of water conditioning (Figure 11). Further water ageing resulted in additional stress: after 2016 h (84 days) stress level increased up to −1.6 MPa (Figure 11).

The highest contraction stress was observed for SmartCem 2 amounting up to 15.1 MPa. The contraction stress of SmartCem 2 after 2016 h (84 days) of water storage reduced up to 1.6 MPa (Figure 13).

4. Discussion

High configuration factor (C-factor) and the low viscosity of resin cements may generate relatively high contraction stress. This stress may cause debonding of the luting material, thereby increasing microleakage [14]. Our previous study (using an epoxy resin plate) [18,24], demonstrated that the photoelastic method can be used to evaluate the effect of water sorption on stress reduction at the tooth-restoration interface. This method shows that the contraction stress of dental resins may be partially relieved by the water uptake [18]. However, the in-depth analysis of the shrinkage stress values in various resin cement materials after water ageing is also highly demanded.

The overall results showed the development of the initial stress in the compressive direction during photopolymerization. The composition of resin cements affected the sorption and solubility processes which, in turn, exerted influence on the hygroscopic expansion and plasticization. Thus, the compensatory effect was composition-dependent [26]. This study confirmed the lower water sorption for composite resin cements as compared with self-adhesive resin cements that underwent water ageing. The presence of hydroxyl, carboxyl, and phosphate groups in monomers made them more hydrophilic and, supposedly, more prone to water sorption [27].

Variolink Esthetic DC and NX3 do not contain adhesive monomers. In the present study they exhibited sorption similar to composite materials [18]. Variolink Esthetic DC showed a high solubility value and the lowest decrease in contraction stress (of about 70%). The water immersion of resin materials might result in dissolving and leaching of some components (unreacted monomers or fillers) out of the material [28]. Variolink Esthetic DC contains a modified polymer matrix and nanofiller. The lowest contraction stress might result from a small hydrolysis and plasticization effect of the modified resin matrix.

Cement It is a composite resin cement which, in comparison with NX3 and Variolink Esthetic DC, showed higher values of water sorption and its total value of stress changes was 12.5 MPa. This could be explained by the composition of the polymer matrix containing bis-GMA and HDDMA. These monomers showed comparable characteristics: high water sorption values [29,30], similar polymer networks, and susceptibility to hydrolysis [31].

The four tested materials did not meet the requirements of ISO 4049, as they showed sorption values above 40 $\mu g/mm^3$ (Breeze and MaxCem Elite Chroma) or the solubility value above 7.5 $\mu g/mm^3$ (Variolink Esthetic DC and Panavia 2.0). The differences in water absorption of the polymer network depending on monomer type were reported. The highest water sorption was observed for MaxCem Elite Chroma (Figure 15). This material consists of HEMA and GDM that have one of the highest hydrophilicities among dental resins. HEMA was shown to induce water sorption, leading to the expansion of the polymer matrix [32]. Resin-modified glass-ionomer cements (RMGICs) absorbed more water due to hydroxyethyl methacrylate content, present in the hydrogel form in the polymerized matrices [33]. HEMA might be present either as a separate component or a grafted component into the structure of the polyacrylic acid backbone. The polymerized matrices of these materials were very hydrophilic and might include an interpenetrating network of poly(HEMA), copolymers of grafted HEMA, and polyacid salts that were more prone to water uptake [34]. Park et al. [35] showed that GDM exhibited the highest water sorption in comparison to bis-GMA, HEMA, EGDM, DEGDM, TEGDMA, GDM, and GTM. In the present study, the decrease in contraction stress after 2016 h (84 days) of water immersion varied significantly between tested materials. Figures 2–16 showed that the expansion dynamics also differed substantially. All studied materials exhibited contraction stress relief during water immersion. The value of stress decreased up to 0 MPa in different times depending on the material and its composition.

To sum up, the phenomenon of hydroscopic expansion after compensation of contraction stress should be emphasized more and evaluated. Such over-compensation could lead to internal expansion stress [36]. Hygroscopic stress could result in micro-cracks or even cusp fractures in the restored tooth [37], poorer mechanical properties [38,39], hydrolytic degradation of bonds particularly at the resin–filler interface [40], polymer plasticization leading to hardness reduction and glass transition temperature [40], and impaired wear resistance [41]. Excessive water sorption is not desired as it causes an outward movement of residual monomers and ions due to material solubility. Furthermore, water sorption might generate peeling stress in bonded layers of polymers that may cause serious clinical consequences [42], which may occur especially when prosthetic restorations are adhesively cemented [42].

The present study demonstrated that self-adhesive cements, i.e., Maxcem Elite Chroma, Speed Cem Plus, Cement It, Panavia SA Plus, Breeze, and Panavia 2.0 exhibited high stress values due to water expansion (from 0 up to almost 7 MPa). Water expansion stress of Maxcem Elite Chroma and Breeze amounted to up to ~6–7 MPa which could be associated with their composition, particularly with acidic monomer 4-MET in Breeze and HEMA, and GDM and tetramethylbutyl hydroperoxide in Maxcem Elite Chroma. The monomers, mentioned above, were responsible for water uptake and stress built-up associated with hydroscopic expansion [35]. According to the literature such high stress values were not desirable. Huang et al. [33] found that a giomer material exhibited extensive hygroscopic expansion (due to osmotic effect) enabling enclosing glass cylinders to crack after two weeks of immersion in water. Cusp fracture in endodontically-treated teeth was attributed to hygroscopic expansion of a temporary filling material [33], while cracks in all-ceramic crowns were associated with hygroscopic expansion of compomer and resin-modified glassionomer materials used as core build-up and/or luting cements [33]. Three-year clinical performance study also suggested hygroscopic expansion as a possible cause of cusp fracture in 19% of teeth restored with an ion-releasing composite [43].

Thus, the positive influence of water sorption on contraction stress relief in the case of luting cements, particularly self-adhesive materials, should be considered carefully. Shrinkage occurred within seconds, but water sorption took days and weeks. The rate of hygroscopic shear stress relief depended on the resin volume and its accessibility to water [11]. The contraction stress relief rates observed in luting resin cements could be much lower than in composite resin restorative materials. The composite restorations usually have a relatively large surface exposed to water in comparison to the overall surface of the luting material. As far as luting cements are concerned, the surface exposed to oral fluids is extremely small, while the pathway is extremely long. The consequences (slower compensation of contraction stress) might be less severe if water sorption is also possible from the dentin (dentin exposed to oral environment) [26].

The precise effect of water absorption depends on many factors including not only the material characteristics, the rate and amount of water absorbed, but also the mechanism of absorption [44]. Absorption leads to dimensional changes and has potentially important clinical implications. The positive effect of water absorption on composite restorative materials can be described as the mechanism for the compensation of polymerization shrinkage and the relaxation of stress. In clinical conditions, water absorption may help in the closure of contraction gaps around composite filling materials. It is worth emphasizing that the absorption can, in some cases, result in significant hydroscopic expansion and, thus, be damaging to the resin material and bonded tooth structure.

5. Conclusions

Among all studied resin cements, self-adhesive cements exhibited the highest water sorption due to acid monomer content, which affected the formation of hydroscopic expansion stress. The presence of this type of stress might pose a threat to prosthetic restorations. Therefore, there is still a need for research that would precisely illustrate the generated stress in clinical conditions.

Tested resin cements generated differentiated contraction stress during photopolymerization. The dynamic of hydroscopic compensation (resulting from water sorption) or over-compensation of the contraction stress is also material characteristic-dependent.

Author Contributions: M.-L.S., K.B., and J.S. conceived and designed the experiments; A.S., B.L., and K.K. performed the experiments; M.D. and G.S. analyzed the data; and G.S., A.S., and K.B. wrote the paper.

References

1. Christensen, G.J. Why use resin cements? *J. Am. Dent. Assoc.* **2010**, *141*, 204–206. [CrossRef] [PubMed]
2. Diaz-Arnold, A.M.; Vargas, M.A.; Haselton, D.R. Current status of luting agents for fixed prosthodontics. *J. Prosthet. Dent.* **1999**, *81*, 135–141. [CrossRef]
3. Radovic, I.; Monticelli, F.; Goracci, C.; Vulicevic, Z.R.; Ferrari, M. Self-adhesive resin cements: A literature review. *J. Adhes. Dent.* **2008**, *10*, 251–258. [CrossRef] [PubMed]
4. Sunico-Segarra, M.; Segarra, A. *A Practical Clinical Guide to Resin Cements*; Springer: Berlin/Heidelberg, Germany, 2015; pp. 9–23.
5. Rawls, H.R.; Shen, C.; Anusavice, K.J. Dental Cements. In *Phillips' Science of Dental Materials*; Saunders: Philadelphia, PA, USA, 2013; pp. 307–339.
6. Hill, E.E.; Lott, J. A clinically focused discussion of luting materials. *Aust. Dent. J.* **2011**, *56* (Suppl. S1), 67–76. [CrossRef] [PubMed]
7. El-Mowafy, O. The use of resin cements in restorative dentistry to overcome retention problems. *J. Can. Dent. Assoc.* **2001**, *67*, 97–102. [PubMed]
8. Vrochari, A.D.; Eliades, G.; Hellwig, E.; Wrbas, K.T. Curing efficiency of four self-etching, self-adhesive resin cements. *Dent. Mater.* **2009**, *25*, 1104–1108. [CrossRef] [PubMed]
9. Turkistani, A.; Sadr, A.; Shimada, Y.; Nikaido, T.; Sumi, Y.; Tagami, J. Sealing performance of resin cements before and after thermal cycling: Evaluation by optical coherence tomography. *Dent. Mater.* **2014**, *30*, 993–1004. [CrossRef] [PubMed]
10. Hitz, T.; Stawarczyk, B.; Fischer, J.; Hämmerle, C.H.F.; Sailer, I. Are self-adhesive resin cements a valid alternative to conventional resin cements? A laboratory study of the long-term bond strength. *Dent. Mater.* **2012**, *28*, 1183–1190. [CrossRef] [PubMed]
11. Feilzer, A.J.; De Gee, A.J.; Davidson, C.L. Increased Wall-to-Wall Curing Contraction in Thin Bonded Resin Layers. *J. Dent. Res.* **1989**, *68*, 48–50. [CrossRef] [PubMed]
12. Al Sunbul, H.; Silikas, N.; Watts, D.C. Polymerization shrinkage kinetics and shrinkage-stress in dental resin-composites. *Dent. Mater.* **2016**, *32*, 998–1006. [CrossRef] [PubMed]
13. Spinell, T.; Schedle, A.; Watts, D.C. Polymerization shrinkage kinetics of dimethacrylate resin-cements. *Dent. Mater.* **2009**, *25*, 1058–1066. [CrossRef] [PubMed]
14. Frassetto, A.; Navarra, C.O.; Marchesi, G.; Turco, G.; Di Lenarda, R.; Breschi, L.; Ferracane, J.L.; Cadenaro, M. Kinetics of polymerization and contraction stress development in self-adhesive resin cements. *Dent. Mater.* **2012**, *28*, 1032–1039. [CrossRef] [PubMed]
15. Shiozawa, M.; Takahashi, H.; Asakawa, Y.; Iwasaki, N. Color stability of adhesive resin cements after immersion in coffee. *Clin. Oral Investig.* **2015**, *19*, 309–317. [CrossRef] [PubMed]
16. Petropoulou, A.; Vrochari, A.D.; Hellwig, E.; Stampf, S.; Polydorou, O. Water sorption and water solubility of self-etching and self-adhesive resin cements. *J. Prosthet. Dent.* **2015**, *114*, 674–679. [CrossRef] [PubMed]
17. Marghalani, H.Y. Sorption and solubility characteristics of self-adhesive resin cements. *Dent. Mater.* **2012**, *28*, e187–e198. [CrossRef] [PubMed]
18. Bociong, K.; Szczesio, A.; Sokolowski, K.; Domarecka, M.; Sokolowski, J.; Krasowski, M.; Lukomska-szymanska, M. The Influence of Water Sorption of Dental Light-Cured Composites on Shrinkage Stress. *Materials* **2017**, *10*, 1142. [CrossRef] [PubMed]
19. *Stomatologia—Materiały Polimerowe do Odbudowy*; PN-EN ISO 4049:2010; Polski Komitet Normalizacyjny: Warszawa, Poland, 2010.

20. Li, L.; Chen, M.; Zhou, X.; Lu, L.; Li, Y.; Gong, C.; Cheng, X. A case of water absorption and water/fertilizer retention performance of super absorbent polymer modified sulphoaluminate cementitious materials. *Constr. Build. Mater.* **2017**, *150*, 538–546. [CrossRef]
21. Müller, J.A.; Rohr, N.; Fischer, J. Evaluation of ISO 4049: Water sorption and water solubility of resin cements. *Eur. J. Oral Sci.* **2017**, *125*, 141–150. [CrossRef] [PubMed]
22. Bociong, K. Naprężenia skurczowe generowane podczas fotoutwardzania eksperymentalnego kompozytu stomatologicznego. Cz. II. *Przem. Chem.* **2017**, *1*, 72–74. [CrossRef]
23. Bociong, K.; Krasowski, M.; Domarecka, M.; Sokołowski, J. Wpływ metody fotopolimeryzacji kompozytów stomatologicznych na bazie zywic dimetakrylanowych na naprężenia skurczowe oraz wybrane właściwości utwardzonego materiału. *Polimery* **2016**, *61*, 499–508. [CrossRef]
24. Domarecka, M.; Sokołowski, K.; Krasowski, M.; Szczesio, A.; Bociong, K.; Sokołowski, J.; Łukomska-Szymańska, M. Influence of water sorption on the shrinkage stresses of dental composites. *J. Stomatol.* **2016**, *69*, 412–419.
25. Timoshenko, S.; Goodier, J.N. *Theory of Elasticity*, 2nd ed.; McGraw-Hill: New York, NY, USA, 1951.
26. Feilzer, A.J.; de Gee, A.J.; Davidson, C.L. Relaxation of polymerization contraction shear stress by hygroscopic expansion. *J. Dent. Res.* **1990**, *69*, 36–39. [CrossRef] [PubMed]
27. Santerre, J.P.; Shajii, L.; Leung, B.W. Relation of dental composite formulations to their degradation and the release of hydrolyzed polymeric-resin-derived products. *Crit. Rev. Oral Biol. Med.* **2001**, *12*, 136–151. [CrossRef] [PubMed]
28. Mahajan, R.P.; Shenoy, V.U.; MV, S.; Walzade, P.S. Comparative Evaluation of Solubilities of Two Nanohybrid Composite Resins in Saliva Substitute and Distilled Water: An in vitro Study. *J. Contemp. Dent.* **2017**, *7*, 82–85.
29. Siswomihardjo, W.; Sunarintyas, S.; Matinlinna, J.P. The influence of resin matrix on the water sorption of fiber-reinforced composites for DENTAL use. *J. Eng. Appl. Sci.* **2016**, *11*, 2678–2682.
30. Sideridou, I.; Tserki, V.; Papanastasiou, G. Study of water sorption, solubility and modulus of elasticity of light-cured dimethacrylate-based dental resins. *Biomaterials* **2003**, *24*, 655–665. [CrossRef]
31. Ling, L.; Xu, X.; Choi, G.Y.; Billodeaux, D.; Guo, G.; Diwan, R.M. Novel F-releasing composite with improved mechanical properties. *J. Dent. Res.* **2009**, *88*, 83–88. [CrossRef] [PubMed]
32. Malacarne, J.; Carvalho, R.M.; de Goes, M.F.; Svizero, N.; Pashley, D.H.; Tay, F.R.; Yiu, C.K.; de Oliveira Carrilho, M.R. Water sorption/solubility of dental adhesive resins. *Dent. Mater.* **2006**, *22*, 973–980. [CrossRef] [PubMed]
33. Huang, C.; Kei, L.; Wei, S.H.Y.; Cheung, G.S.P.; Tay, F.R.; Pashley, D.H. The influence of hygroscopic expansion of resin-based restorative materials on artificial gap reduction. *J. Adhes. Dent.* **2002**, *4*, 61–71. [PubMed]
34. Wilson, A.D. Resin-modified glass-ionomer cements. *Int. J. Prosthodont.* **1990**, *3*, 425–429. [PubMed]
35. Park, J.; Eslick, J.; Ye, Q.; Misra, A.; Spencer, P. The influence of chemical structure on the properties in methacrylate-based dentin adhesives. *Dent. Mater.* **2013**, *31*, 1713–1723. [CrossRef] [PubMed]
36. Wei, Y.J.; Silikas, N.; Zhang, Z.T.; Watts, D.C. Diffusion and concurrent solubility of self-adhering and new resin–matrix composites during water sorption/desorption cycles. *Dent. Mater.* **2011**, *21*, 97–205. [CrossRef] [PubMed]
37. Rüttermann, S.; Krüger, S.; Raab, W.H.M.; Janda, R. Polymerization shrinkage and hygroscopic expansion of contemporary posterior resin-based filling materials—A comparative study. *J. Dent.* **2007**, *35*, 806–813. [CrossRef] [PubMed]
38. Musanje, L.; Shu, M.; Darvell, B.W. Water sorption and mechanical behaviour of cosmetic direct restorative materials in artificial saliva. *Dent. Mater.* **2001**, *17*, 394–401. [CrossRef]
39. Bastioli, C.; Romano, G.; Migliaresi, C. Water sorption and mechanical properties of dental composites. *Biomaterials* **1990**, *11*, 219–223. [CrossRef]
40. Ferracane, J.L. Hygroscopic and hydrolytic effects in dental polymer networks. *Dent. Mater.* **2006**, *22*, 211–222. [CrossRef] [PubMed]
41. Göhring, T.N.; Besek, M.J.; Schmidlin, P.R. Attritional wear and abrasive surface alterations of composite resin materials in vitro. *J. Dent.* **2002**, *30*, 119–127. [CrossRef]
42. Kalachandra, S.; Turner, D.T. Water sorption of polymethacrylate networks: Bis-GMA/TEGDM copolymers. *J. Biomed. Mater. Res.* **1987** *21*, 329–338. [CrossRef] [PubMed]

43. Versluis, A.; Tantbirojn, D.; Lee, M.S.; Tu, L.S.; Delong, R. Can hygroscopic expansion compensate polymerization shrinkage? Part I. Deformation of restored teeth. *Dent. Mater.* **2011**, *27*, 126–133. [CrossRef] [PubMed]
44. McCabe, J.F.; Rusby, S. Water absorption, dimensional change and radial pressure in resin matrix dental restorative materials. *Biomaterials* **2004**, *25*, 4001–4007. [CrossRef] [PubMed]

9

Degree of Conversion and BisGMA, TEGDMA, UDMA Elution from Flowable Bulk Fill Composites

Edina Lempel [1,*], Zsuzsanna Czibulya [2,3], Bálint Kovács [2,3], József Szalma [4], Ákos Tóth [5], Sándor Kunsági-Máté [2,3], Zoltán Varga [1] and Katalin Böddi [6]

1 Department of Restorative Dentistry and Periodontology, University of Pécs, 5 Dischka Gy Street, Pécs H-7621, Hungary; varga.zoltan@gmail.com
2 Department of General and Physical Chemistry, University of Pécs, 6 Ifjúság Street, Pécs H-7624, Hungary, czibulya.zsuzsanna@gmail.com (Z.C.); balint621@gmail.com (B.K.); kunsagi@gamma.ttk.pte.hu (S.K.-M.)
3 János Szentágothai Research Center, University of Pécs, 20 Ifjúság Street, Pécs H-7624, Hungary
4 Department of Oral and Maxillofacial Surgery, University of Pécs, 5 Dischka Gy Street, Pécs H-7621, Hungary; szalma.jozsef@pte.hu
5 Faculty of Sciences, University of Pécs, 6 Ifjúság Street, Pécs H-7621, Hungary; totha@gamma.ttk.pte.hu
6 Department of Biochemistry and Medical Chemistry, University of Pécs, 12 Szigeti Street, Pécs H-7624, Hungary; katalin.boddi@aok.pte.hu
* Correspondence: lempel.edina@pte.hu

Abstract: The degree of conversion (DC) and the released bisphenol A diglycidyl ether dimethacrylate (BisGMA), triethylene glycol dimethacrylate (TEGDMA) and urethane dimethacrylate (UDMA) monomers of bulk-fill composites compared to that of conventional flowable ones were assessed using micro-Raman spectroscopy and high performance liquid chromatography (HPLC). Four millimeter-thick samples were prepared from SureFil SDR Flow (SDR), X-tra Base (XB), Filtek Bulk Fill (FBF) and two and four millimeter samples from Filtek Ultimate Flow (FUF). They were measured with micro-Raman spectroscopy to determine the DC% of the top and the bottom surfaces. The amount of released monomers in 75% ethanol extraction media was measured with HPLC. The differences between the top and bottom DC% were significant for each material. The mean DC values were in the following order for the bottom surfaces: SDR_4mm_20s > FUF_2mm_20s > XB_4mm_20s > FBF_4mm_20s > XB_4mm_10s > FBF_4mm_10s > FUF_4mm_20s. The highest rate in the amount of released BisGMA and TEGDMA was found from the 4 mm-thick conventional flowable FUF. Among bulk-fills, FBF showed a twenty times higher amount of eluted UDMA and twice more BisGMA; meanwhile, SDR released a significantly higher amount of TEGDMA. SDR bulk-fill showed significantly higher DC%; meanwhile XB, FBF did not reach the same level DC, as that of the 2 mm-thick conventional composite at the bottom surface. Conventional flowable composites showed a higher rate of monomer elution compared to the bulk-fills, except FBF, which showed a high amount of UDMA release.

Keywords: bulk-fill composite; degree of conversion; monomer elution; micro-Raman spectroscopy; HPLC

1. Introduction

The evolution led to contemporary resin-based composites (RBCs) showing high clinical success and survival rates [1–4]. However, despite the continuous development of RBCs, there are some shortcomings, such as polymerization volume shrinkage, incomplete degree of conversion (DC) of the matrix monomers and their release into the oral cavity and pulp space. The degree of conversion of an RBC is an important factor in determining the mechanical properties of the material and its biocompatibility [5,6]. A lower conversion rate will influence the physical performance of the RBC, and increased elution of monomers have been reported [7,8]. However, the DC% for adequate clinical performance has not yet been determined; only a negative correlation of *in vivo* abrasive wear depth with DC has been established in the range of 55–65 DC% [9,10]. To prevent clinical failures and decrease the elution of unreacted monomers, some practical strategies are recommended, including alternative light curing protocols [11], the use of flowable cavity liners [12] and incremental filling techniques [13]. The generally-accepted maximal layer thickness that provides adequate light penetration and photo-polymerization is 2 mm [7,14–16]. However, restoring cavities with RBC increments of 2 mm in thickness is time consuming; voids may be included; and this implies a risk of contaminations between the increments [17]. Thus, bulk-fill RBCs were developed to avoid the aforementioned disadvantages [18]. Literature data suppose better light transmittance of these materials to allow for a reported depth of cure in excess of 4 mm [19–21]. According to the manufacturer's recommendation, bulk-fill materials are indicated as basing materials or permanent restorative materials. *In vitro* studies showed that the application of one thicker increment of bulk-fill composite could be equally successful in marginal adaptation, cavity-bottom adhesion and in depth of cure as the conventional layering technique [20,22]. Bulk-fill materials showed lower shrinkage stress and exhibited an acceptable creep deformation and reduced cuspal deflection when compared to conventional RBCs [17,23,24]. In a recent investigation, mechanical properties, including degree of cure, were shown to be constant within the 4-mm increment [25]. In the dental literature, studies investigated the amount of eluted monomers; thus, the biocompatibility and clinical performance of bulk-fill flowable RBC base materials are limited [20–22,24,26]. Biocompatibility depends on the quality and quantity of released monomers and their derivates, which can irritate the pulp, the soft tissues of the oral cavity and may lead eventually to a toxic reaction [27,28]. Several factors, such as the DC, the specimen thickness, the chemical composition, the filler particle type and content, the porosity and the solvent can influence the amount of released monomers [29].

The aim of this study was to assess the DC and the amount of released BisGMA, TEGDMA and UDMA monomers of some low-viscosity bulk-fill composite materials in a 4-mm layer thickness compared to that of conventional flowable one in a 2-(positive control) and a 4-mm (negative control) thickness, using micro-Raman spectroscopy and HPLC.

2. Results

2.1. Degree of Conversion-Micro-Raman Spectroscopy

The top and bottom surface DC values of the materials are presented in Figures 1 and 2.

The mean DC values on the top surface of the materials were in the following order: SDR_4mm_20s > FBF_4mm_20s > FUF_4mm_2mm > FUF_4mm_20s > FBF_4mm_10s > XB_4mm_20s > XB_4mm_10s; however, the order of the mean DC values on the bottom surface was significantly different from the top surface: SDR_4mm_20s > FUF_2mm_20s > XB_4mm_20s > FBF_4mm_20s > XB_4mm_10s > FBF_4mm_10s > FUF_4mm_20s. Dunnett's *t*-test showed that all of the investigated materials had statistically significant differences in DC% at the bottom surface when compared to each other, except between FBF_4mm_20s and XB_4mm_20s ($p = 0.221$). On the contrary, between FUF_2mm_20s and FUF_4mm_20s ($p = 0.306$), FUF_2mm_20s and FBF_4mm_20s ($p = 1.000$), FUF_4mm_20s and FBF_4mm_20s ($p = 0.241$), FUF_4mm_20s and FBF_4mm_10s ($p = 0.059$) and between XB_4mm_20s and FBF_4mm_10s ($p = 0.063$), Dunnett's *t*-test did not show significant difference in DC% at the top surface. The conventional flowable composite FUF_4mm_20s had the lowest DC value at the bottom (16.53%), while SDR_4mm_20s (50.05%) had the highest DC value not only at the bottom, but at the top surface, as well. The extended curing time of FBF and XB from 10–20 s significantly increased the DC%, especially at the bottom surface.

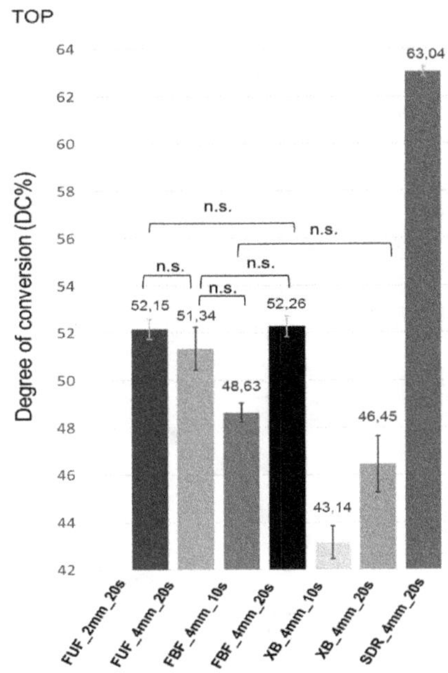

Figure 1. Mean DC% and 95% confidence intervals of the top surface of the samples (abbreviations: DC, degree of conversion; n.s., not significant difference; FUF_2mm_20s, Filtek Ultimate Flow in a 2-mm layer thickness cured for 20 s; FUF_4mm_20s, Filtek Ultimate Flow in a 4-mm layer thickness cured for 20 s; FBF_4mm_10s, 4 mm-thick Filtek Bulk Fill light cured for 10 s; FBF_4mm_20s, 4 mm-thick Filtek Bulk Fill light cured for 20 s; XB_4mm_10s, 4 mm-thick X-tra Base light cured for 10 s; XB_4mm_20s, 4 mm-thick X-tra Base light cured for 20 s; SDR_4mm_20s, SureFil SDR Flow in a 4-mm layer thickness cured for 20 s).

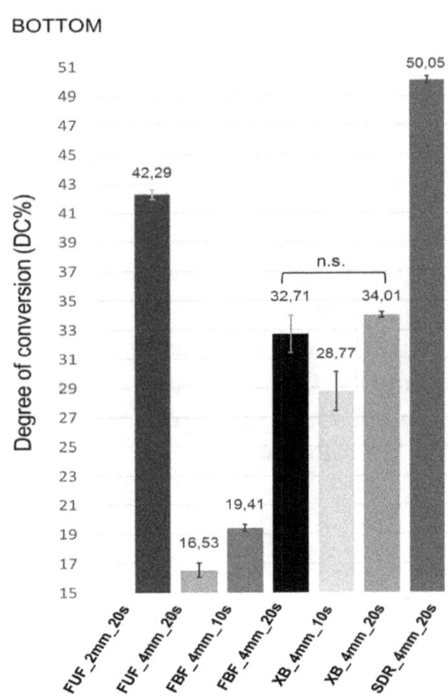

Figure 2. Mean DC% and 95% confidence intervals of the bottom surface of the samples (abbreviations: DC, degree of conversion; n.s., not significant difference; FUF_2mm_20s, Filtek Ultimate Flow in a 2-mm layer thickness cured for 20 s; FUF_4mm_20s, Filtek Ultimate Flow in a 4-mm layer thickness cured for 20 s; FBF_4mm_10s, 4 mm-thick Filtek Bulk Fill light cured for 10 s; FBF_4mm_20s, 4 mm-thick Filtek Bulk Fill light cured for 20 s; XB_4mm_10s, 4 mm-thick X-tra Base light cured for 10 s; XB_4mm_20s, 4 mm-thick X-tra Base light cured for 20 s; SDR_4mm_20s, SureFil SDR Flow in a 4-mm layer thickness cured for 20 s).

2.2. Monomer Elution: HPLC

Figure 3 shows the amount of eluted BisGMA, UDMA and TEGDMA from the 2 mm- and 4 mm-thick conventional flowable and the bulk-fill flowable RBC materials.

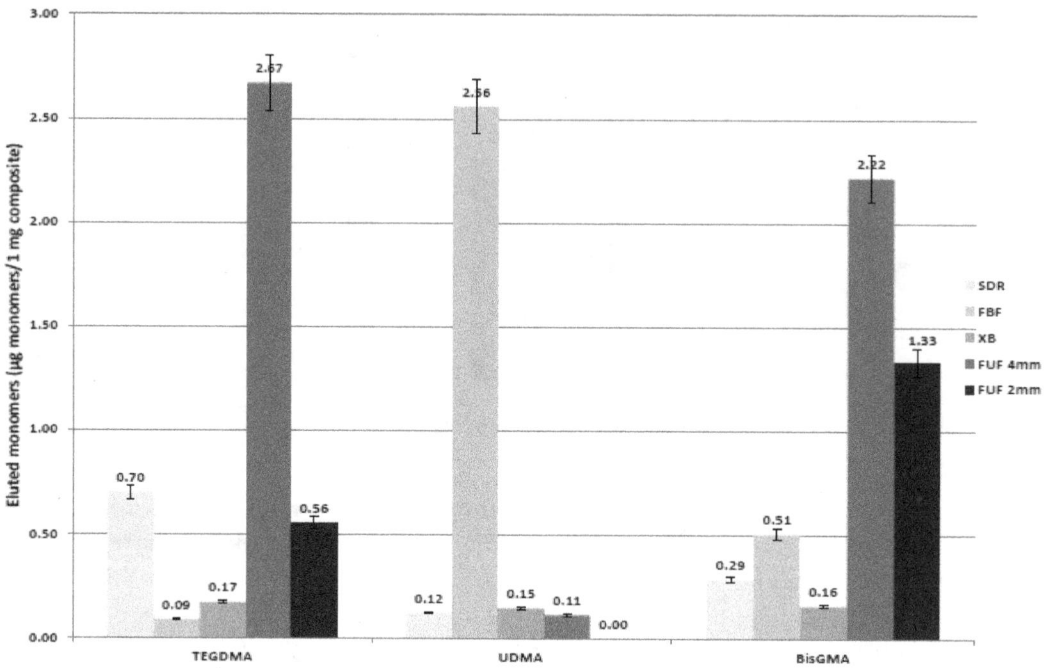

Figure 3. Amount of eluted monomers from bulk-fill and conventional flowable composites. (Abbreviations: SDR, SureFil SDR Flow in a 4-mm layer thickness light cured for 20 s; FBF, Filtek Bulk Fill in a 4-mm layer thickness light cured for 10 s; XB, X-tra Base in a 4-mm layer thickness light cured for 10 s; FUF 4 mm, Filtek Ultimate Flow in a 4-mm layer thickness light cured for 20 s; FUF 2 mm, Filtek Ultimate Flow in a 2-mm layer thickness light cured for 20 s).

In spite of the fact that there is no BisGMA in SDR and XB according to the manufacturer's information, there was a detectable amount of this monomer from these bulk-fill materials, such as TEGDMA from XB. In comparison, with Dunnett's *t*-test, there were significant differences between the groups. More than a five-times higher elution rate was found in the amount of released BisGMA in the case of the 4 mm-thick conventional flowable FUF when this material was compared to the bulk-fill materials, and the difference in BisGMA release between the 2 mm- and 4 mm-thick FUF was almost twice ($p < 0.001$). The leached BisGMA from bulk-fill RBCs showed the following order: FBF > SDR > XB; the differences were statistically significant ($p < 0.001$). The FUF_4mm_20s had a statistically-significant higher rate of TEGDMA elution, as well, compared to the other materials ($p < 0.001$). Among bulk-fills, SDR showed a seven-times higher amount of TEGDMA elution. More than a twenty-times higher amount of eluted UDMA was observed in the case of FBF compared to SDR, XB and FUF; meanwhile, UDMA was not listed in the FUF's technical product profile.

In the case of FUF and FBF, a high intensity peak was detected on the HPLC chromatogram at a different retention time than that of the above-mentioned three monomers, which was not identified and quantified in the lack of a standard monomer. However, according to the manufacturer's information, it is probably the peak of procrylate monomer.

3. Discussion

In this study, the DC and the elution of unreacted monomers of different bulk fill and commercial flowable dental composites were assessed using micro-Raman spectroscopy and HPLC.

The setting process has a major influence on the mechanical and biological properties of RBCs [30]. Resin polymerization depends on the chemical structure of the monomer, filler characteristics, the photoinitiator concentration and the polymerization conditions [31]. Since polymerization conditions, such as layer thickness, intensity of the curing unit and exposure time, were standardized in this study, differences in the DC value of conventional and bulk-fill RBCs can be attributed to the different composition of the materials, mostly to variations in the chemistry of their resin matrix and the filler loading. In general, the manufacturers of bulk-fill RBCs were able to improve polymerization depth by the use of potent photoinitiator systems along with an increased translucency [18,32]. As light transmission is strongly dependent on material opacity [33], the observed higher DC% at a 4-mm specimen thickness for the investigated bulk-fills compared to the 4 mm-thick conventional flowable RBC might be a result of their reduced opacity. However, when the DC% of bulk fills was compared to the 2 mm-thick conventional flow, only SDR_4mm_20s produced a higher conversion rate. Higher translucency can also be achieved by the reduction in filler content [34]. It has been demonstrated by Halvorson *et al.* that increasing the filler-matrix ratio progressively decreases conversion, because an increased amount of filler particles is an obstacle for polymeric chain propagation [35]. According to Nomoto and Hirasawa [36], the depth of cure and, thus, the DC are affected by the filler's light permeability, the monomer composition, the type and concentration of the initiator and the inhibitor/accelerator systems in the RBCs. In the present study, a significantly higher DC value was observed with the SDR_4mm_20s, and a tendency for a higher DC value was detected in FBF in comparison to XB cured for both 10 and 20 s. This finding is supported by other investigators [19,37–39] and might be explained by the higher filler content of XB, which may increase light scattering, causing a concurrent decrease of translucency for blue light [18].

Due to the presence of a photo-active modulator in the matrix system and the increased translucency, the manufacturer's recommendation for the exposure time is 10 s for the universal shades, with the intensity of the curing unit ranging from 550–1000 $mW\cdot cm^{-2}$, while 20 s for SDR and FUF irrespective of the output intensity of the curing unit. Based on this fact, 5.5–10 $J\cdot cm^2$ of delivered energy should be enough for the adequate polymerization of bulk-fills. For a conventional RBC, the recommendation of a 21-$J\cdot cm^2$ and a 24-$J\cdot cm^2$ energy density has been made for the satisfactory conversion of a 2 mm-thick composite specimen [40]. Thus, as was expected, a 20-$J\cdot cm^2$ energy density was not enough for the acceptable polymerization rate of conventional flowable restorative samples in a 4-mm layer thickness; meanwhile, the decrease of layer thickness to 2 mm increased the polymerization rate with 61.5%. In the case of bulk fill XB and FBF, the extended curing time resulted in a 15.5% and a 40.7% increase in the rate of polymerization. In contrast with our findings, Finan *et al.* [19] observed higher DC% for SDR (59%) and XB (48%) using a quartz tungsten halogen (QTH) light curing unit (LCU) for polymerization, which operates at an output intensity of 650 mW/cm^2 for 20 s; while Zorzin *et al.* [41] measured a 52% DC value for SDR, 63% for XB, 66% for FBF and 66% for FUF at a 4-mm layer thickness cured with an LED unit (1200 mW/cm^2) for 20 s in the case of A2 shades. The possible explanation for this difference may be that wider samples in diameter were used to allow a higher degree of light penetration for polymerization or that Fourier transform infrared spectrophotometer was used to analyze the DC of RBC samples. However, Zorzin *et al.* concluded that extended curing time (30 s) had a positive effect on polymerization properties, so enhanced light curing of bulk-fills in deep cavities is recommended [41]. Similarly to our study, Li *et al.* [39] used micro-Raman spectroscopy to map the DC along a cross-section of bulk-fill and a conventional composite block. They measured 80% mean maximum DC for FBF and 77.3% for SDR; however, their study design was different from our design, as the investigators tested the curing profile of a thicker (16 mm × 6 mm × 12 mm) rectangular bulk-fill RBC block.

Besides the filler-matrix ratio, the DC is affected by the viscosity and reactivity of the polymerizable monomer, as well [42]. The DC of different monomer systems increases in the following order: BisGMA < BisEMA < UDMA < TEGDMA [43]. BisGMA is considered the most viscous monomer due to the strong intramolecular hydrogen bonding, which can decrease the reactivity and mobility of the monomer during the polymerization process. This might be one of the explanations for the significantly lower DC of the conventional flowable FUF_4mm_20s than that of other materials, as FUF contains the highest amount of BisGMA monomer in the resin matrix. In our study, the investigated bulk-fill RBCs are UDMA-based materials in combination with different types of monomers. Sideridou *et al.* found that UDMA, combining relatively high molecular weight with a high concentration of double bonds and low viscosity, was shown to reach higher final DC% values than BisGMA [43]. Low viscosity has a high impact on free radical migration. It was proven that the DC of RBC monomers is strongly influenced by the nature of the polymerizing monomers, for example more flexible monomers increase the rate of conversion [44]. Although the viscosity of UDMA is much lower than that of BisGMA, when it is mixed with the high molecular weight BisEMA or EBPADMA, it can significantly restrict the mobility of UDMA monomers and decrease their reactivity and conversion value [37,45]. This may explain the significantly lower DC value of FBF and XB cured for both 10 and 20 s than that of SDR_4mm_20s, as was reported by Alshali *et al.* [37]. SDR is similarly an UDMA/EBPADMA-based bulk-fill flowable composite; however, it contains TEGDMA, which has a synergistic effect on the rate of polymerization, and thus, the DC value of this monomer is significantly higher than that of the other investigated bulk-fill materials.

In addition, according to the manufacturer's technical information, a photo-active modulator in SDR may cooperate with camphorquinone (CQ), thereby facilitating polymerization.

In the present study, monomer elution from RBC was quantified using HPLC. This is a standard method used for the determination of monomer elution from RBCs [46]. The release of components has a potential effect on the structural stability and wear rate, as well as the biocompatibility of the material. The analysis of the elution of selected unreacted BisGMA, TEGDMA and UDMA will not provide an absolute measure of the quality of released components; thus, it is a limitation of this study.

Several factors may influence the monomer elution, such as the rate of polymerization, the chemical features of the solvent and the chemical nature of the leached components [5,47]. In the present study, 75% ethanol was used to extract most of the examined unreacted monomers from the polymerized composite samples in order to identify monomer quantity. The elution pattern of unreacted monomers is higher in ethanol than in water storage medium, because of their hydrophobic character, which can significantly reduce and rationalize examination periods. Water storage may simulate oral conditions better than ethanol; however, changeful oral parameters (pH, temperature, enzyme activities) are hardly simulated in water medium. According to our results there was a strong correlation between DC% and the amount of eluted monomers in the case of the conventional flowable RBC (FUF). This is a BisGMA/TEGDMA/procrylate-based material, and the highest amount of leached TEGDMA and BisGMA was observed with the lowest DC%. Meanwhile, the reduced layer thickness decreased the amount of released TEGDMA and BisGMA by five- and two-times, respectively. The possible reasons for the different values for these monomers could be the chemical nature, the different molecular weight and the reactivity of the molecules. Tanaka *et al.* [48] found that TEGDMA has higher mobility caused by its low molecular weight, resulting in a higher and faster rate of elution than the larger BisGMA and UDMA [47,48]. As a TEGDMA/UDMA-based material, SDR showed a high amount of TEGDMA release following FUF_4mm_20s. Similar to our findings, Cebe *et al.* also found a higher amount of eluted TEGDMA monomers than from the other bulk-fills, and the cumulative amount of eluted TEGDMA increased with time [49]. In their study, Łagocka *et al.* detected lower (8.4 μg/g) TEGDMA elution from SDR during the first 24 h of storage in 75% ethanol solvent; however, the elution rate rapidly decreased with time [50]. The reason for the increased elution of the high molecular weight BisGMA could be the low rate of polymerization explained by the hampered light penetration and the decreased photoinitiator activation in the conventional flowable composite at a 4-mm layer thickness. Among bulk-fill composites, FBF showed the highest rate of released UDMA and BisGMA. Cebe *et al.* also detected a higher rate of eluted BisGMA from FBF, especially at the 30-day time interval [49].

Considering the filler content, FBF has the lowest filler value among the investigated bulk-fill materials, which may influence the release of unreacted monomers. Comparing the molecular weight of BisGMA and UDMA, BisGMA has a higher weight; thus, there is quicker and more substantial

UDMA release in a certain time interval. Among bulk fills, XB showed a significantly lower rate of eluted monomers. The lower solubility might be based on the higher (75%) filler content in contrast with the other bulk-fills. There are reports that illustrate a lower absorption rate in composite materials with high filler contents compared to materials with lower filler content [51–53]. The results of the present study, which are in line with these reports, showed a lower monomer elution rate from XB with higher filler content compared to the other investigated bulk-fills. The possible explanation might be the lower solvent absorption in XB samples, which resulted in less leachable component elution. This leads to the conclusion that the elution mechanism is complex and cannot be explained only by the degree of conversion. On the other hand, Sideridou *et al.* concluded that higher silane content has a positive effect on interfacial adhesion between filler and matrix [54]. As the filler particles are chemically bonded to the matrix monomers and oligomers by the silane coupling agent, their higher volume fraction can provide a more stable ligation for the unreacted, leachable monomers, decreasing their release into the solvent. The structure of the silane coupling agent and its bonding to the filler particle has a high impact on the solubility of the RBC [55].

The detected BisGMA from the XB samples might be impurities of the monomer matrix complex.

Considering the BisEMA content in the investigated bulk-fill materials, there was no information from the degree of ethoxylation of the bisphenol A molecule; therefore, it was not possible to identify in the lack of standard monomer. Compared to other composite resin monomers, BisEMA is not a single monomer molecule, rather belonging to a large series of ethoxylated bisphenol A-based dimethacrylates with an ethoxylation reaction of a very reactive ethylene oxide [56,57]. Therefore, the ethoxylation reaction is unselective and difficult to control, leading to different ethoxylated products and byproducts, which must be separated analytically [58].

4. Materials and Methods

BisGMA (98%), UDMA (⩾97%) and TEGDMA (95%) (Sigma-Aldrich, Steinheim, Germany) were used as standard materials for the identification of the monomer peaks in the chromatograms. Filtek Ultimate Flow flowable nanocomposite samples were prepared as references. The investigated materials were the following: SureFil SDR Flow, X-tra Base and Filtek Bulk Fill. Table 1 shows the composition of the materials. All samples were stored in a 75% ethanol/water solution (Spektrum-3D, Debrecen, Hungary). Acetonitrile (ACN) (VWR International, Leuven, Belgium) was used for the preparation of the mobile phase for the HPLC separation.

Table 1. Materials, manufactures and composition.

Group	Material	Code	Manufacturer	Shade	Organic Matrix	Filler	Filler Loading	LOT Number
Bulk-fill composite	SureFil SDR Flow	SDR	Dentsply Caulk, Milford, DE, USA	U	Modified UDMA, EBPADMA, TEGDMA	Ba-Al-F-B silicate glass, Sr-Al-F silicate glass	68 wt %	1202174
	x-tra base	XB	Voco, Cuxhaven, Germany	U	UDMA, BisEMA	no information	75 wt %	1305261
	Filtek Bulk Fill	FBF	3M ESPE, St Paul, MN, USA	U	BisGMA, UDMA, BisEMA(6), TEGDMA, substituated dimethacrylate, Procrylat resin	silane treated zirconia/silica, ytterbium trifluoride	64.5 wt %	N414680
Conventional flowable composite	Filtek Ultimate Flow	FUF	3M ESPE, St Paul, MN, USA	A2	BisGMA, TEGDMA, substituated dimethacrylate, Procrylat resin	silane treated zirconia/silica, ytterbium trifluoride	65 wt %	N652740

Abbreviations: U, universal; UDMA, urethane dimethacrylate; EBPADMA, ethoxylated Bisphenol A dimethacrylate; TEGDMA, triethylene glycol dimethacrylate; BisEMA, Bisphenol A polyethylene glycol diether dimethacrylate; BisGMA, Bisphenol A diglycidil ether dimethacrylate; Procrylate, reacted polycaprolactone polymer. Missing entries are not specified by the manufacturer.

4.1. Preparation of the Composite Resin Specimens

The flowable bulk-fill RBCs (SDR, XB, FBF) were poured into a stainless steel mold with a size of 3 mm in diameter × 4 mm in thickness ($n = 3 \times 5$) and positioned on a glass slide. As the negative control, conventional flowable composite (FUF) samples were used also with a size of 3 mm in diameter × 4 mm in thickness ($n = 5$) to be comparable with bulk-fill RBCs and with a size of 3 mm in diameter × 2 mm in thickness ($n = 5$) as a positive control. During preparation, each sample was measured to obtain samples of similar weight and volume. The top and the bottom of the RBC were covered with a polyester (Mylar, Dentamerica Inc., San Jose Ave, CA, USA) strip in order to avoid contact with oxygen, which is an inhibitor of the polymerization. The specimens were irradiated with a light-emitting diode (LED) curing unit (λ = 420–480 nm; LED.C, Woodpecker, Guilin, China) with the recommended exposure time at a light intensity of 1100 mW$\cdot$cm^{-2} with an irradiated diameter of 10 mm. The manufacturer's instruction for curing time at a 4-mm thickness and universal shades is 10 s in FBF and XB bulk-fill RBCs. In the case of these two materials, the effect of extended curing time (20 s) was also investigated. For SDR, the recommended exposure time is 20 s without giving a suggested value for the light intensity. In the case of A2 shade conventional flowable RBC, a 20-s exposure time at a 2-mm thickness is recommended; however, to investigate and to compare the DC value and the amount of released monomers, this product was also used in a 4-mm thickness and was irradiated only for 20 s. Table 2 summarizes the abbreviations of the prepared samples.

Table 2. Sample preparation with layer thickness and exposure time.

Abbreviation	Material	Layer Thickness (mm)	Exposure Time (s)
FUF_2mm_20s	Filtek Ultimate Flow	2	20
FUF_4mm_20s	Filtek Ultimate Flow	4	20
FBF_4mm_10s	Filtek Bulk Fill	4	10
FBF_4mm_20s	Filtek Bulk Fill	4	20
XB_4mm_10s	X-tra Base	4	10
XB_4mm_20s	X-tra Base	4	20
SDR_4mm_20s	SureFil SDR Flow	4	20

A radiometer (SDS, Kerr, Danbury, CT, USA) was used to control the intensity of the curing unit before and after the light exposition. The tip of the curing light guide was positioned parallel and 1 mm above the composite sample. One day after polymerization, the specimens were measured with micro-Raman spectroscopy. For the dissolution of the unreacted monomers the specimens were stored in 1 mL of 75% ethanol/water solution for 72 h in darkness at room temperature. After 3 days, the amount of dissolved unpolymerized monomers was analyzed with reverse-phase high-performance liquid chromatography (RP-HPLC) from the ethanol solutions.

4.2. Micro-Raman Spectroscopy Measurement

The polymerized composite samples were examined using a Labram HR 800 Confocal Raman spectrometer (HORIBA JobinYvon S.A.S., Longjumeau Cedex, France) 24 h after polymerization. During the micro-Raman measurements, a 20-mW He-Ne laser with a 632.817-nm wavelength was applied; the spatial resolution was ~1.5 μm; the spectral resolution was ~2.5 cm^{-1}; with magnification of 100× (Olympus UK Ltd., London, UK), applying a D 0.3 filter (~1.98 mW on the sample). The spectra were taken on the top and also on the bottom surface of the composite specimens at three random locations. The integration time was 10 s, and ten acquisitions were averaged for each geometrical point. Uncured composite spectra were measured as a reference. These samples were placed between two non-fluorescent glass slides. Post-processing of spectra was performed using the dedicated software LabSpec 5.0 (HORIBA JobinYvon S.A.S., Longjumeau Cedex, France), and the Levenberg–Marquardt non-linear peak fitting method was applied for the best fit [59,60]. The following equation was used to calculate the ratio of the double-bond content of monomer to polymer in the composite:

$$DC\% = \left(1 - \left(\frac{R_{\text{cured}}}{R_{\text{uncured}}}\right)\right) \times 100 \quad (1)$$

where R is the ratio of aromatic and aliphatic C=C bonds at peak intensities of 1639 cm^{-1} and 1609 cm^{-1} in cured and uncured composite samples, respectively [43,61].

4.3. RP-HPLC Measurements

The RP-UHPLC system (Dionex Ultimate 3000, Thermo Fisher Scientific Inc, Sunnyvale, CA, USA) consists of a Dionex LPG 3400 SD gradient pump, Dionex ACC 3000 autosampler and a Dionex UWD 3400 RS UV–VIS detector (Dionex GmbH, Germering, Germany). Data acquisition was completed using Chromeleon software integrated in Hystar (version: 3.2). The separations were performed on a Synergi HYDRO-RP (particle size: 4 μm; pore size: 8) (Phenomenex, Gen-Lab, Budapest, Hungary) column (150 mm × 2.00 mm) with gradient elution. The composition of Eluent "A" was 40% *v*/*v* ACN in bidistilled water, whereas Mobile Phase "B" was composed of 95% *v*/*v* ACN and 5% bidistilled water. During the 30-min chromatographic separation, the "B" eluent content increased from 20%–100%. The low rate was 0.3 mL· min^{-1}. As the regeneration of the stationary phase, Mobile Phase B content was decreased from 100% down to 20% in 1 min, and after 31–46 min, the system was washed with 20% "A".

The detection of the eluted monomers was at the following wavelengths: 205, 215, 227 and 254 nm. Two hundred five nanometers was found to be optimal; therefore, the evaluation relied on the data collected at this wavelength. Each separation was implemented at room temperature.

The amount of the eluted monomers was calculated by the calibration curve with the areas under the curve of peaks produced by the monomers, respectively. The TEGDMA, UDMA and BisGMA standard solutions had retention times of 2.95, 5.08 and 6.88 min, respectively, whereas the peaks were well separated from each other.

4.4. Validation of the Monomer Determination the Limit of Detection and the Limit of Quantification

The detection limit (determined as the amount of monomers giving a peak height 5-times higher than the noise level) of TEGDMA is 0.018 pmol (5.19 pg), UDMA, 0.015 pmol (7.196 pg), and BisGMA, 0.007 pmol (3.556 pg). The quantification limit of the method (the peak height of the monomers 10-times higher than the noise level) was low for TEGDMA is 0.036 pmol (10.382 pg), for UDMA, 0.031 pmol (14.392 pg), and for BisGMA, 0.014 pmol (7.1120 pg). Calibration was carried out in the range of 1–50.0 μg· mL^{-1} monomers, respectively. A calibration curve was plotted by the measurement of standard solutions at 205 nm (R^2) 0.9924 for TEGDMA, 0.9966 for UDMA and 0.9996 for BisGMA, respectively. All injections were repeated three times.

4.5. Statistical Analysis

The statistical analysis was performed using SPSS (Statistical Package for Social Science, SPSS Inc., Chicago, IL, USA) software for Windows. The values for the degree of conversion and for residual monomers between the studied test groups were compared by a one-way analysis of variance (ANOVA) test followed by Dunnett's t-test at the $\alpha = 0.05$ level.

5. Conclusions

Within the limitation of the present study, the following can be concluded:

(1) Among the investigated low viscosity bulk fill and conventional flowable RBCs, SDR showed the highest DC value at the top and bottom surface of the samples.
(2) The DC values of the 4 mm-thick bulk-fill composites SDR, FBF, XB were significantly higher than that of the 4 mm-thick conventional composite (negative control) studied; meanwhile, only

SDR bulk-fill resulted in a higher DC value compared to that of the 2 mm-thick conventional flowable RBC (positive control).

(3) Although the recommended exposure time by the manufacturers for the universal shade FBF and XB is 10 s (with a 1000-mW/cm^2 curing unit), extended (20 s) curing time significantly increased the DC% value.

(4) The amount of released BisGMA and TEGDMA monomers from the bulk-fill composite materials was generally lower than from the conventional composite.

(5) Among bulk fills, in spite of the highest DC%, SDR showed the highest rate of TEGDMA elution; meanwhile, the highest amount of UDMA was eluted from FBF.

Acknowledgments: This work was supported by Pécsi Tudományegyetem Általános Orvostudományi Kar-Kutatási Alap 2013/5 and Pécsi Tudományegyetem Általános Orvostudományi Kar-Kutatási Alap-2016/1 Research Grants. The present scientific contribution is dedicated to the 650th anniversary of the foundation of the University of Pécs, Hungary.

Author Contributions: Edina Lempel conceived of and designed the experiments and wrote the paper. Zsuzsanna Czibulya and Bálint Kovács performed the micro-Raman spectroscopy measurements. József Szalma and Ákos Tóth analyzed the data. Sándor Kunsági-Máté contributed analysis tools. Zoltán Varga prepared the samples. Katalin Böddi designed experiments and performed the HPLC measurements.

Abbreviations

DC	degree of conversion
HPLC	high performance liquid chromatography
RP-HPLC	reverse-phase high-performance liquid chromatography
SDR	SureFil SDR Flow
XB	X-tra Base
FBF	Filtek Bulk Fill
FUF	Filtek Ultimate Flow
FUF_2mm_20s	Filtek Ultimate Flow in a 2-mm layer thickness cured for 20 s
FUF_4mm_20s	Filtek Ultimate Flow in a 4-mm layer thickness cured for 20 s
FBF_4mm_10s	4 mm-thick Filtek Bulk Fill light cured for 10 s
FBF_4mm_20s	4 mm-thick Filtek Bulk Fill light cured for 20 s
XB_4mm_10s	4 mm-thick X-tra Base light cured for 10 s
XB_4mm_20s	4 mm-thick X-tra Base light cured for 20 s
SDR_4mm_20s	SureFil SDR Flow in a 4-mm layer thickness cured for 20 s
UDMA	urethane dimethacrylate
BisGMA	bisphenol A diglycidyl ether dimethacrylate
TEGDMA	triethylene glycol dimethacrylate
BisEMA	bisphenol A polyethylene glycol diether dimethacrylate
EBPADMA	ethoxylated bisphenol A dimethacrylate
RBC	resin-based composite
SD	standard deviation
QTH	quartz tungsten halogen
LCU	light curing unit
CQ	camphorquinone
CAN	acetonitrile
LED	light emitting diode
LOD	limit of detection
LOQ	limit of quantification

1. Da Rosa Rodolpho, P.A.; Donassollo, T.A.; Cenci, M.S.; Loguércio, A.D.; Moraes, R.R.; Bronkhorst, E.M.; Opdam, N.J.M.; Demarco, F.F. 22-year clinical evaluation of the performance of two posterior composites with different filler characteristics. *Dent. Mater.* **2011**, *27*, 955–963. [CrossRef] [PubMed]
2. Lempel, E.; Tóth, Á.; Fábián, T.; Krajczár, K.; Szalma, J. Retrospective evaluation of posterior direct composite restorations: 10-Year findings. *Dent. Mater.* **2015**, *31*, 115–122. [CrossRef] [PubMed]
3. Opdam, N.J.M.; Bronkhorst, E.M.; Loomans, B.A.; Hujsmans, M.C. 12-year survival of composite *vs.* amalgam restorations. *J. Dent. Res.* **2010**, *89*, 1063–1067. [CrossRef] [PubMed]
4. Pallesen, U.; van Dijken, J.W.V.; Halken, J.; Hallosten, A.L.; Höigaard, R. Longevity of posterior resin composite restorations in permanent teeth in Public Dental Health Service: A prospective 8 years follow up. *J. Dent.* **2013**, *41*, 297–306. [CrossRef] [PubMed]
5. Ferracane, J.L. Elution of leachable components from composites. *J. Oral Rehabil.* **1994**, *21*, 441–452. [CrossRef] [PubMed]
6. Ferracane, J.L.; Greener, E.H. The effect of resin formulation on the degree of conversion and mechanical properties of dental restorative resins. *J. Biomed. Mater. Res.* **1986**, *20*, 121–131. [CrossRef] [PubMed]
7. Lempel, E.; Czibulya, Z.; Kunsági-Máté, S.; Szalma, J.; Sümegi, B.; Böddi, K. Quantification of conversion degree and monomer elution from dental composite using HPLC and micro-raman spectroscopy. *Chromatographia* **2014**, *77*, 1137–1144. [CrossRef]
8. Poggio, C.; Lombardini, M.; Gaviati, S.; Chiesa, M. Evaluation of Vickers hardness and depth of cure of six composite resins photo-activated with different polymerization modes. *J. Conserv. Dent.* **2012**, *15*, 237–241. [CrossRef] [PubMed]
9. Silikas, N.; Eliades, G.; Watts, D.C. Light intensity effects on resin-composite degree of conversion and shrinkage strain. *Dent. Mater.* **2000**, *16*, 292–296. [CrossRef]
10. Turssi, C.P.; Ferracane, J.L.; Vogel, K. Filler features and their effects on wear and degree of conversion of particulate dental resin composites. *Biomaterials* **2005**, *26*, 4932–4937. [CrossRef] [PubMed]
11. Ilie, N.; Jelen, E.; Hickel, R. Is the soft-start polymerization concept still relevant for modern curing units? *Clin. Oral Investig.* **2011**, *15*, 21–29. [CrossRef] [PubMed]
12. Alomari, Q.D.; Reinhardt, J.W.; Boyer, D.B. Effect of liners on cusp deflection and gap formation in composite restorations. *Oper. Dent.* **2001**, *26*, 406–411. [PubMed]
13. Park, J.; Chang, J.; Ferracane, J.; Lee, I.B. How should composite be layered to reduce shrinkage stress: Incremental or bulk filling. *Dent. Mater.* **2008**, *24*, 1501–1505. [CrossRef] [PubMed]
14. Obici, A.C.; Sinhoreti, M.A.C.; Frollini, E.; Correr-Sobrinho, L.; Fernando de Goes, M.; Henriques, G.E.P. Monomer conversion at different dental composite depths using six light-curing methods. *Polym. Test.* **2006**, *25*, 282–288. [CrossRef]
15. Watts, D.C.; Cash, A.J. Analysis of optical transmission by 400–500 nm visible light into aesthetic dental biomaterials. *J. Dent.* **1994**, *22*, 112–117. [CrossRef]
16. Flury, S.; Hayoz, S.; Peutzfeldt, A.; Hüsler, J.; Lussi, A. Depth of cure of resin composites: Is the ISO 4049 method suitable for bulk fill materials? *Dent. Mater.* **2012**, *28*, 521–528. [CrossRef] [PubMed]
17. El-Safty, S.; Silikas, N.; Watts, D.C. Creep deformation of restorative resin-composites intended for bulk-fill placement. *Dent. Mater.* **2012**, *28*, 928–935. [CrossRef] [PubMed]
18. Bucuta, S.; Ilie, N. Light transmittance and micro-mechanical properties of bulk fill vs. conventional resin based composites. *Clin. Oral Investig.* **2014**, *18*, 1991–2000. [CrossRef] [PubMed]
19. Finan, L.; Palin, W.M.; Moskwa, N.; McGinley, E.L.; Fleming, G.J.P. The influence of irradiation potential on the degree of conversion and mechanical properties of two bulk-fill flowable RBC base materials. *Dent. Mater.* **2013**, *29*, 906–912. [CrossRef] [PubMed]
20. Van Ende, A.; De Munch, J.; Van Landuyt, K.L.; Poitevin, A.; Peumans, M.; Van Meerbeek, B. Bulk-filling of high C-factor posterior cavities, effect on adhesion to cavity bottom dentin. *Dent. Mater.* **2013**, *29*, 269–277. [CrossRef] [PubMed]
21. Campodonico, C.E.; Tantbirojn, D.; Olin, P.S.; Versluis, A. Cuspal deflection and depth of cure in resin-based composite restorations filled by using bulk; incremental and transtooth illumination techniques. *J. Am. Dent. Assoc.* **2011**, *142*, 1176–1182. [CrossRef] [PubMed]

22. Roggendorf, M.J.; Kramer, N.; Appelt, A.; Naumann, M.; Frankenberger, R. Marginal quality of flowable 4-mm base vs conventionally layered resin composite. *J. Dent.* **2011**, *39*, 643–647. [CrossRef] [PubMed]
23. Ilie, N.; Hickel, R. Investigations on a methacrylate-based flowable composite based on the SDR™ technology. *Dent. Mater.* **2011**, *27*, 348–355. [CrossRef] [PubMed]
24. Moorthy, A.; Hogg, C.H.; Dowling, A.H.; Grufferty, B.F.; Benetti, A.R.; Fleming, G.J.P. Cuspal deflection and microleakage in premolar teeth restored with bulk-fill flowable resin-based composite base materials. *J. Dent.* **2012**, *40*, 500–505. [CrossRef] [PubMed]
25. Czasch, P.; Ilie, N. *In vitro comparison* of mechanical properties and degree of cure of *bulk fill* composites. *Clin. Oral Investig.* **2013**, *17*, 227–235. [CrossRef] [PubMed]
26. Van Dijken, J.W.V.; Pallesen, U. A randomized controlled three year evaluation of "bulk-filled" posterior resin restorations based on stress decreased resin technology. *Dent. Mater.* **2014**, *30*, 245–251. [CrossRef] [PubMed]
27. Goldberg, M. *In vitro* and *in vivo* studies on the toxicity of dental resin components, a review. *Clin. Oral Investig.* **2008**, *12*, 1–8. [CrossRef] [PubMed]
28. Bakopoulou, A.; Mourelatos, D.; Tsiftsoglou, A.S.; Giassin, N.P.; Mioglou, E.; Garefis, P. Genotoxic and cytotoxic effects of different types of dental cement on normal cultured human lymphocytes. *Mutat. Res.* **2009**, *672*, 103–112. [CrossRef] [PubMed]
29. Silva, G.S.; Almeida, G.S.; Poskus, L.T.; Guimarães, J.G. Relationship between the degree of conversion; solubility and salivary sorption of a hybrid and nanofilled resin composite: Influence of the light activation mode. *Appl. Oral Sci.* **2008**, *16*, 161–166. [CrossRef]
30. Cramer, N.B.; Stansbury, J.W.; Bowman, C.N. Recent advances and developments in composite dental restorative materials. *J. Dent. Res.* **2011**, *90*, 402–416. [CrossRef] [PubMed]
31. Leprince, J.G.; Palin, W.M.; Hadis, M.A.; Devaux, J.; Leloup, G. Progress in dimethacrylate-based dental composite technology and curing efficiency. *Dent. Mater.* **2013**, *29*, 139–156. [CrossRef] [PubMed]
32. Alrahlah, A.; Silikas, N.; Watts, D.C. Post-cure depth of cure of bulk fill dental resin-composites. *Dent. Mater.* **2014**, *30*, 149–154. [CrossRef] [PubMed]
33. Shortall, A.C. How light source and product shade influence cure depth for a contemporary composite. *J. Oral Rehabil.* **2005**, *32*, 906–911. [CrossRef] [PubMed]
34. Lee, Y.K. Influence of filler on difference between the transmitted and reflected colors of experimental resin composites. *Dent. Mater.* **2008**, *24*, 1243–1247. [CrossRef] [PubMed]
35. Halvorson, R.H.; Erickson, R.L.; Davidson, C.L. The effect of filler and silane content on conversion of resin-based composite. *Dent. Mater.* **2003**, *19*, 327–333. [CrossRef]
36. Nomoto, R.; Hirasawa, T. Residual monomer and pendant methacryloyl group in light-cured composite resins. *Dent. Mater. J.* **1992**, *11*, 177–188. [CrossRef] [PubMed]
37. Alshali, R.Z.; Silikas, N.; Satterthwaite, J.D. Degree of conversion of bulk-fill compared to conventional resin-composites at two time intervals. *Dent. Mater.* **2013**, *29*, 213–217. [CrossRef] [PubMed]
38. Tarle, Z.; Attin, T.; Marovic, D.; Andermatt, L.; Ristic, M.; Tauböck, T.T. Influence of irradiation time on subsurface degree of conversion and microhardness of high-viscosity bulk-fill resin composites. *Clin. Oral Investig.* **2015**, *19*, 831–840. [CrossRef] [PubMed]
39. Li, X.; Pongprueksa, P.; van Meerbeek, B.; de Munk, J. Curing profile of bulk-fill resin-based composites. *J. Dent.* **2015**, *43*, 664–672. [CrossRef] [PubMed]
40. Emami, N.; Söderholm, K.J.M. How light irradiance and curing time affect monomer conversion in light-cured resin composites. *Eur. J. Oral Sci.* **2003**, *111*, 536–542. [CrossRef] [PubMed]
41. Zorzin, J.; Maier, E.; Harre, S.; Fey, T.; Belli, R.; Lohbauer, U.; Petschelt, A.; Taschner, M. Bulk-fill resin composites: Polymerization properties and extended light curing. *Dent. Mater.* **2015**, *31*, 293–301. [CrossRef] [PubMed]
42. Baroudi, K.; Saleh, A.M.; Silikas, N.; Watts, D.C. Shrinkage behaviour of flowable resin-composites related to conversion and filler-fraction. *J. Dent.* **2007**, *35*, 651–655. [CrossRef] [PubMed]
43. Sideridou, I.D.; Karabela, M.M. Effect of the amount of 3-methacryloxypropyltrimethoxysilane coupling agent on physical properties of dental resin nanocomposites. *Dent. Mater.* **2009**, *25*, 1315–1324. [CrossRef] [PubMed]
44. Asmussen, E.; Peutzfeldt, A. Influence of UEDMA, BisGMA and TEGDMA on selected mechanical properties of experimental resin composites. *Dent. Mater.* **1998**, *14*, 51–56. [CrossRef]

45. Khatri, C.A.; Stansbury, J.W.; Schultheisz, C.R.; Antonucci, J.M. Synthesis characterization and evaluation of urethane derivates of Bis-GMA. *Dent. Mater.* **2003**, *19*, 584–588. [CrossRef]
46. Uzunova, Y.; Lukanov, L.; Filipov, I.; Vladimirov, S. High-performance liquid chromatographic determination of unreacted monomers and other residues contained in dental composites. *J. Biomech. Biophys. Methods* **2008**, *70*, 883–888. [CrossRef] [PubMed]
47. Caughmann, W.F.; Caughmann, G.B.; Shiflett, R.; Rueggeberg, F.; Schuster, G. Correlation of cytotoxicity, filler loading and curing time of dental composites. *Biomaterials* **1991**, *12*, 737–740. [CrossRef]
48. Tanaka, K.; Taira, M.; Shintani, H.; Wakasa, K.; Yamaki, M. Residual monomers (TEGDMA and Bis-GMA) of a set visible-light-cured dental composite resin when immersed in water. *J. Oral Rehabil.* **1991**, *18*, 353–362. [CrossRef] [PubMed]
49. Cebe, M.A.; Cebe, F.; Cengiz, M.F.; Cetin, A.R.; Arpag, O.F.; Ozturk, B. Elution of monomer from different bulk fill dental composite resin. *Dent. Mater.* **2015**, *31*, 141–149. [CrossRef] [PubMed]
50. Łagocka, R.; Jakubowska, K.; Chlubek, D.; Buczkowska-Radlińska, J. Elution study of unreacted TEGDMA from bulk-fill composite (SDR™ Dentsply) using HPLC. *Adv. Med. Sci.* **2015**, *60*, 191–198. [CrossRef] [PubMed]
51. Ortengren, U.; Wellendorf, H.; Karlsson, S.; Ruyter, IE. Water sorption and solubility of dental composites and identification of monomers released in an aqueous environment. *J. Oral Rehabil.* **2001**, *28*, 1106–1115. [CrossRef] [PubMed]
52. Braden, M.; Clarke, R.L. Water absorption characteristics of dental microfine composite filling materials. I. Proprietary materials. *Biomaterials* **1984**, *5*, 369–372. [CrossRef]
53. Braden, M.; Davy, K.W.M. Water absorption characteristics of some unfilled resins. *Biomaterials* **1986**, *7*, 474–475. [CrossRef]
54. Sideridou, I.; Tserki, V.; Papanastasiou, G. Effect of chemical structure on degree of conversion in light-cured dimethacrylate-based dental resins. *Biomaterials* **2002**, *23*, 1819–1829. [CrossRef]
55. Karabela, M.M.; Sideridou, I.D. Effect of the structure of silane coupling agent on sorption characteristics of solvents by dental resin-nanocomposites. *Dent. Mater.* **2008**, *24*, 1631–1639. [CrossRef] [PubMed]
56. Alshali, R.Z.; Salim, N.A.; Sung, R.; Satterthwaite, J.D.; Silikas, N. Qualitative and quantitative characterization of monomers of uncured bulk-fill and conventional resin-composites using liquid chromatography/mass spectrometry. *Dent. Mater.* **2015**, *31*, 711–720. [CrossRef] [PubMed]
57. Smith, M.B.; March, J. *March's Advanced Organic Chemistry, Reactions, Mechanisms and Structure*, 6th ed.; John Wiley & Sons: Hoboken, NJ, USA, 2007.
58. Durner, J.; Schrickel, K.; Watts, D.C.; Ilie, N. Determination of homologous distributions of BisEMAdimethacrylates in bulk-fill resin-composites by GC-MS. *Dent. Mater.* **2015**, *31*, 473–480. [CrossRef] [PubMed]
59. Marquardt, D.W. An algorithm for least-squares estimation of nonlinear parameters. *J. Soc. Ind. Appl. Math.* **1963**, *11*, 431–441. [CrossRef]
60. Santini, A.; Miletic, V.; Koutsaki, D. Degree of conversion of three fissure sealants cured by different light curing units using micro-Raman spectroscopy. *J. Dent. Sci.* **2012**, *7*, 26–32. [CrossRef]
61. Ogliari, F.A.; Ely, C.; Zanchi, C.H.; Fortes, C.B.B.; Samuel, S.M.W.; Demarco, F.F.; Petzhold, C.L.; Piva, E. Influence of chain extender length of aromatic dimethacrylates on polymer network development. *Dent. Mater.* **2008**, *20*, 165–171. [CrossRef] [PubMed]

10

Modified Polymeric Nanoparticles Exert In Vitro Antimicrobial Activity Against Oral Bacteria

Manuel Toledano-Osorio [1], Jegdish P. Babu [2], Raquel Osorio [1,*], Antonio L. Medina-Castillo [3], Franklin García-Godoy [2] and Manuel Toledano [1]

1 Dental School, University of Granada, Campus de Cartuja s/n, 18071 Granada, Spain; toledano@correo.ugr.es (M.T.-O.); toledano@ugr.es (M.T.)
2 College of Dentistry, University of Tennessee Health Science Center, 875 Union Avenue, Memphis, TN 381632110, USA; jbabu@uthsc.edu (J.P.B.); fgarciagodoy@gmail.com (F.G.-G.)
3 NanoMyP, Spin-Off Enterprise from University of Granada, Edificio BIC-Granada, Av. Innovación 1, Armilla, 18016 Granada, Spain; amedina@nanomyp.com
* Correspondence: rosorio@ugr.es

Abstract: Polymeric nanoparticles were modified to exert antimicrobial activity against oral bacteria. Nanoparticles were loaded with calcium, zinc and doxycycline. Ions and doxycycline release were measured by inductively coupled plasma optical emission spectrometer and high performance liquid chromatography. *Porphyromonas gingivalis*, *Lactobacillus lactis*, *Streptoccocus mutans*, *gordonii* and *sobrinus* were grown and the number of bacteria was determined by optical density. Nanoparticles were suspended in phosphate-buffered saline (PBS) at 10, 1 and 0.1 mg/mL and incubated with 1.0 mL of each bacterial suspension for 3, 12, and 24 h. The bacterial viability was assessed by determining their ability to cleave the tetrazolium salt to a formazan dye. Data were analyzed by ANOVA and Scheffe's F ($p < 0.05$). Doxycycline doping efficacy was 70%. A burst liberation effect was produced during the first 7 days. After 21 days, a sustained release above 6 μg/mL, was observed. Calcium and zinc liberation were about 1 and 0.02 μg/mL respectively. The most effective antibacterial material was found to be the Dox-Nanoparticles (60% to 99% reduction) followed by Ca-Nanoparticles or Zn-Nanoparticles (30% to 70% reduction) and finally the non-doped nanoparticles (7% to 35% reduction). *P. gingivalis*, *S. mutans* and *L. lactis* were the most susceptible bacteria, being *S. gordonii* and *S. sobrinus* the most resistant to the tested nanoparticles.

Keywords: antibacterial; calcium; doxycycline; nanoparticles; zinc

1. Introduction

Bacteria are the main cause of prevalent oral diseases as caries and periodontitis. Oral administration of antibacterial agents presents an important limitation, as it is accessing the dentin interface, the radicular canal or the subgingival pockets where these bacteria grow. In these cases, benefits of local versus systemic delivery routes are clear [1]. This work explores the design of nanoparticles (NPs) that locally administered will exert therapeutic antibacterial properties against oral bacteria.

Resin-based restorative materials are commonly employed in clinical treatments to seal the interfaces and as a result, bonding to dentin is challenging [2]. Gaps at these bonded interfaces lead to microleakage, which also facilitate the invasion of cariogenic pathogens to cause secondary caries infections [2,3]. Therefore, in order to minimize the incidence of secondary caries, it would be desirable the existence of an antibacterial agent able to inhibit cariogenic pathogens at the dentin interface [4]. For this purpose, studying antibacterial effects against *Streptococcus mutans* (*Sm*), *Streptococcus gordonii* (*Sg*), *Streptococcus sobrinus* (*Ss*), and *Lactobacillus lactis* (*Ll*) have been recommended [3].

In endodontic treatment, elimination of bacteria in the root canal system, is a major challenge. Microorganisms remained after canal treatment will impair periapical healing and will facilitate developing apical lesions [5]. *Porphyromonas gingivalis* (*Pg*) is a major etiologic agent not only in the recurrent infections after endodontic treatment [6], but also in the development and progression of periapical lesions and periodontitis [7]. Biomaterials design leading to minimize the incidence of persistent or recurrent infections of the root canal system and apical periodontitis would also be desirable [8]. It is important to note that the biosafety of sodium hypochlorite during root canal treatment has been recently questioned [9].

Endogenous matrix metalloproteinases (MMPs) are interstitial collagenases present in radicular dentin, periodontal tissue and periapical bone [10–14]. MMPs have been related to chronic inflammation processes and abscesses at apical level [10,12]. Then MMPs inhibition will improve the prognosis of endodontic treatments [11]. Moreover, if resin-based materials are used for dentin bonding and tooth restoring, collagen degradation by MMPs will occur at the dentin interface jeopardizing restorations longevity [15]. When bonding to dentin in restorative dentistry, if dentin is infiltrated by MMP inhibitors, crystallite-sparse collagen fibrils of the scaffold could be protected from degradation facilitating further remineralization [2,16,17]. Metal nanoparticles (i.e., silver, gold, or zinc oxide . . .) have been previously introduced in restorative dentistry, mainly due to their antibacterial or MMPs inhibition properties [18–20].

Novel polymeric nanoparticles (NPs), about 100 nm in diameter, have been synthetized and previously tested at the resin-dentin bonded interface [17,21]. NPs have been shown to inhibit dentin MMPs collagen degradation [22], and to facilitate mineral growth at the interface without impairing bond strength [21,22]. Sequences of anionic carboxylate (i.e., COO^-) are along the backbone of the polymeric NPs. These functional groups permit the possibility of calcium and zinc quelation (1 μg Ca/mg NPs and 2.2 μg Zn/mg NPs) [23]. Cationic metals, loaded onto particles surfaces, if released, may provide for antimicrobial activity. Both metal cations have been demonstrated to have significant antibacterial effects [24,25]. Moreover, when NPs are larger than 10 nm, they do not penetrate bacteria membranes and are thought to exert further antimicrobial effects through accumulation on cell membranes [26]. At this stage, the bacterial membrane permeability may become compromised rendering the cell unable to regulate transport through it, and eventually causing cell death [27]. Doxycycline hyclate is also an antibacterial [28] and potent MMPs inhibitor [29] that is proposed to be immobilized on presented NPs.

Proposed NPs may be employed in three different dental clinical applications: (1) during the dentin bonding process, to exert antibacterial activity at the resin–dentin bonded interface [17,21]; (2) inside the radicular canal, during the endodontic treatment, to facilitate bacterial elimination; and (3) at the periodontal pocket, onto the cementum surface, to directly exert antibacterial activity [23].

Thus, the purpose of this *in vitro* study was to design and synthetize NPs doped with calcium/zinc ions or with immobilized doxycycline able to exert antibacterial activity against *Sm*, *Sg*, *Ss*, *Ll* and *Pg*. The null hypotheses to be tested are that: (1) Calcium, zinc and doxycycline are not liberated from NPs, and (2) NPs, calcium, zinc and doxycycline doped NPs do not affect bacterial viability.

2. Results

1. *Loading efficacy and release of doxycycline hyclate from NPs:* The amount of doxycycline in the aqueous solution before NPs immersion was 1333 μg/mL (per mg of NPs). In the supernatant, after NPs immersion, doxycycline concentration was 399.5 μg/mL (per mg of NPs). Loading efficacy was around 70%. Mean and standard deviation of doxycycline liberation (μg/mL) and cumulative liberation (%), per 10 mg of NPs at each time point are presented in Table 1. Doxycycline liberation was 106 μg/mL (per mg of NPs) at 12 h. A burst effect with rapid doxycycline liberation was observed from 12 h until the first week of storage. After 7 days, the antibiotic release was above 20 μg/mL (per mg of NPs). After 21 days, doxycycline liberation was stably sustained, being 8 and 6 μg/mL (per mg of NPs) at 21 and 28 days, respectively. After 24 h, a 57% of the immobilized doxycycline was

liberated, and after 7 days and 28 days, 72% and 80% of loaded antibiotic was respectively released (Table 1).

Table 1. Mean and standard deviation (SD) of Ca^{2+}, Zn^{2+} and doxycycline liberation in µg. Cumulative liberation (CL) was expressed in percentages. Values are obtained per 10 mg of NPs, at each time point.

Time	Ca^{2+} (µg)	Ca^{2+} CL (%)	Zn^{2+} (µg)	Zn^{2+} CL (%)	Doxycycline (µg)	Doxycycline CL (%)
12 h	1.006 (0.002)	11	0.025 (0.001)	0.1	1211.29 (166.32)	30
24 h	1.007 (0.001)	21	0.025 (0.001)	0.2	1065.98 (146.15)	57
48 h	0.909 (0.003)	30	0.023 (0.002)	0.3	458.08 (63.5)	68
7 days	0.856 (0.001)	39	0.021 (0.001)	0.4	210.81 (28.33)	74
21 days	2.082 (0.05)	61	0.024 (0.002)	0.5	81.85 (10.97)	78
28 days	2.031 (0.02)	82	0.044 (0.005)	0.8	63.23 (9.01)	80

2. *Calcium and zinc liberation from NPs:* Mean and standard deviation of Ca^{2+} and Zn^{2+} liberation (µg) and cumulative liberation (%), per 10 mg of NPs at each time point are presented in Table 1. Calcium liberation ranged from 0.856 to 1.007 µg (per 10 mg of NPs) during the first week. This calcium release was doubled after 21 d, being around 2 µg (per 10 mg of NPs). Zn-NPs maintained a sustained zinc liberation that ranged from 0.021 to 0.025 µg (per 10 mg of NPs) between 12 to 21 days. A double fold increase was observed at day 28, when 0.044 µg were released per each 10 mg of NPs.

3. *MTT assay:* Mean and standard deviations of the different bacteria survival values expressed as number of viable cells after 3, 12 and 24 h of exposure to the distinct NPs and control PBS are shown in Figures 1–5.

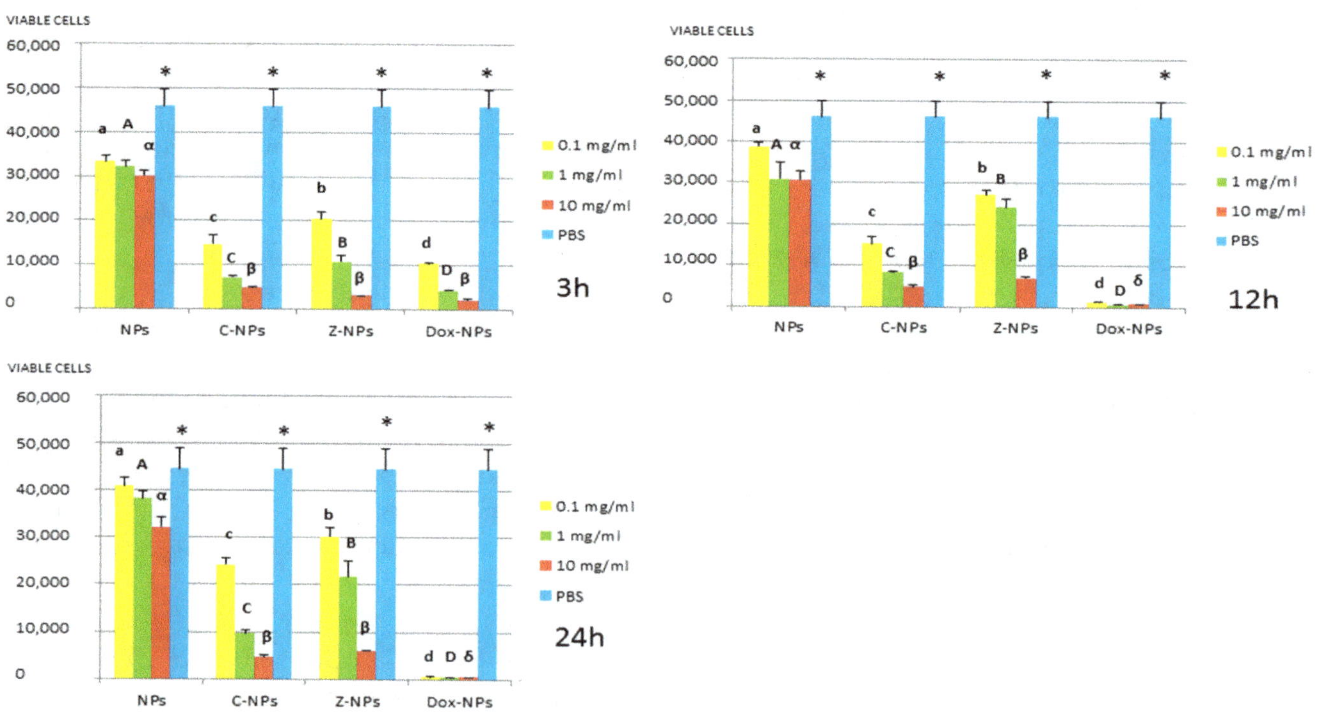

Figure 1. *P. gingivalis* survival (number of viable cells) after 3 h, 12 h, and 24 h of different concentration NPs exposure. Same letter or symbol indicates no significant difference of viable bacteria between different NPs concentrations ($p < 0.05$).

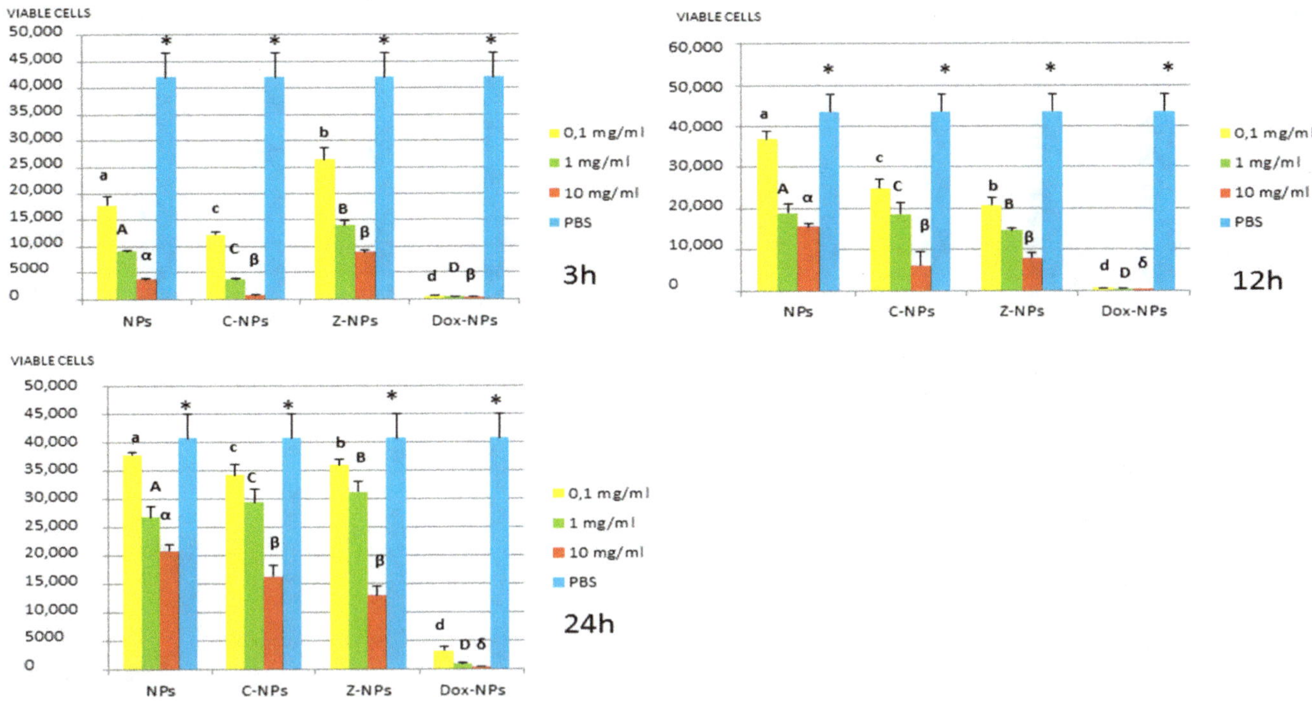

Figure 2. *S. mutans* survival (number of viable cells) after 3 h, 12 h, and 24 h of different concentration NPs exposure. Same letter or symbol indicates no significant difference of viable bacteria between different NPs concentrations ($p < 0.05$).

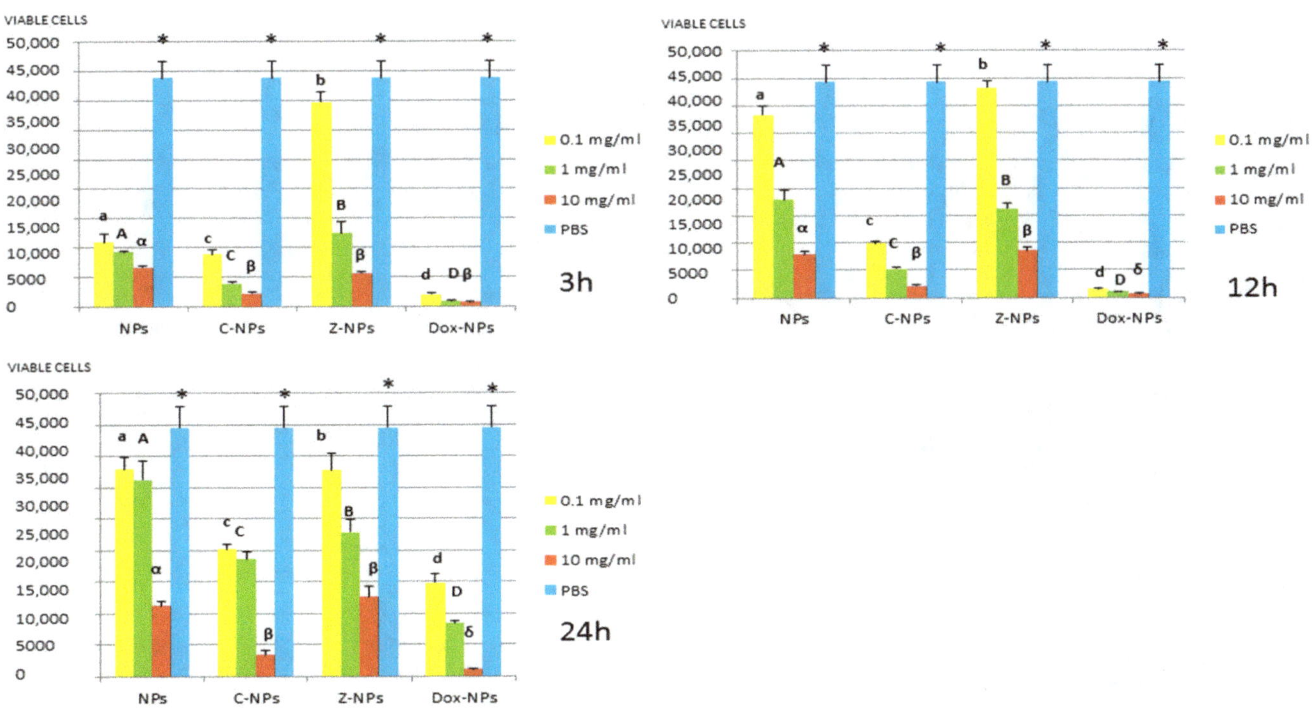

Figure 3. *L. lactis* survival (number of viable cells) after 3 h, 12 h, and 24 h of different concentration NPs exposure. Same letter or symbol indicates no significant difference of viable bacteria between different NPs concentrations ($p < 0.05$).

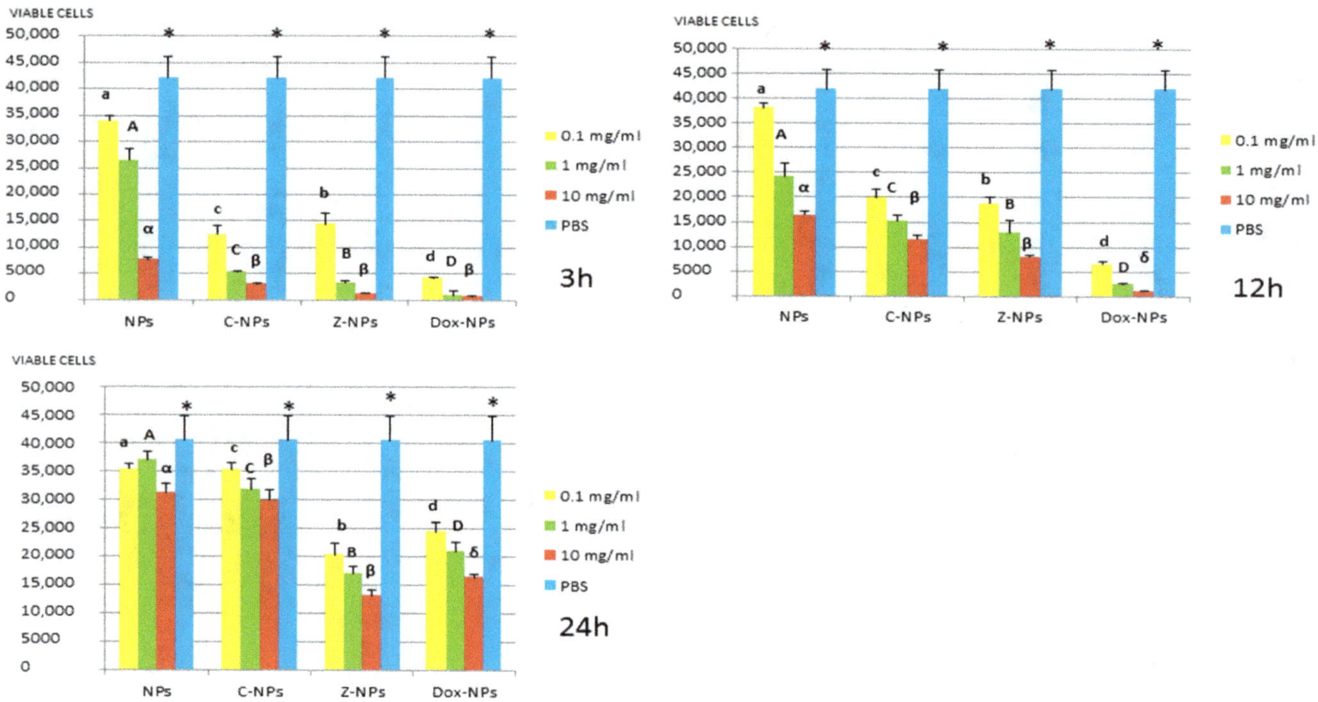

Figure 4. *S. gordonii* survival (number of viable cells) after 3 h, 12 h, and 24 h of different concentration NPs exposure. Same letter or symbol indicates no significant difference of viable bacteria between different NPs concentrations ($p < 0.05$).

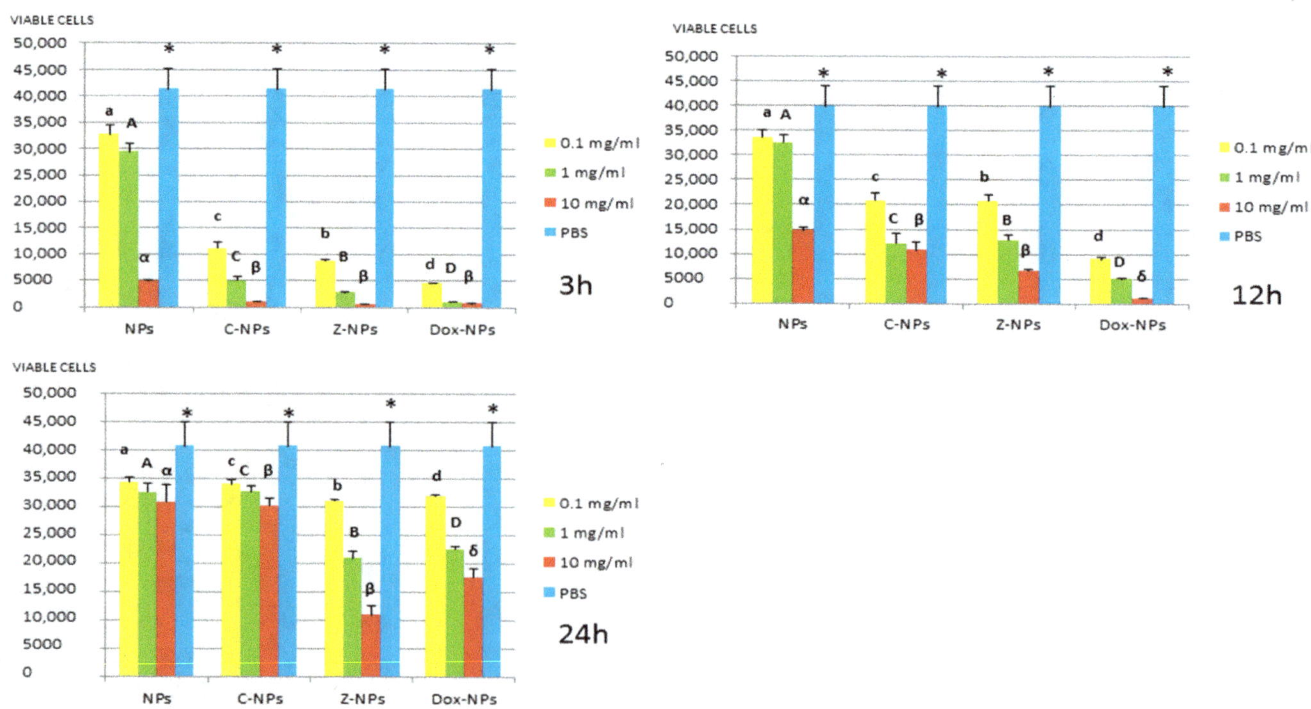

Figure 5. *S. sobrinus* survival (number of viable cells) after 3 h, 12 h, and 24 h of different concentration NPs exposure. Same letter or symbol indicates no significant difference of viable bacteria between different NPs concentrations ($p < 0.05$).

In general, all tested NPs affected the viability of bacterial suspension. The most effective were the Dox-NPs followed by Ca-NPs or Zn-NPs and finally non-doped NPs that attained the most variable and least reduction in bacterial survival (8% to 70% after 24 h).

The viability of tested bacteria following the incubation with NPs depends on the type of NPs. The two bacteria, *S. gordonii* and *S. sobrinus* were found to be the most resistant to the tested NPs. After 24 h, they were only affected by Zn-NPs (70% reduction in bacterial viability) and by Dox-NPs (60% reduction). For *P. gingivalis*, *S. mutans* and *L. lactis*, Dox-NPs reduced the bacterial viability by 60% to 99%, after 24 h depending on the concentration of doxycycline. Meanwhile the reduction in bacterial viability were from 20% to 60% for *S. gordonii* and *S. sobrinus*. The *P. gingivalis*, *L. lactis* and *S. mutans* Dox-NPs effect was not variable during the time of the study. Only in the cases of *S. gordonii* and *S. sobrinus* cultures a drop in Dox-NPs efficacy was observed after 24 h. At 24 h, for *P. gingivalis* all tested concentrations of Dox-NPs attained above 98% bacterial death. In general, most effective dosage of Dox-NPs was found to be 10 mg/mL.

When testing Ca, Zn-doped or even undoped-NPs for *S. mutans* and *L. lactis*, bacterial viability was significantly affected in doses and time dependent manners. After 24 h, only those NPs contained 10 mg/mL were effective. Both bacteria were equally susceptible to Zn-NPs (68% cells reduction). When considering Ca-NPs or undoped-NPs, *L. lactis* was more susceptible (reduction values for Ca-NPs: 90%, for unloaded NPs: 70%) than *S. mutans* (reduction values for Ca-NPs: 60%, for unloaded NPs: 50%).

Testing of NPs doped with Ca and Zn-doped NPs at 0.1 mg/mL against *P. gingivalis*, bacterial viability was significantly affected and bacterial death ranges between 55% to 27%. However, at the most effective concentration -10 mg/mL, bacterial reduction ranges were from 80% to 93%, without significant differences between both ion-doped NPs. *P. gingivalis* incubated with unloaded NPs attained low but dose and time-dependent percentages of bacterial survival reduced, from 34.3% to 7.2%.

3. Discussion

There are several in vitro testing models for the efficacy of antibacterial agents, which may involve single or multispecies bacteria. This microcosm model is the most clinically relevant, but attained results are often difficult to interpret as there is no way to control for the behavior of individual bacterial species. It is also difficult to decide which species are appropriate in each experiment and their relative amounts [3]. Using biofilm models is also challenging as the results may also be different on various materials surfaces with different chemistry and/or topography [30]. Therefore, when analyzing novel antibacterial agents planktonic monoculture tests are necessary to facilitate results interpretation. Further studies need to be conducted on clinical isolates and multi-species biofilms on different material surfaces or interfaces, which may express resistance trait against tested antibacterial effect.

P. gingivalis was selected for the present study as it is one of the most frequently detected anaerobic microorganisms in subgingival plaque samples from periodontal-endodontic combined lesions and necrotic pulp [6]. *S. mutans*, *S. gordonii*, *S. sobrinus* and *L. lactis* were used as are the most frequently detected microorganisms in cariogenic plaque [3]. *P. gingivalis* is a Gram-negative bacteria, *S. mutans*, *S. gordonii*, *S. sobrinus* and *L. lactis* are Gram positive. *P. gingivalis* has an asymmetric distribution of lipids at their cell walls, the outer face contains lipopolysaccharide (LPS), and the inner face has phospholipids [8]. *S. gordonii*, *S. sobrinus S. mutans* and *L. lactis* also have LPS at their membranes, which exhibits anionic charge, as a result it may facilitate cationic groups to bond and exert antimicrobial activity [8]. This may be a reason for observing low antibacterial activity of tested non-loaded NPs, as they are also anionic (potential zeta is -41 ± 5 mV measured in water at pH = 7) [20], and will not be attracted to tested bacteria which posse a zeta potential of approximately -25 mV at pH = 7 [31].

Ca-NPs and Zn-NPs exerted antibacterial activity, at 10 mg/mL 80% to 93% bacterial reduction after 48 h, was encountered (Figure 1) as a possible result of liberated calcium and zinc from NPs. After 48 h, 0.9 and 0.02 μg per 10 mg of NPs of calcium and zinc are respectively released

(Table 1). Cationic metals as calcium or zinc have been shown to be potent antimicrobials [24,25,27]. Calcium release from NPs was estimated to be 0.08 and 0.1 μg/mL (per mg of NPs) from 12 h up to 7 days, while zinc release was around 0.02 μg/mL (per mg of NPs) at the same time-points. Cummulative liberation of both ions is 30% for calcium and 0.3% for zinc after 48 h. It has been shown that lipopolysaccharides at the outer membrane of Gram-negative bacteria possess magnesium and calcium ions that bridge to negatively-charged phosphor-sugars [8]. Therefore, cationic elements may also displace these metal ions damaging the outer membrane, leading to cell death [8,26]. It has also been previously shown that zinc ions markedly enhanced the adhesion and accumulation of salivary and serum proteins on cells of *P. gingivalis* and inhibited their coaggregation when growing on biofilms [27].

Zinc has a known inhibitory effect on glycolysis and proteinase activity in many oral bacteria [27]. Zinc may affect *S. mutans* viability by inhibiting glycolysis [32]. Kinetic studies of the glucosyltransferases of *S. sobrinus* by Devulapalle and Mooser [33] showed that the Zn ion acts as a reversible, competitive inhibitor at the fructose subsite within the active site of the glucosyltransferase. This observation may well explain the reported dose-dependent effects of zinc on the tested bacteria. Even when the exact antibacterial mechanism of zinc has not been clearly identified yet, covalently or oxidatively induced damage has been claimed [32]. Zinc ions are considered useful for limiting the settlement/colonization of *P. gingivalis* in the gingival sulcus with the goal of preventing periodontal disease [27] and in the case of *S. mutans* preventing carious disease [32]. Zinc has long been known as a plaque-inhibiting compound and also can influence acid production by different microbes [32]. In addition, zinc is able to depolarize the membrane potential, it does not always cause the bacterial cell membrane to rupture and leak, but alters permeability that is closely related to the sensitivity of bacteria to ionic environment [30]. Ion homeostasis affects the proliferation, communication and metabolism of bacteria; then, zinc may sometimes produce an inhibitive instead of destructive effect against bacteria [30].

Dox-NPs exerted the highest antibacterial activity to all the tested concentrations (80% to 97% bacterial reduction after 24 h). Following our results, doxycycline was found to be released at sustained levels for over 28 days, with a significant burst effect at 24 h. It is liberated at concentrations high above to those considered effective against bacteria at any time point of the present study. For each mg of NPs 121, 106 and 46 μg/mL of doxycycline will be liberated at 12, 24 and 48 h, respectively. A burst effect with rapid doxycycline liberation was observed from 12 h until the first week of storage. After 7 days time-point, antibiotic release was maintained above 20 μg/mL (per mg of NPs). As bacterial susceptibility to doxycycline is obtained around 0.1 to 0.2 μg/mL [28], doxycycline is then liberated from NPs at concentrations high above to those considered effective against most of the tested bacteria. It was shown that doxycycline at a concentration between 0.5 and 1 μg/mL is bactericidal against different *Pg* strains [34], and between 0.1 and 6.0 μg/mL is effective against *Pg* and other putative periodontal pathogens [35,36]. It should be stressed that tested Dox-NPs after 28 days are able to liberate doxycycline concentrations above 6 μg/mL.

Doxycycline is a polar and amphoteric compound. Doxycycline as a salt (hyclate) is water soluble. Doxycycline is known to act against most bacteria by inhibiting the microbial protein synthesis that requires access into the cell wall and lipid solubility [37]. Doxycycline binds the ribosome to prevent ribonucleic acid synthesis by avoiding addition of more amino acid to the polypeptide [37]. Doxycycline is also known to provoke a potent and long-lasting inhibition of dentin matrix metalloproteinases [29] that are related to chronic inflammation processes and abscesses at apical level [10]. It may explain how long-term administration of a sub-antimicrobial dose of doxycycline, to dogs with periodontitis, is regarded as an effective treatment for periodontal inflammation, even when it does not induce antimicrobial effects [38]. It is also important to note that MMPs inhibition may also prevent collagen degradation at the resin bonded dentin interface [15]. It will also probably reduce secondary caries formation, as MMPs activity is augmented at caries affected dentin [39].

The reported doxycycline liberation data are high and sustained, if compared to the release profile of other previously proposed compounds as a cellulose-acetate-loaded doxycycline formulation studied by Tonetti et al. [40]. Kim et al. [28] introduced a biodegradable doxycycline gel and reported a mean local concentration of 20 mg/mL, after 15 min; values that were lowered to 577 μg/mL after 3 days and to 16 μg/mL after 12 days. Deasy et al. [41] used tetracycline hydrochloride in poly(hydroxybutyric acid) as a biodegradable polymer matrix and showed sustained release just over 4 to 5 days, with a significant burst effect at 24 h. Previously introduced materials are then able to liberate doxycycline at higher concentrations, but in shorter periods of time, denoting accentuated burst effects.

In general, tested NPs had little effect on the growth of (*S. sobrinus* and *S. gordonii*) and specially Dox-NPs after 24 h, which greatly affected *P. gingivalis*, *S. mutans* and *L. lactis* survival rates (at least at the evaluated time points and concentrations). Recent results on advanced caries lesions in young human teeth, using bacterial sequence analysis methods are consistent and indicate that *S. gordonii* diminishes greatly in caries-associated plaque biofilm, while *S. mutans* persists [42]. It means that NPs may selectively inhibit cariogenic and periodontal bacteria, while leaving commensal microbes. However, it should be assayed in properly designed multibacteria biofilms models in future studies. It is to be noted that the tested NPs are biocompatible against human fibroblasts [23], and the application of antibacterials is crucial if regenerative/revascularization processes are performed for the endodontic treatment [43], these NPs may be an interesting tool.

Two important limitations are recognized for the present Dox-NPs: (1) antibiotics may produce bacterial strain resistance, which is a current global concern; therefore, further research is needed. (2) The bacteria grow in biofilms, and are known to be more resistant to antimicrobial treatment than the planktonic cultures used for the present antimicrobial susceptibility testing [44]. Then, it is imperative to include the biofilm mode of growth of bacteria when testing treatments for bonded dentin interfaces, endodontic and periapical diseases. But these tests are difficult to control, in terms of knowing specifically how bacteria are involved in the process [3]. It will not be possible to ascertain if a specific toxicity of NPs against individual bacteria is being produced [44], or just a biofilm disruption interfering with first colonizers bacteria attachment to dentin.

It may be concluded after this in vitro study that experimental NPs loaded with zinc, calcium or doxycycline are effective to eradicate tested oral bacteria. For clinical applications, using these NPs at the resin-bonded interface as cavity liners may be recommended. As it was shown before, that NPs do not affect bond efficacy and improve dentin remineralization [17,21,22]. The same beneficial effect may be found if NPs are used in endodontics, before resin sealant cement application. However, as recognized in the study limitations, further investigations into antibacterial effects through biofilm models of multiple bacterial species should be implemented.

4. Material and Methods

1. *Preparation of Nanoparticles (NPs):* PolymP-*n* Active NPs were acquired (NanoMyP, Granada, Spain). Particles are fabricated trough polymerization precipitation. Main components of NPs are 2-hydroxyethyl methacrylate, ethylene glycol dimethacrylate and methacrylic acid; these compounds are the backbone monomer, the cross-linker and the functional monomer respectively.

Calcium-loaded NPs (Ca-NPs) and Zinc-loaded NPs (Zn-NPs) were produced. Zinc and calcium complexation was obtained immersing 30 mg of NPs during 3 days, under continuous shaking in aqueous solutions of $ZnCl_2$ or $CaCl_2$, at room temperature. Fifteen mL of the solutions containing zinc or calcium at 40 ppm were employed (pH 6.5). Then, the adsorption equilibrium of metal ions was reached [23]. To separate the NPs from the supernatant, the suspensions were centrifuged. 0.96 ± 0.04 μg Ca/mg NPs and 2.15 ± 0.05 μg Zn/mg NPs were the attained ion complexation values [23]. NPs loaded with doxycycline hyclate were also produced. An 18-mL aqueous solution, with 40 mg/mL of doxycycline hyclate (Sigma-Aldrich, Darmstadt, Germany) was prepared, and 30 mg of NPs were immersed in the solution for 4 h, under continuous shaking. Then, to separate NPs from the supernatant the suspensions were centrifuged. Following groups were tested: (1) NPs (NPs), (2) NPs loaded with Ca (Ca-NPs), (3) NPs loaded with Zn (Zn-NPs), and (4) NPs with immobilized doxycycline hyclate (Dox-NPs).

2. *Loading efficacy and release of doxycycline from NPs:* For loading efficacy 18 mL of 40 mg/mL aqueous solution of doxycycline hyclate was prepared and the amount of doxycycline in the initial aqueous solution was assessed in triplicate samples of 100 μL and recorded as initial doxycycline concentration (1333 μg Dox/mL). Three different samples containing 1 mg of NPs and 0.6 mL of the doxycycline solution were incubated for 4 h, under continuous shaking. Then, the suspensions were centrifuged and the particles were separated from the supernatant, 100 μL of each supernatant was analyzed for final doxycycline concentration. Final doxycycline concentration was subtracted from initial values to calculate loading efficacy [45]. To ascertain for doxycycline liberation, 30 mg of doxycycline loaded-NPs were suspended in 3 mL of phosphate buffer saline (PBS, pH 7.4, Fisher Scientific SL, Madrid, Spain), three different eppendorf tubes containing 1 mL of the Dox-NPs suspension were stored at 37 °C. After 12 h, suspensions were centrifuged and the particles were separated from the supernatant. An aliquot (0.1 mL) of each supernatant was analyzed for doxycycline concentration. NPs were washed and 1 mL of fresh PBS was used to resuspend the NPs at 10 mg/mL until the next supernatant collection. Seven different time-points were tested: 12, 24, 48 h, 7, 14, 21 and 28 days. Supernatans were stored at −20 °C until doxycycline concentration measuring [45]. The amount of doxycycline was assayed by high performance liquid chromatography (HPLC) (Waters Alliance 2690, Waters Corporation, Milford, MA, USA) equipped with a UV-Vis detector. A binary mobile phase consisting of solvent systems A and B was used in an isocratic elution with 80:20 A:B. Mobile phase A was 50 mM $KHPO_4$ in distilled H_20 and mobile phase B was 100% acetonitrile. The HPLC flow rate was 1.0 mL/min and the total run time was 10 min. The retention time was 4.85 min. The concentration of doxycycline was calculated based on a standard curve of known levels of doxycycline at 273 nm [45].

3. *Calcium and zinc liberation from NPs:* 150 mg of zinc and 150 mg of calcium loaded-NPs were suspended in 15 mL of deionized water. Three different eppendorf tubes containing 5 mL of the Ca-NPs suspensions and other 3 with Zn-NPs were stored at 37 °C. After 12 h, suspensions were centrifuged and the particles separated from the supernatant; 5 mL of each supernatant was analyzed for calcium and zinc concentration. NPs were washed and 5 mL of fresh deionized water was used to resuspend the NPs at 10 mg/mL until the next supernatant collection. Seven different time points were tested: 12 h, 24 h, 48 h, 7 d, 14 d, 21 d and 28 d. Supernatans were stored at −20 °C until testing. Calcium and zinc concentrations were analyzed through an inductively coupled plasma (ICP) optical emission spectrometer (ICP-OES Optima 8300, Perkin-Elmer, MA, USA) [23].

4. *Bacteria: P. gingivalis* 33,277, *S. mutans* 700,610, *S. sobrinus* 33,478, *S. gordonii* 10,558 and *L. lactis* 12,315 were obtained from ATCC (Bethesda, MD, USA). The anaerobic organism, *Pg* was grown in Tryptic Soy broth (TSB) supplemented with yeast extract (5 g/L), Hemin (5 mg/L), Menadione (1 mg/L), for 72 h. Strict anaerobic conditions were employed, *Thermo Scientific* Oxoid *AnaeroGen* (Thermo Fisher Scientific, Waltham, MA, USA) was used in an anaerobic jar, which provides 7–15% CO_2 and <0.1% O_2. The remaining test bacteria were grown in TSB for 24 h at 37 °C. The bacterial cells were harvested by centrifugation and re-suspended in the same growth media. The number of bacteria per mL was determined by measuring the optical density at 600 nm and adjusting it to a standard bacterial suspension of 1×10^7 CFU/mL [46].

5. *MTT assay:* The NPs were suspended in PBS at three different concentrations (10 mg/mL, 1 mg/mL and 0.1 mg/mL). NPs were placed into Eppendorf tubes with bacterial broths (1×10^7 CFU/mL for each 0.45 mL of NPs suspensions) and incubated for 3, 12 and 24 h at 37 °C. Sterile pipetting was used throughout the study. Susceptibility testing of *P. gingivalis* was conducted in an anaerobic jar as described above. At the end of each incubation period, the effect of the NPs on bacteria was evaluated by the ability of viable bacteria to cleave the tetrazolium salt (3-[4,5-dimethylthiazol-2-yl]-2,5-diphenyl tetrazolium bromide) (MTT) to a formazan

dye (Sigma-Aldrich, Darmstadt, Germany). 96-well flat-bottom microtiter plates were used to place the suspensions in. The plates were incubated for 4 h at 37 °C, after the MTT labeling agent addition to each culture well. Then, the solubilizing agent that was provided by the manufacturer was added and an overnight incubation at room temperature was performed. An enzyme-linked immunosorbent assay (ELISA) reader (Spectrostar Nano, BMG Labtech, Cary, NC, USA) was employed, the purple formazan color that was produced from the MTT by viable cells, was read (560 nm) [46]. Assays were performed with three determinants, and experiments were performed in triplicate. Data expressed as mean ± standard deviation were analyzed by one-way analysis of variance (ANOVA) and the post hoc comparisons Scheffe's F tests, at $p < 0.05$, using SPSS Statistic 20.

Author Contributions: Conceptualization, M.T.-O., J.B., F.G., M.T. and R.O.; Methodology, M.T.-O., J.B., F.G., A.M., M.T. and R.O.; Software, M.T.-O., J.B.; Formal Analysis, M.T.-O., J.B., F.G., A.M., M.T. and R.O.; Investigation, M.T.-O., J.B., F.G., A.M., M.T. and R.O.; Resources, M.T.-O., J.B., A.M.; Data Curation, M.T.-O., J.B., F.G., A.M., M.T. and R.O.; Writing—Original Draft Preparation, M.T.-O., J.B., F.G., A.M., M.T. and R.O.; Writing—Review & Editing, M.T.-O., J.B., F.G., M.T. and R.O.; Supervision, J.B., F.G., M.T. and R.O; Project Administration, R.O. and M.T.; Funding Acquisition, M.T. and R.O.

Acknowledgments: The research project MAT2017-85999-P was funded by the Spanish Ministry of Economy and Competitiveness (MINECO) and European Regional Development Fund (FEDER). No funds were received to cover publication costs.

References

1. Chaves, P.; Oliveira, J.; Haas, A.; Beck, R.C.R. Applications of polymeric nanoparticles in oral diseases: A review of recent findings. *Curr. Pharm. Des.* **2018**. [CrossRef] [PubMed]
2. Spencer, P.; Ye, Q.; Park, J.; Topp, E.M.; Misra, A.; Marangos, O.; Wang, Y.; Bohaty, B.S.; Singh, V.; Sene, F.; et al. Adhesive/Dentin Interface: The Weak Link in the Composite Restoration. *Ann. Biomed. Eng.* **2010**, *38*, 1989–2003. [CrossRef] [PubMed]
3. Ferracane, J.L. Models of Caries Formation around Dental Composite Restorations. *J. Dent. Res.* **2017**, *96*, 364–371. [CrossRef] [PubMed]
4. Hirose, N.; Kitagawa, R.; Kitagawa, H.; Maezono, H.; Mine, A.; Hayashi, M.; Haapasalo, M.; Imazato, S. Development of a Cavity Disinfectant Containing Antibacterial Monomer MDPB. *J. Dent. Res.* **2016**, *95*, 1487–1493. [CrossRef] [PubMed]
5. Albuquerque, M.T.P.; Evans, J.D.; Gregory, R.L.; Valera, M.C.; Bottino, M.C. Antibacterial TAP-mimic Electrospun Polymer Scaffold—Effects on *P. gingivalis*-Infected Dentin Biofilm. *Clin. Oral Investig.* **2016**, *20*, 387–393. [CrossRef] [PubMed]
6. Kim, R.J.; Kim, M.O.; Lee, K.S.; Lee, D.Y.; Shin, J.H. An in vitro evaluation of the antibacterial properties of three mineral trioxide aggregate (MTA) against five oral bacteria. *Arch. Oral Biol.* **2015**, *60*, 1497–1502. [CrossRef] [PubMed]
7. Rôças, I.N.; Siqueira, J.F.; Santos, K.R.; Coelho, A.M. "Red complex" (*Bacteroides forsythus*, *Porphyromonas gingivalis*, and *Treponema denticola*) in endodontic infections: A molecular approach. *Oral Surg. Oral Med. Oral Pathol. Oral Radiol. Endod.* **2001**, *91*, 468–471. [CrossRef] [PubMed]
8. Wang, L.; Xie, X.; Weir, M.D.; Fouad, A.F.; Zhao, L.; Xu, H.H. Effect of bioactive dental adhesive on periodontal and endodontic pathogens. *J. Mater. Sci. Mater. Med.* **2016**, *27*, 168. [CrossRef] [PubMed]
9. Gu, L.; Huang, X.; Griffin, B.; Bergeron, B.R.; Pashley, D.H.; Niu, L.; Tay, F.R. Primum non nocere—The effects of sodium hypochlorite on dentin as used in endodontics. *Acta Biomater.* **2017**, *61*, 144–156. [CrossRef] [PubMed]
10. Letra, A.; Ghaneh, G.; Zhao, M. MMP-7 and TIMP-1, New Targets in Predicting Poor Wound Healing in Apical Periodontitis. *J. Endod.* **2013**, *39*, 1141–1146. [CrossRef] [PubMed]
11. Menezes-Silva, R.; Khaliq, S.; Deeley, K.; Letra, A.; Vieira, A.R. Genetic Susceptibility to Periapical Disease: Conditional Contribution of MMP2 and MMP3 Genes to the Development of Periapical Lesions and Healing Response. *J. Endod.* **2012**, *38*, 604–607. [CrossRef] [PubMed]

12. Paula-Silva, G.F.W.; Bezerra da Silva, L.A.; Kapila, L.Y. Matrix Metalloproteinase Expression in Teeth with Apical Periodontitis Is Differentially Modulated by the Modality of Root Canal Treatment. *J. Endod.* **2010**, *36*, 231–237. [CrossRef] [PubMed]
13. Ahmed, G.M.; El-Baz, A.A.; Hashem, A.A.; Shalaan, A.K. Expression levels of matrix metalloproteinase-9 and gram-negative bacteria in symptomatic and asymptomatic periapical lesions. *J. Endod.* **2013**, *39*, 444–448. [CrossRef] [PubMed]
14. Accorsi-Mendonca, T.; Silva, E.J.; Marcaccini, A.M.; Gerlach, R.F.; Duarte, K.M.; Pardo, A.P.; Line, S.R.; Zaia, A.A. Evaluation of gelatinases, tissue inhibitor of matrix metalloproteinase-2, and myeloperoxidase protein in healthy and inflamed human dental pulp tissue. *J. Endod.* **2013**, *39*, 879–882. [CrossRef] [PubMed]
15. Osorio, R.; Yamauti, M.; Osorio, E.; Ruiz-Requena, M.E.; Pashley, D.; Tay, F.R.; Toledano, M. Effect of dentin etching and chlorhexidine application on metalloproteinase-mediated collagen degradation. *Eur. J. Oral Sci.* **2011**, *119*, 79–85. [CrossRef] [PubMed]
16. Liu, Y.; Mai, S.; Li, N. Differences between top-down and bottom-up approaches in mineralizing thick, partially-demineralized collagen scaffolds. *Acta Biomater.* **2011**, *7*, 1742–1751. [CrossRef] [PubMed]
17. Toledano, M.; Osorio, R.; Osorio, E.; Medina-Castillo, A.L.; Toledano-Osorio, M.; Aguilera, F.S. Ions-modified nanoparticles affect functional remineralization and energy dissipation through the resin-dentin interface. *J. Mech. Behav. Biomed. Mater.* **2017**, *68*, 62–79. [CrossRef] [PubMed]
18. Zhu, J.; Liang, R.; Sun, C.; Xie, L.; Wang, J.; Leng, D.; Wu, D.; Liu, W. Effects of nanosilver and nanozinc incorporated mesoporous calcium-silicate nanoparticles on the mechanical properties of dentin. *PLoS ONE* **2017**, *12*, e0182583. [CrossRef] [PubMed]
19. Zhang, K.; Cheng, L.; Imazato, S.; Antonucci, J.M.; Lin, N.J.; Lin-Gibson, S.; Bai, Y.; Xu, H.H.K. Effects of dual antibacterial agents MDPB and nano-silver in primer on microcosm biofilm, cytotoxicity and dentin bond properties. *J. Dent.* **2013**, *41*, 464–474. [CrossRef] [PubMed]
20. Hashimoto, M.; Sasaki, J.I.; Yamaguchi, S.; Kawai, K.; Kawakami, H.; Iwasaki, Y.; Imazato, S. Gold Nanoparticles Inhibit Matrix Metalloproteases without Cytotoxicity. *J. Dent. Res.* **2015**, *94*, 1085–1091. [CrossRef] [PubMed]
21. Osorio, R.; Cabello, I.; Medina-Castillo, A.L.; Osorio, E.; Toledano, M. Zinc-modified nanopolymers improve the quality of resin-dentin bonded interfaces. *Clin. Oral Investig.* **2016**, *20*, 2411–2420. [CrossRef] [PubMed]
22. Osorio, R.; Osorio, E.; Medina-Castillo, A.L.; Toledano, M. Polymer nanocarriers for dentin adhesion. *J. Dent. Res.* **2014**, *93*, 1258–1263. [CrossRef] [PubMed]
23. Osorio, R.; Alfonso-Rodríguez, C.A.; Medina-Castillo, A.L.; Alaminos, M.; Toledano, M. Bioactive Polymeric Nanoparticles for Periodontal Therapy. *PLoS ONE* **2016**, *7*, e0166217. [CrossRef] [PubMed]
24. Munchow, E.A.; Albuquerque, M.T.; Zero, B.; Kamocki, K.; Piva, E.; Gregory, R.L.; Bottino, M.C. Development and characterization of novel ZnO-loaded electrospun membranes for periodontal regeneration. *Dent. Mater.* **2015**, *31*, 1038–1051. [CrossRef] [PubMed]
25. Munchow, E.A.; Pankajakshan, D.; Albuquerque, M.T.; Kamocki, K.; Piva, E.; Gregory, R.L.; Bottino, M.C. Synthesis and characterization of CaO-loaded electrospun matrices for bone tissue engineering. *Clin. Oral Investig.* **2016**, *27*, 1921–1933. [CrossRef] [PubMed]
26. Vargas-Reus, M.A.; Memarzadeh, K.; Huang, J.; Ren, G.G.; Allaker, R.P. Antimicrobial activity of nanoparticulate metal oxides against peri-implantitis pathogens. *Int. J. Antimicrob. Agents* **2012**, *40*, 135–139. [CrossRef] [PubMed]
27. Tamura, M.; Ochiai, K. Zinc and copper play a role in coaggregation inhibiting action of *Porphyromonas gingivalis*. *Mol. Oral Microbiol.* **2009**, *24*, 56–63. [CrossRef]
28. Kim, T.S.; Bürklin, T.; Schacher, B.; Ratka-Krüger, P.; Schaecken, M.T.; Renggli, H.H.; Fiehn, W.; Eickholz, P. Pharmacokinetic profile of a locally administered doxycycline gel in crevicular fluid, blood, and saliva. *J. Periodontol.* **2002**, *73*, 1285–1291. [CrossRef] [PubMed]
29. Osorio, R.; Yamauti, M.; Osorio, E.; Ruiz-Requena, M.E.; Pashley, D.H.; Tay, F.R.; Toledano, M. Zinc reduces collagen degradation in demineralized human dentin explants. *J. Dent.* **2011**, *39*, 148–153. [CrossRef] [PubMed]
30. Fan, W.; Sun, Q.; Li, Y.; Tay, F.R.; Fan, B. Synergistic mechanism of Ag^{+}–Zn^{2+} in anti-bacterial activity against *Enterococcus faecalis* and its application against dentin infection. *J. Nanobiotechnol.* **2018**, *16*, 10. [CrossRef] [PubMed]

31. Cowan, M.M.; Van der Mei, H.C.; Stokroos, I.; Busscher, H.J. Heterogeneity of surfaces of subgingival bacteria as detected by zeta potential measurements. *J. Dent. Res.* **1992** *71*, 1803–1806. [CrossRef] [PubMed]
32. Wunder, D.; Bowen, W.H. Action of agents on glucosyltransferases from Streptococcus mutans in solution and adsorbed to experimental pellicle. *Arch. Oral Biol.* **1999**, *44*, 203–214. [CrossRef]
33. Devulapalle, K.S.; Mooser, G. Subsite specificity of the active site of glucosyltransferases from *Streptococcus sobrinus*. *J. Biol. Chem.* **1994**, *269*, 11967–11971. [PubMed]
34. Larsen, T. Susceptibility of *Porphyromonas gingivalis* in biofilms to amoxicillin, doxycycline and metronidazole. *Oral Microbiol. Immunol.* **2002**, *17*, 267–271. [CrossRef] [PubMed]
35. Slots, J.; Rams, T.E. Antibiotics in periodontal therapy: Advantages and disadvantages. *J. Clin. Periodontol.* **1990**, *17*, 479–493. [CrossRef] [PubMed]
36. Larsen, T. In vitro release of doxycycline from bioabsorbable materials and acrylic strips. *J. Periodontol.* **1990**, *61*, 30–34. [CrossRef] [PubMed]
37. Gamal, A.Y.; Kumper, R.M.A. Novel Approach to the Use of Doxycycline-Loaded Biodegradable Membrane and EDTA Root Surface Etching in Chronic Periodontitis: A Randomized Clinical Trial. *J. Periodontol.* **2012**, *83*, 1086–1094. [CrossRef] [PubMed]
38. Kim, S.E.; Hwang, S.Y.; Jeong, M. Clinical and microbiological effects of a subantimicrobial dose of oral doxycycline on periodontitis in dogs. *Vet. J.* **2016**, *208*, 55–59. [CrossRef] [PubMed]
39. Toledano, M.; Nieto-Aguilar, R.; Osorio, R.; Campos, A.; Osorio, E.; Tay, F.R.; Alaminos, M. Differential expression of matrix metalloproteinase-2 in human coronal and radicular sound and carious dentine. *J. Dent.* **2010**, *38*, 635–640. [CrossRef] [PubMed]
40. Tonetti, M.S.; Lang, N.P.; Cortellini, P.; Suvan, J.E.; Eickholz, P.; Fourmousis, I.; Topoll, H.; Vangsted, T.; Wallkamm, B. Effects of a single topical doxycycline administration adjunctive to mechanical debridement in patients with persistent/recurrent periodontitis but acceptable oral hygiene during supportive periodontal therapy. *J. Clin. Periodontol.* **2012**, *39*, 475–482. [CrossRef] [PubMed]
41. Deasy, P.B.; Collins, A.E.; MacCarthy, D.J.; Russell, R.J. Use of strips containing tetracycline hydrochloride or metronidazole for the treatment of advanced periodontal disease. *J. Pharm. Pharmacol.* **1989**, *41*, 694–699. [CrossRef] [PubMed]
42. Gross, E.L.; Leys, E.J.; Gasparovich, S.R.; Firestone, N.D.; Schwartzbaum, J.A.; Janies, D.A.; Asnani, K.; Griffen, A.L. Bacterial 16S sequence analysis of severe caries in young permanent teeth. *J. Clin. Microbiol.* **2010**, *48*, 4121–4128. [CrossRef] [PubMed]
43. Yassen, G.H.; Vail, M.M.; Chu, T.G.; Platt, J.A. The effect of medicaments used in endodontic regeneration on root fracture and microhardness of radicular dentine. *Int. Endod. J.* **2013**, *46*, 688–695. [CrossRef] [PubMed]
44. Garrett, T.R.; Bhakoo, M.; Zhang, Z.B. Bacterial adhesion and biofilms on surfaces. *Prog. Nat. Sci.* **2008**, *18*, 1049–1056. [CrossRef]
45. Palasuk, J.; Windsor, L.J.; Platt, J.A.; Lvov, Y.; Geraldeli, S.; Bottino, M.C. Doxycycline-loaded nanotube-modified adhesives inhibit MMP in a dose-dependent fashion. *Clin. Oral Investig.* **2018**, *22*, 1243–1252. [CrossRef] [PubMed]
46. Banzi, E.C.; Costa, A.R.; Puppin-Rontani, R.M.; Babu, J.P.; García-Godoy, F. Inhibitory effects of a cured antibacterial bonding system on viability and metabolic activity of oral bacteria. *Dent. Mater.* **2014**, *30*, e238–e244. [CrossRef] [PubMed]

11

Human In Situ Study of the effect of Bis(2-Methacryloyloxyethyl) Dimethylammonium Bromide Immobilized in Dental Composite on Controlling Mature Cariogenic Biofilm

Mary Anne S. Melo [1,*], Michael D. Weir [1], Vanara F. Passos [2], Juliana P. M. Rolim [3], Christopher D. Lynch [4], Lidiany K. A. Rodrigues [2,*] and Hockin H. K. Xu [1,5,6,*]

1 Department of Advanced Oral Sciences and Therapeutics, University of Maryland School of Dentistry, Baltimore, MD 21201, USA; Mweir@umaryland.edu

2 Postgraduate Program in Dentistry, Faculty of Pharmacy, Dentistry and Nursing, Federal University of Ceara, Fortaleza, CE 60430-355, Brazil; vanarapassos@hotlmail.com

3 Faculty of Dentistry UniChristus, Fortaleza, CE 60160-230, Brazil; julianapml@unichristus.br

4 Restorative Dentistry, University Dental School and Hospital, University College Cork, Wilton T12 K8AF, Ireland; chris.lynch@ucc.ie

5 Center for Stem Cell Biology & Regenerative Medicine, University of Maryland School of Medicine, Baltimore, MD 21201, USA

6 Marlene and Stewart Greenebaum Cancer Center, University of Maryland School of Medicine, Baltimore, MD 21201, USA

* Correspondence: mmelo@umaryland.edu (M.A.S.M.); lidianykarla@ufc.br (L.K.A.R.); HXu@umaryland.edu (H.H.K.X.)

Abstract: Cariogenic oral biofilms cause recurrent dental caries around composite restorations, resulting in unprosperous oral health and expensive restorative treatment. Quaternary ammonium monomers that can be copolymerized with dental resin systems have been explored for the modulation of dental plaque biofilm growth over dental composite surfaces. Here, for the first time, we investigated the effect of bis(2-methacryloyloxyethyl) dimethylammonium bromide (QADM) on human overlying mature oral biofilms grown intra-orally in human participants for 7–14 days. Seventeen volunteers wore palatal devices containing composite specimens containing 10% by mass of QADM or a control composite without QADM. After 7 and 14 days, the adherent biofilms were collected to determine bacterial counts via colony-forming unit (CFU) counts. Biofilm viability, chronological changes, and percentage coverage were also determined through live/dead staining. QADM composites caused a significant inhibition of *Streptococcus mutans* biofilm formation for up to seven days. No difference in the CFU values were found for the 14-day period. Our findings suggest that: (1) QADM composites were successful in inhibiting 1–3-day biofilms in the oral environment in vivo; (2) QADM significantly reduced the portion of the *S. mutans* group; and (3) stronger antibiofilm activity is required for the control of mature long-term cariogenic biofilms. Contact-killing strategies using dental materials aimed at preventing or at least reducing high numbers of cariogenic bacteria seem to be a promising approach in patients at high risk of the recurrence of dental caries around composites.

Keywords: antibacterial; biofilm; caries; dental composite; quaternary ammonium monomers; human in situ study

1. Introduction

In the past decade, dental materials research has intensified attempts at reducing or modulating dental plaque biofilm growth over dental composite surfaces [1] because recurrent caries around restorations (CARS) are identified as some of the major reasons for the failure of composite restorations [2,3]. Replacement rates of failed restorations have been reported to be 37–70%, with consequences that can seriously compromise oral health status [4,5]. CARS are frequently located at the gingival margins of the proximal restorations, which are common areas for food impaction [6]. Patients consider the cleaning of dental biofilm at the proximal space challenging, and very often fail to control biofilm build-up over time.

Dental caries are marked by continuous mineral loss promoted by organic acids released by bacteria after sugar metabolization [7], mainly streptococci from the *mutans* group. Cariogenic bacteria are characterized as pathologically shifted species, with the ability to generate large amounts of acid and to survive in acidic microenvironments [8]. The introduction of novel treatment approaches, supplementary to conventional therapeutic strategies, is thus considered as crucial for the efficient control of CARS. Cariogenic oral biofilms influence the initiation and progression of carious lesions not just in their primary development but also in their recurrence [9]. Reports in the literature have stated a temporal relationship between changes in biofilm composition and enamel demineralization following exposure to sucrose [10,11]. An undisturbed dental biofilm exposed to frequent sucrose leads to enamel demineralization after seven days of biofilm accumulation [10]. As the cariogenic biofilm becomes more mature, some acidogenic and aciduric bacteria become dominant in the biofilm [12].

Resin composites facilitate cariogenic biofilm growth [13]. Dental monomers such as bisphenol A-glycidyl dimethacrylate (BisGMA) and triethylene glycol dimethacrylate (TEGMA) may alter the metabolism and promote the proliferation of *Streptococcus mutans* [14]. Therefore, the synthesis of free radical monomers that have quaternary ammonium groups in their chemical structures paved the way for a noninvasive, biofilm-targeted method that can be used against oral biofilms [15]. Reactive and easily miscible quaternary ammonium monomers have the advantage of copolymerizing with the current dental resin systems through covalent bonding with the polymer network. These polymers are referred to as nonleaching antimicrobial or contact-killing agents. The antibacterial action results from the direct contact of the polymer with the microorganisms, with no release of active molecules. Although the exact antimicrobial mechanism of action has not been fully elucidated, the predominant mode of action is disruption of the cell membrane [16]. This imparts a durable and permanent antibacterial capability to dental composites.

Studies have presented different positions of the functional groups and alkyl chain length for improved balance between mechanical properties, antibacterial effects, and biocompatibility [17]. The majority of the synthetic quaternary ammonium monomers have only one methacrylate group, as monomethacrylates. Incorporating a high content of monomethacrylates could compromise the overall cross-linked polymer matrix [18].

Several in vitro studies have investigated the antibacterial performance of bis(2-methacryloyloxyethyl) dimethylammonium bromide (QADM), a quaternary ammonium monomer containing two methacrylate groups [18]. QADM was loaded at 10 wt % into different parental formulations, such as commercial and experimental adhesive systems [19,20] and nanocomposites [21], rendering reductions in *S. mutans* and total micro-organisms. Overall, these studies achieved a significant reduction of biofilm viability, metabolic activity, lactic acid, and bacterial counts using a 48-h human saliva microcosm biofilm model [22]. The incorporation of QADM also did not compromise the mechanical or bonding performance of the parental materials, and its antibacterial and mechanical properties were long-term and maintained after a one-year follow-up [23].

Although encouraging results were found in vitro [19–22], only a few studies have used native in situ dental plaque to study the effects of quaternary ammonium methacrylate [24,25]. In these studies, bacterial colonization over a short period (from hours to three days) was assessed. Antibacterial dental composites using QADM on an overlying mature cariogenic biofilm formed over seven days have not been studied to date. A longer-term in situ study would give insight into the in vivo antibacterial performance of this material in challenging conditions that mimic the clinical scenario of retentive proximal areas where the biofilm could not be removed in patients with a high risk of caries. Moreover, over a seven-day period, dysbiosis was present due to the proliferation or overgrowth of cariogenic bacteria in a low-pH econiche, and enamel was prone to demineralization.

In light of the evidence available to support quaternary ammonium monomers on initial oral biofilm, the present study for the first time evaluated the antibacterial performance of QADM in a relatively long-term study (beyond three days) by challenging the effectiveness of QADM-containing materials against mature oral biofilms formed in situ. Intact oral biofilms were grown under a cariogenic challenge in situ on composites within the oral cavity for 7 and 14 days. In addition to the determination of bacterial counts, the chronological changes in the biofilm were also visualized by live/dead staining, and the percentages were measured.

2. Results

All 17 volunteers completed the study, and no protocol deviation was identified. Treatment compliance was satisfactory. The mean and standard deviation values of colony-forming unit (CFU) counts of biofilms collected at 7 and 14 days are plotted in Figure 1A,B. The QADM composite had a significant effect on the viability of *S. mutans* at the 7 days ($p = 0.0303$). This effect corresponded to a 43% reduction of both solutions compared with the control. The QADM composite's effect on the viability of total streptococci, lactobacilli, and total microorganisms on the in situ biofilms was measured. However, no statistical significance was observed between the groups ($p > 0.05$). During the 14-day period, the microbiological composition of the biofilms formed on restoration was statistically similar for all evaluated conditions ($p > 0.5$).

Figure 2A shows the statistically significant difference between the tested groups ($p = 0.0385$) at the 7-day period, expressed by the variable percentage of mutans streptococci related to total streptococci (MS/TS). However, the percentage of mutans streptococci related to total micro-organisms was similar during the same period. These variables showed no difference during the 14-day period (Figure 3B).

Figure 3A–D,F–I shows live/dead staining images of biofilms grown on the QADM and control composites on the 1st, 3rd, 7th, and 14th days. Biofilms grown on the control composite on the 1st and 3rd days were primarily alive, which was indicated by continuous green staining (Figure 3A,B). Widespread bacterial cell killing was more pronounced on the 1st and 3rd day of biofilm accumulation on the QADM composite (Figure 3). At the 7th and 14th day, the overly mature biofilm structure was compact, with numerous layers showing a mushroom-like configuration with channels in the outer layer (Figure 3C,D for the control composites and Figure 3G,H for the QADM composites). Complete coverage of the composite surface was observed after seven days. No significant difference between the control and the QADM was observed.

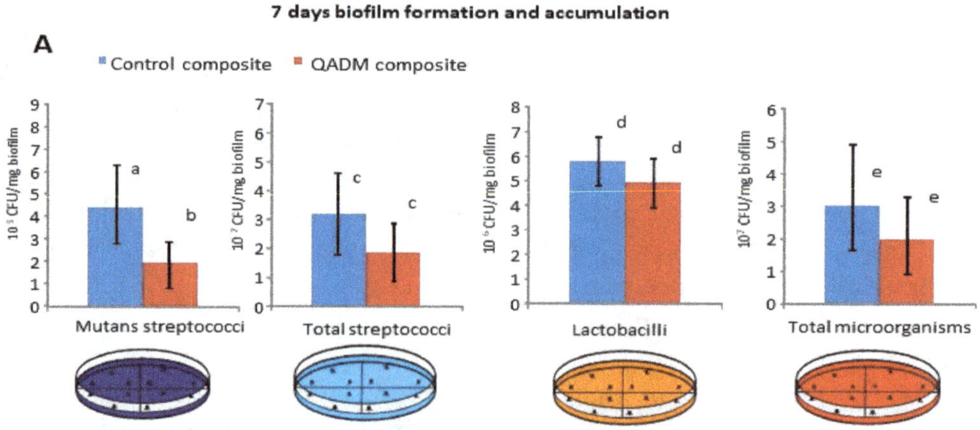

Figure 1. *Cont.*

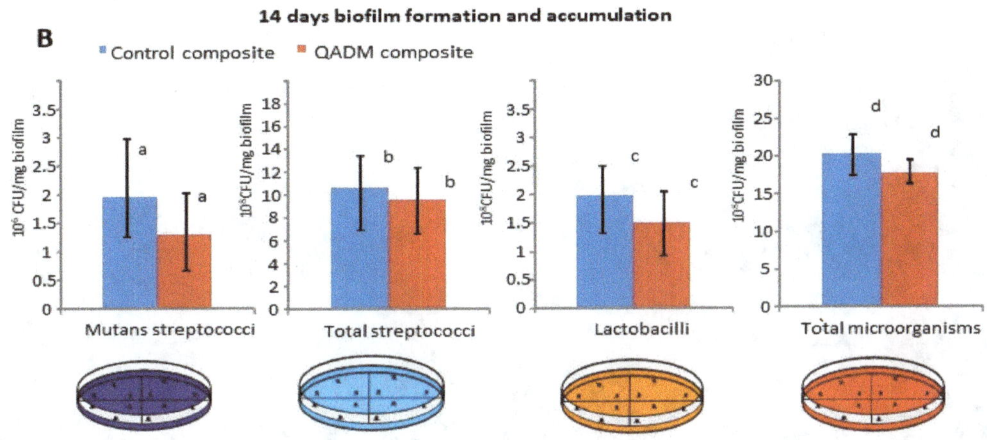

Figure 1. (**A**) Colony-forming unit (CFU) counts for the viability of mutans streptococci (MS), total streptococci (TS), lactobacilli, and total microorganisms (TM) present in the biofilms formed in situ after a 7-day and (**B**) 14-day period. Error bars represent the standard deviation of the mean, and data followed by different letters differed statistically ($p < 0.05$). The reduction in CFU counts from biofilms adherent to the QADM (bis(2-methacryloyloxyethyl) dimethylammonium bromide) composites was significantly different from the control for *Streptococcus mutans* after 7 days of growth. After 14 days, no further reduction was observed for *S. mutans*.

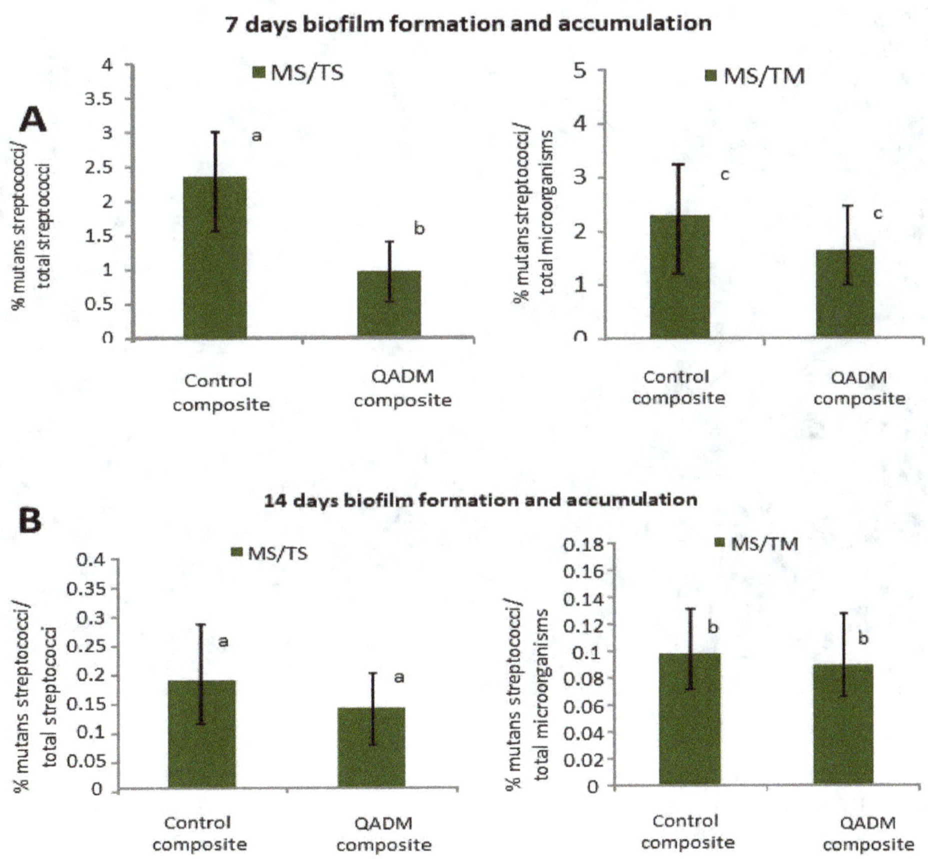

Figure 2. (**A**) The percentage of mutans streptococci related to total streptococci (MS/TS) and the percentage of mutans streptococci related to total micro-organisms (MS/TM) present in biofilms formed in situ after a 7-day and (**B**) 14-day period. The MS/TS was greatly reduced for biofilms adherent to the QADM composite in relation to the control at the 7-day period. Error bars represent SD, and data followed by different letters differed statistically ($p < 0.05$).

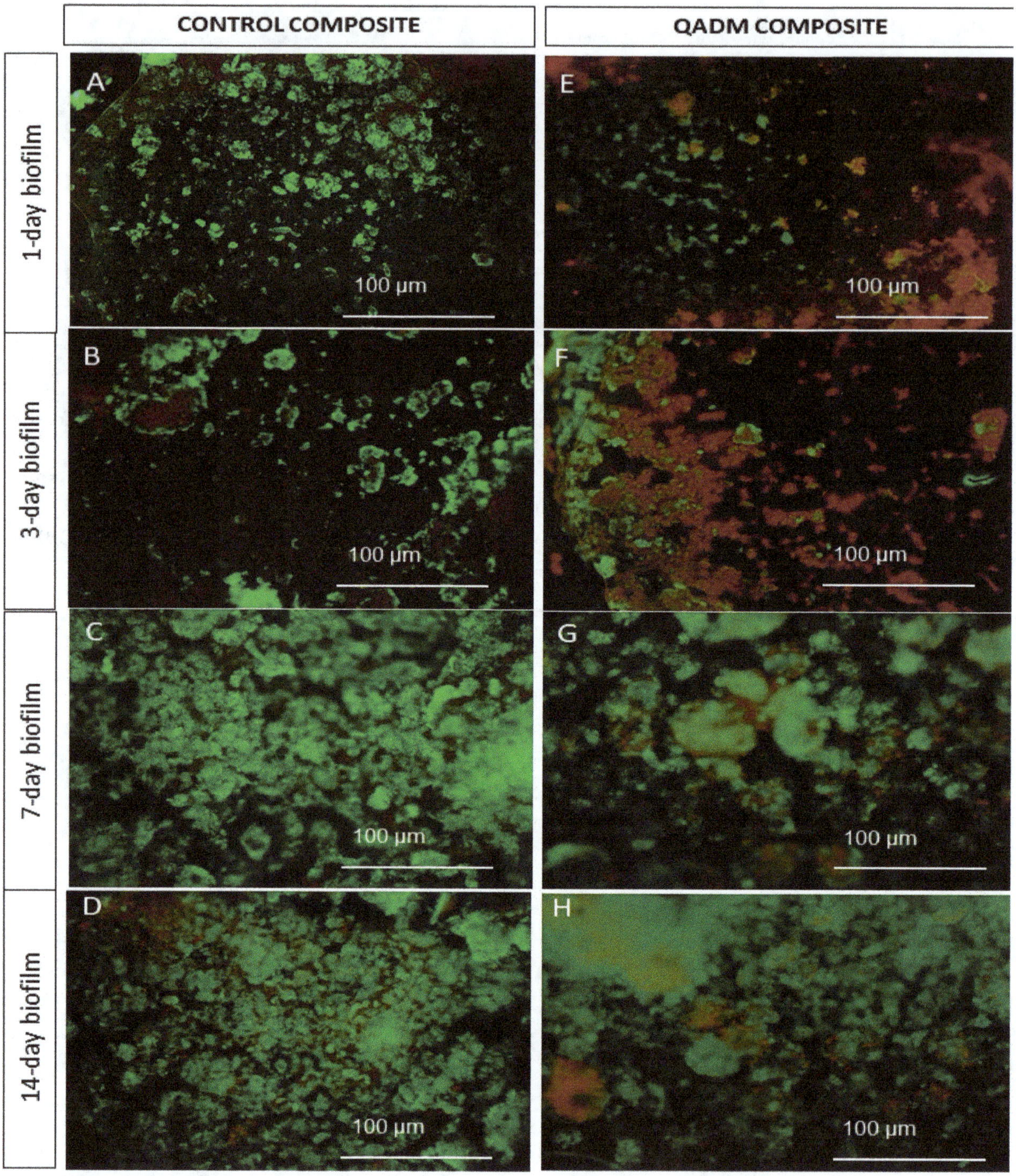

Figure 3. Live/dead staining images of biofilms grown on the QADM and control composites during the 1-, 3-, 7-, and 14-day periods. (**A**,**B**) Biofilms grown on the control composite on the 1st and 3rd days were primarily alive with continuous green staining. (**E**,**F**) Widespread cell-killing of bacteria was more pronounced on the 1- and 3-day biofilm accumulation on the QADM composite. On the 7th and 14th day, the overly mature biofilm structure was compact, with numerous layers presenting a mushroom-like configuration with channels in the outer layer: (**C**,**D**) for the control and (**G**,**H**) for the QADM.

Figure 4 image analyses show that the living cells grown over control composites accounted for 93% ± 3% (±SD) and 93% ± 7% (±SD) of the total biofilm cells for the 1- and 3-day biofilms.

Percentages of living cells (46% ± 8% for the first day and 37% ± 3% for the third day) were determined on the QADM-containing composites for the same time. They were inactive and dead.

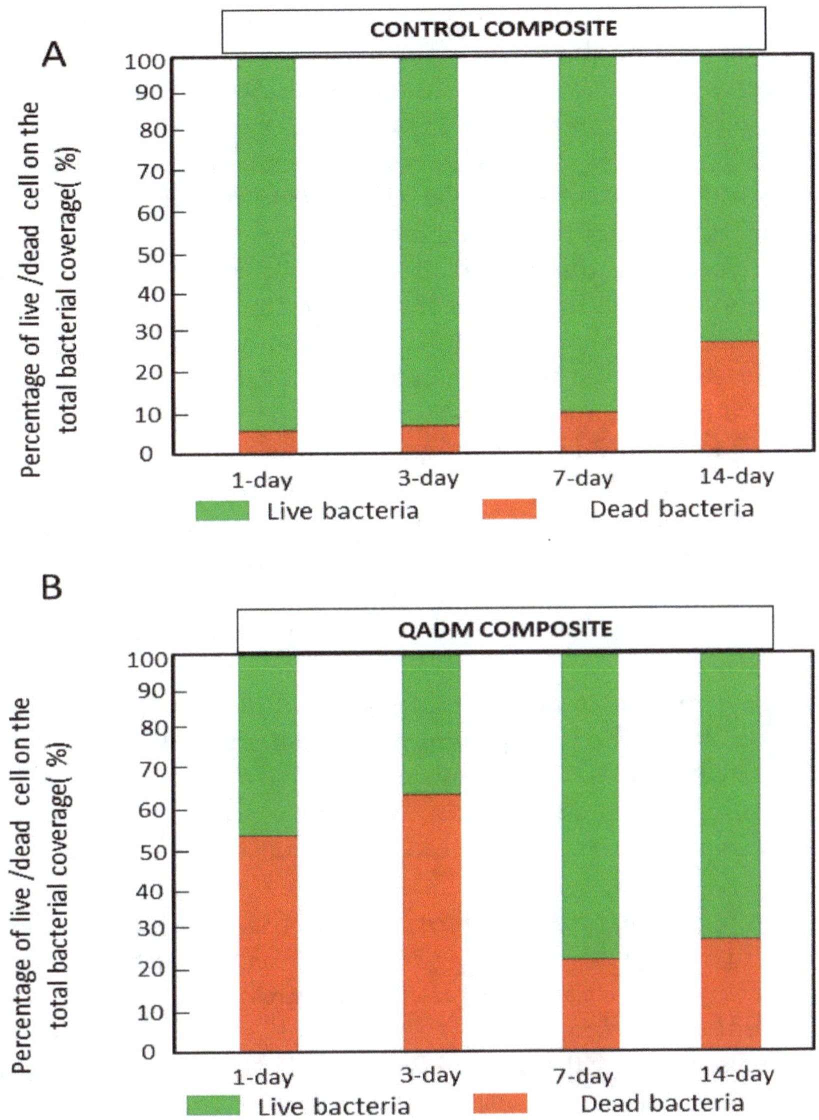

Figure 4. The percentage of live/dead bacterial cells found for the total biofilm coverage over the (**A**) control and (**B**) QADM composites. An increase in the dead percentage was observed for the biofilm grown over the QADM composite during the first and third day.

3. Discussion

Bacterial attachment to dental composite surfaces and subsequent cariogenic biofilm formation is a complex process [26]. There is an interplay between biological factors (i.e., the bacterial ability to rapidly convert dietary sugars to acids lowers the pH and demineralizes the tooth structure), patient-related factors, and physicochemical factors such as surface topography, surface charge, and surface energy of the dental materials [27,28]. Typical treatment for biofilm-mediated recurrence of caries lesions around the composite restorations involves operative replacement of composites, which incurs additional healthcare costs and additional loss of tooth structure.

To avoid biofilms on dental materials, an attractive alternative and complementary method to dental caries management is the use of biomaterials that possess antibacterial surfaces [27]. The contact-active antibacterial material is effective in preventing biofilm formation by killing bacteria [29], reducing bacteria amounts in the surrounding microenvironment, and extending the material's service life.

Antibiofilm effects of new dental materials with releasing fillers or ions were also investigated in the literature [30]. The incorporation of silver nanoparticles was among the bioactive compounds investigated that could provide antibacterial effects on oral bacteria. However, long-term release kinetics have challenged this approach's use in dental materials [31,32].

As contact-killing agents, the quaternary ammonium monomers for dental applications have been intensely investigated in vitro in the past years, with a positive outcome overall. Investigations have shown immediate and robust antibacterial effects (more than 3 log reductions) against oral micro-organisms [21,23,25]. QADM di-functional monomers are effective in producing active surfaces with high densities of immobilized antimicrobial agents [33,34]. For the specific quaternary ammonium used in our study, the previous in vitro studies showed reductions of 68% and 79% in biofilm CFU counts and lactic acid production, respectively, on cured primers specimens [20].

For this in situ study, for the first time we challenged the antibacterial performance of a dual methacrylate group QADM incorporated into composites against overly mature oral biofilms formed inside the oral cavity for up to 14 days in an acidogenic biofilm structure capable of causing substantial mineral loss and deep lesions on the enamel surface. This approach has high clinical relevance since anti-caries therapies aimed at controlling the assembly of cariogenic biofilms should contribute to the prevention of the onset of early carious lesions, clinically known as white spots.

The data revealed that QADM compromised the *S. mutans* group's biofilm accumulation during the 7-day period. The two most common species constantly linked to caries formation are *S. mutans* and *S. sobrinus* [35]. The cariogenic potential of *S. mutans* is accentuated when sucrose is available [36]. Sucrose-mediated biofilm formation creates spatial organizations expressed by a complex network of microcolonies, which modulate the development of compartmentalized acidic microenvironments across the 3D biofilm architecture [37]. Furthermore, within 3D biofilms, *S. mutans* display properties that are dramatically distinct from their planktonic counterparts, including much higher resistance to antibacterial approaches, which makes the biofilm much more difficult to kill than planktonic bacteria [35].

Although our research revealed the inhibitory effect of QADM on *S. mutans* biofilms, the exact mechanism of this inhibition is still unclear. The antibacterial efficacy may be related to the contact-killing mechanism of quaternization of the amino groups of QADM available on the bottom layer of the biofilm adjacent to the composite. The negatively charged counter-ions that stabilize the bacterial membrane were displaced by the positively charged cationic N^+ sites in the chemical structure of the quaternary ammonium-based resin. Indeed, the live/dead images obtained at the initial period of biofilm formation showed the presence of a higher proportion of nonviable bacteria (the red-orange color areas). Previous studies have highlighted the similar viability of biofilms growing on resin-based materials containing quaternary ammonium monomers [35,36,38,39]. Beyth and co-workers have suggested an intracellularly mediated death program, in which the bacterial lysis promoted by the presence of quaternary ammonium on the resin surface functions as a stressful condition triggering programmed cell death in the bacteria further away in the biofilm [25,40].

No expressive microbial reduction results on CFU values or micro-organism proportions were observed for *S. mutans*. These results point out the challenge faced by anti-caries approaches against mature biofilms. The bacterial adhesion processes under in vivo and in vitro conditions differ considerably [33]. Bacteria in biofilms are far less sensitive to antibacterial agents because of the exopolymeric matrix, extracellular polysaccharides, specific gene expression, and metabolic activity, all factors that protect antibacterial therapies to reach target bacteria [41]. The live/dead images of biofilms show a well-developed dense and compact extracellular polymeric substance - EPS matrix and the presence of bacterial cell clusters or microcolonies (Figure 4C,D for the control composites and Figure 4G,H for the QADM composites). The relative alteration of the proportion of live/dead found in the 7–14-day images was related to the uneven spatial distribution of vital and dead microorganisms found in matured and thick dental biofilms, with decreased vitality toward the outer layers [41]. Tawakoli et al. [42] also supported the high variability of the live/dead distribution and the CFU counts as challenges found in in situ biofilm models. Recently, new investigations have started to emerge using nanoparticles to improve the penetration of therapeutic agents into the biofilm matrix of oral cariogenic biofilms [43].

Another aspect to consider is the spatial arrangement, charge density, and counter-anion of the quaternary ammonium monomers and their antibacterial activity [32]. Previous studies have designed antibacterial monomers containing an eight-carbon or longer chain, which has correlated with significant antibacterial activity in vitro [44]. Surface charge density has displayed antibacterial performance in vitro. These monomers need to translate their antibacterial performance from in vitro to a human in vivo [45–48]. Future studies are warranted, especially to investigate whether the charge density is a relevant factor in the antibacterial effect of these new quaternary ammonium monomers.

In summary, the findings in this paper demonstrate that QADM composites at 10% promote a substantial bacterial reduction of *S. mutans* biofilm. This was achieved in the initial days of contact and also reached a 7-day period, an interval where patients at high risk of caries would develop initial enamel carious lesions. However, dental caries result from interactions over time. An undisturbed cariogenic biofilm well-established on the composite surface over long periods is extremely difficult to eradicate. Its inhibition should not rely only on contact with an antibacterial surface. Removing or disturbing biofilm from all tooth and composite surfaces and reducing sugar intake within three days is expected to control carious lesions. Concomitant and multitargeting strategies are needed against mature long-term cariogenic biofilms.

4. Materials and Methods

4.1. Study Design and Participants

This study involved a prospective, randomized, single-blind, split-mouth in situ design conducted according to the code of ethics of the World Medical Association (Declaration of Helsinki) for experiments involving humans. The region's ethical committee (protocol #1232012) also approved it. Seventeen healthy volunteers of both genders, aged from 21 to 36 years, accepted participation in this study, fulfilling the required criteria. Inclusion criteria were a normal salivary flow rate, good general and oral health with no active caries lesions or periodontal treatment needs, an ability to comply with the experiment protocol, no use of antibiotics during the three months before the study, and no use of fixed or removable orthodontic devices. Exclusion criteria were failing to use the device according to the established protocol and taking medication interfering with saliva flow rate or containing antimicrobial agents. The sample size was determined by a power analysis and was based on previous data [25]. Seventeen volunteers were recruited: 16 for the study and 1 volunteer to allow temporal visualization of the biofilm formation through live/dead staining. After being screened, the volunteers were verbally informed about the study aims and procedures, and received written information and the informed consent form. At the next appointment, maxillary alginate impressions were made for the fabrication of the palatal devices.

During the experimental period, each volunteer used a removable acrylic custom-made palatal device containing the tested materials, as shown in Figure 5A. Seven days before the experiment began (i.e., the washout period) and during the whole experiment, the volunteers were asked to use a standard toothbrush and nonfluoridated paste. Each acrylic palatal device enclosed four composite specimens ($5 \times 5 \times 2$ mm^3): two specimens for the control composites and two specimens for the QADM composites. To promote plaque accumulation and to protect it from disarrangement, recessions were created by placing the surface of the composite specimens about 1 mm below the covered plastic mesh (as seen in the details of Figure 1A) [45].

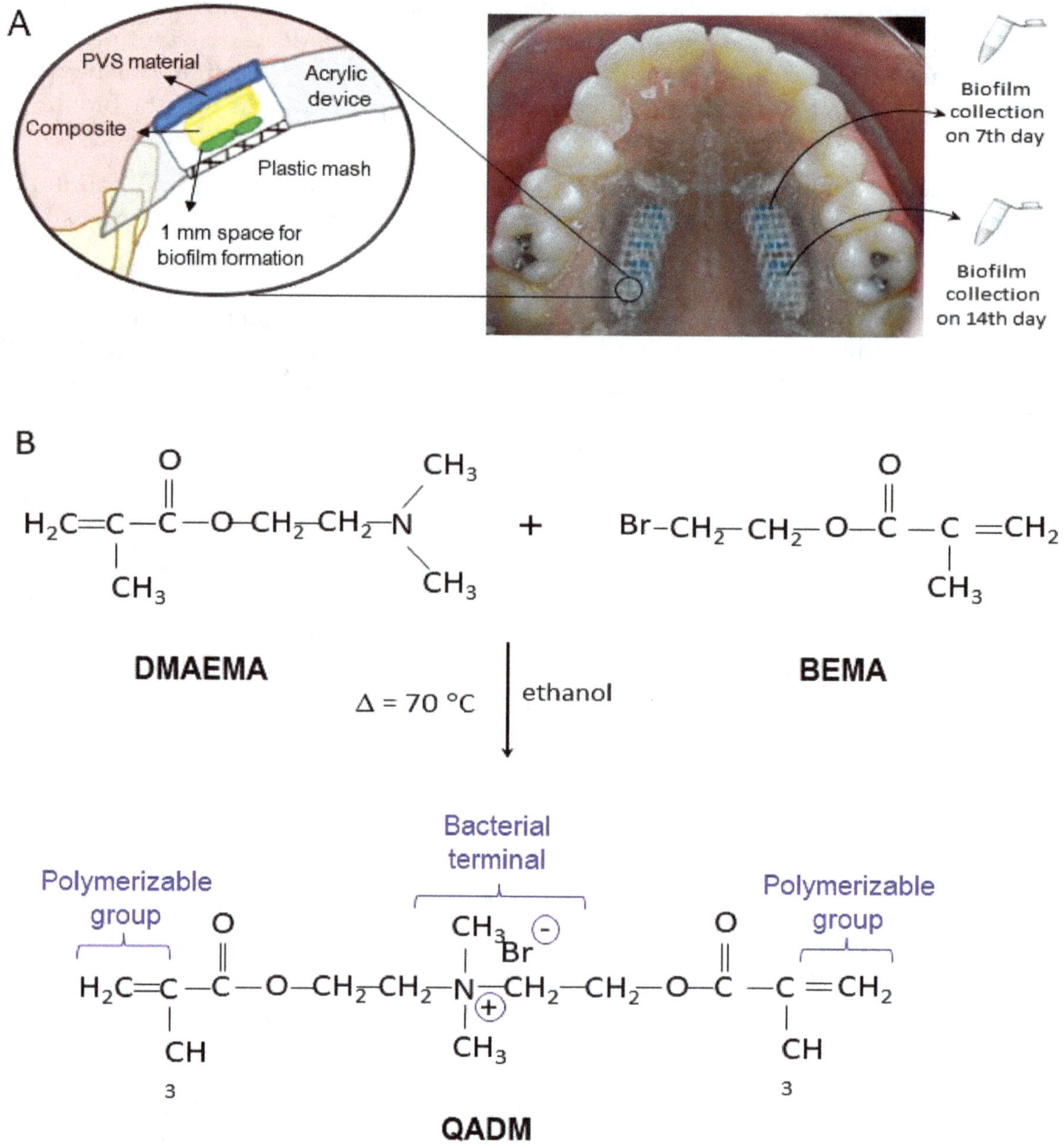

Figure 5. (**A**) In situ palatal devices used by 17 volunteers. Each device contained four slabs, two filled with the QADM composite on one side and two filled with the control composite on the other side. The slabs were held by polyvinyl siloxane (PVS) and covered with a plastic mash to avoid disturbance in the biofilm growth.The biofilm was collected from the surface of the specimens on the 7th and 14th days. The top-left is a magnified description showing details of biofilm formation over the composite specimens inside the device. (**B**) The synthesis route of the bis(2-methacryloyloxyethyl) dimethylammonium bromide monomer via a Menshutkin reaction and the details for dual-polymerizable groups and the bacterial terminal. BEMA: 2-bromoethyl methacrylate; DMAEMA: 2-(*N*,*N*-dimethylamino)ethyl methacrylate.

To divert any possible carry-across effect, the sequence in which the experiment units were assigned in the palatal device took into consideration that antibacterial dental materials should be placed on one side of the palatal appliance and, consequently, that control materials should be placed on the opposite side (Figure 5A). The split-mouth experimental design was a practical approach for testing the effects of various agents on the composition of dental plaque [44]. Within each side of the palatal device, the positions of the specimens were randomly determined according to a computer-generated randomization list [45]. The outcome variables evaluated were colony-forming unit counts for total microorganisms, total streptococci, mutans streptococci, and lactobacilli on the specimens.

4.2. Specimen Preparation

The light-curable composite was made by blending a monomer resin consisting of BisGMA (bisphenol-glycidyl dimethacrylate) and TEGDMA (triethylene glycol dimethacrylate) at a 1:1 ratio (all by mass) with 0.2% camphorquinone and 0.8% ethyl 4-*N*,*N*-dimethylaminobenzoate. As reinforcement co-fillers, barium-boroaluminosilicate glass particles with a median diameter of 1.4 μm (Caulk/Dentsply, Milford, DE, USA) were silanized with 4% 3-methacryloxypropyltrimethoxysilane and 2% *n*-propylamine [21]. The fillers were mixed with the resin at a total filler mass fraction of 60% to form a cohesive paste.

The synthesis of bis(2-methacryloyloxyethyl) dimethylammonium bromide via a modified Menshutkin reaction was previously described [18], and it is summarized in Figure 1B. Briefly, 10 mmol of 2-(*N*,*N*-dimethylamino)ethyl methacrylate (DMAEMA; Sigma-Aldrich, St. Louis, MO, USA) and 10 mmol of 2-bromoethyl methacrylate (BEMA; Monomer-Polymer Labs, Trevose, PA, USA) were combined with 3 g of ethanol in a closed vial. After stirring at 60 °C for 24 h so the reaction could complete, the solvent was removed via evaporation, using a vacuum. This process yielded QADM as a clear and viscous liquid. QADM was mixed with the BisGMA–TEGDMA resin at a QADM mass fraction of 10%. A preliminary study showed that this mass fraction yielded strong antibacterial properties without compromising the resin's mechanical properties [21].

Thirty-six light-curable composite specimens were fabricated for the experimental composition (QADM at 10 wt % each), and a further 36 specimens without antimicrobial monomer served as a control. The composite was inserted and light activated for 20 s using a light-emitting diode (Radii-cal, SDI Limited Victoria, Australia; standard curing mode, irradiance output provided of 689 mW/cm^2). The specimens were mounted in standardized sample chambers inside the device, with an anterior–posterior position, using body impression material (Aquasil Ultra, Dentsply DeTray GmbH, Konstanz, Germany), as demonstrated in Figure 1A.

4.3. Clinical Phase

Audiovisual orientation and written instructions of the in situ protocol were given to the volunteers to assure their adhesion and avoid protocol deviation during the study. To provide a cariogenic challenge during the clinical phase, the application of a 20% sucrose solution extra-orally on the restored specimens was performed by the volunteers eight times per day at predetermined times. According to previous studies, the sucrose was gently dried after 5 min, and the device was reinserted into the mouth [42,44]. No restriction was made about the volunteers' diet, but they were instructed to avoid F-rich food containing bioavailable F, such as black tea. They did, however, drink fluoridated water (about 0.7 ppm fluoride).

4.4. Microbiological and Biochemical Analysis

On the 7th and 14th examination days, the subjects refrained from eating, drinking, and tooth cleaning 12 h after the last application of the sucrose solution and dentifrice before presenting at the clinic (46-48). On the 7th day, the device was removed from the mouth, and the biofilm and one enamel slab from each side were respectively carefully removed and collected (Figure 5B). Then, the device with the remaining specimens was reinserted into the mouth. On the 14th day, a similar process was performed to collect the two residual biofilms from the specimens. After the collection, the biofilm was processed for analysis. First, it was weighed (±1 mg) in preweighed microcentrifuge tubes and agitated during a 2 min period in a Disrupter Genie Cell Disruptor (Precision Solutions, Rice Lake, WI, USA). A 50 μL aliquot of the sonicated suspension was diluted in 0.9% NaCl, and serial decimal dilutions were inoculated in triplicate using the drop-counting technique in the following culture media: (1) in mitis salivarius agar containing 20% sucrose to determine total streptococci (TS), and in mitis salivarius agar plus 0.2 bacitracin/mL to determine mutans streptococci (MS); (2) in Rogosa agar supplemented with 0.13% glacial acetic acid to assess the number of CFU of lactobacilli (LB); and (3) in brain–heart infusion enhanced with 5% sterile defibrinated sheep blood agar plates to determine total micro-organisms (TM). The plates were incubated in 10% CO_2 at 37 °C for 48 h. The CFU were counted, and the results were expressed as CFU/mg biofilm wet weight, the percentage of MS in relation to TM, and the percentage of MS in relation to TS.

4.5. *Live/Dead Assays*

To visualize the micro-organisms during the initial phase of formation as well as during the experimental periods, one volunteer used a palatal device containing eight composite specimens: four specimens for the control composite and four specimens for the QADM composite. One specimen from each group was removed during the 1st, 3rd, 7th, and 14th days. The specimens were immediately washed with phosphate-buffered saline (PBS) and stained using the LIVE/DEAD BacLight Bacterial Viability Kit (Molecular Probes, USA) to qualify bacterial cell viability. This assay employs two nucleic acid stains: the green-fluorescent SYTO 9 stain and the red-fluorescent propidium iodide stain [39]. These stains differ in their ability to penetrate healthy bacterial cells. When used alone, the SYTO 9 stain labels both live and dead bacteria.

In contrast, propidium iodide penetrates only bacteria with damaged membranes, reducing SYTO 9 fluorescence when both dyes are present. Thus, live bacteria with intact membranes fluoresce green, while dead bacteria with damaged membranes fluoresce red. A volume of 100 μL of the previously described fluorescence dyes was pipetted onto the specimens and incubated in a dark chamber for 15 min. The biofilms grown over the specimens were then examined using an epifluorescence microscope (TE2000-U, Nikon, Melville, NY, USA) at a magnification of 100×. Images (n = 4) were acquired and analyzed (NIS Elements software, Nikon Instruments Inc, Melville, NY, USA) for the quantification of live (green fluorescence) and dead (red fluorescence) bacteria.

4.6. *Statistical Analysis*

The assumptions of equality of variances and normal distribution of errors were checked for all the response variables tested, and those that did not satisfy these assumptions were transformed using the Box–Cox power transformation [42]. To determine the differences between test and control values in the in situ experiment, the viable bacteria counts, percent MS/TS, and percent MS/TM were submitted to a two-sample independent Student's t-test. The significance level was set at $\alpha = 0.05$. The statistical appraisal was computed with SPSS for Windows XP 17.0 (SPSS Inc., Chicago, IL, USA).

5. Conclusions

The results of the present in situ study provide a more realistic perspective on the value of integrating bioactive restorative materials with traditional caries management approaches into clinical practice. Contact-killing strategies via dental materials aiming at preventing or at least reducing high numbers of cariogenic bacteria seem to be a promising approach for helping patients at high risk of recurrence of dental caries around composites.

Author Contributions: Conceptualization, M.A.S.M., L.K.A.R. and H.H.K.X.; C.D.L., L.K.A.R. and H.H.K.X; methodology, M.D.W., V.F.P., J.P.M.R.; software, M.A.S.M..; validation, L.K.A.R and H.H.K.X.; formal analysis, M.A.S.M.; investigation, V.F.P., J.P.M.R.; resources, L.K.A.R.; data curation, M.A.S.M.; writing—original draft preparation, M.A.S.M.; writing—review and editing, H.H.K.X.; visualization, M.A.S.M.; supervision, M.A.S.M.; project administration, M.A.S.M.; funding acquisition, H.H.K.X., L.K.A.R., please turn to the CRediT taxonomy for the term explanation. Authorship must be limited to those who have contributed substantially to the work reported.

Acknowledgments: The authors thank the volunteers for their valuable participation and Agostinho Soares de Alcântara Neto (Faculdade de Veterinária, Universidade Estadual do Ceará) for his technical assistance and laboratory facilities for the cell viability assay.

References

1. Hwang, G.; Koltisko, B.; Jin, X.; Koo, H. Nonleachable Imidazolium-Incorporated Composite for Disruption of Bacterial Clustering, Exopolysaccharide-Matrix Assembly, and Enhanced Biofilm Removal. *ACS Appl. Mater. Interfaces* **2017**, *9*, 38270–38280. [CrossRef] [PubMed]
2. Hollanders, A.C.C.; Kuper, N.K.; Maske, T.; Huysmans, M.D.N.J.M. Secondary Caries in situ Models: A Systematic Review. *Caries Res.* **2018**, *52*, 454–462. [CrossRef] [PubMed]
3. Bernardo, M.; Luis, H.; Martin, M.D.; Leroux, B.G.; Rue, T.; Leitao, J. Survival and reasons for failure of amalgam versus composite posterior restorations placed in a randomized clinical trial. *J. Am. Dent. Assoc.* **2007**, *138*, 775–783. [CrossRef] [PubMed]
4. Owen, B.; Guevara, P.H.; Greenwood, W. Placement and replacement rates of amalgam and composite restorations on posterior teeth in a military population. *US Army Med. Dep. J.* **2017**, *2*, 88–94.
5. Roumanas, E.D. The frequency of replacement of dental restorations may vary based on a number of variables, including type of material, size of the restoration, and caries risk of the patient. *J. Evid. Based Dent. Pract.* **2010**, *1*, 23–24. [CrossRef] [PubMed]
6. Mjör, I.A. The location of clinically diagnosed secondary caries. *Quintes Int.* **1998**, *29*, 313–317.
7. Fejerskov, O. Changing paradigms in concepts on dental caries: Consequences for oral health care. *Caries Res.* **2004**, *38*, 182–191. [CrossRef] [PubMed]
8. Marsh, P.D. Are dental diseases examples of ecological catastrophes? *Microbiology* **2003**, *149*, 279–294. [CrossRef] [PubMed]
9. Paes Leme, A.F.; Koo, H.; Bellato, C.M.; Bedi, G.; Cury, J.A. The role of sucrose in cariogenic dental biofilm formation—New insight. *J. Dent. Res.* **2006**, *85*, 878–887. [CrossRef] [PubMed]
10. Vale, G.C.; Tabchoury, C.P.; Arthur, R.A.; Del Bel Cury, A.A.; Paes Leme, A.F.; Cury, J.A. Temporal relationship between sucrose-associated changes in dental biofilm composition and enamel demineralization. *Caries Res.* **2007**, *41*, 406–412. [CrossRef] [PubMed]
11. Cury, J.A.; Tenuta, L.M. Enamel remineralization: Controlling the caries disease or treating early caries lesions? *Braz. Oral Res.* **2009**, *23*, 23–30. [CrossRef] [PubMed]
12. NTakahashi, B. Nyvad. Caries ecology revisited: Microbial dynamics and the caries process. *Caries Res.* **2008**, *42*, 409–418. [CrossRef] [PubMed]
13. Singh, J.; Khalichi, P.; Cvitkovitch, D.G.; Santerre, J.P. Composite resin degradation products from BisGMA monomer modulate the expression of genes associated with biofilm formation and other virulence factors in Streptococcus mutans. *J. Biomed. Mater. Res. A* **2009**, *88*, 551–560. [CrossRef] [PubMed]
14. Sadeghinejad, L.; Cvitkovitch, D.G.; Siqueira, W.L.; Santerre, J.P.; Finer, Y. Triethylene Glycol Up-Regulates Virulence-Associated Genes and Proteins in Streptococcus mutans. *PLoS ONE* **2016**, *11*, 665–760. [CrossRef] [PubMed]
15. Melo, M.A.; Weir, M.D.; Li, F.; Cheng, L.; Zhang, K.; Xu, H.H.K. Control of Biofilm at the Tooth-Restoration Bonding Interface: A Question for Antibacterial Monomers? A Critical Review. *Rev. Adhes. Adhes.* **2017**, *3*, 287–305. [CrossRef]
16. Jiao, Y.; Niu, L.N.; Ma, S.; Li, J.; Tay, F.R.; Chen, J.H. Quaternary ammonium-based biomedical materials: State-of-the-art, toxicological aspects and antimicrobial resistance. *Prog. Pol. Sci.* **2017**, *71*, 53–90. [CrossRef]
17. Zhang, N.; Ma, Y.; Weir, M.; Xu, H.H.K.; Bai, Y.; Melo, M.A. Current Insights into the Modulation of Oral Bacterial Degradation of Dental Polymeric Restorative Materials. *Materials* **2017**, *10*, 507. [CrossRef] [PubMed]
18. Antonucci, J.M.; Zeiger, D.N.; Tang, K.; Lin-Gibson, S.; Fowler, B.O.; Lin, N.J. Synthesis and characterization of dimethacrylates containing quaternary ammonium functionalities for dental applications. *Dent. Mater.* **2012**, *28*, 219–228. [CrossRef] [PubMed]

19. Melo, M.A.S.; Cheng, L.; Weir, M.D.; Hsia, R.; Rodrigues, L.K.A.; Xu, H.H.K. Novel dental bonding agents containing antibacterial agents and calcium phosphate nanoparticles. *J. Biomed. Mater. Res. B Appl. Biomater.* **2013**, *101*, 620–629. [CrossRef] [PubMed]
20. Cheng, L.; Zhang, K.; Melo, M.A.S.; Weir, M.D.; Zhou, X.; Xu, H.H.K. Anti-biofilm dentin primer with quaternary ammonium and silver nanoparticles. *J. Dent. Res.* **2012**, *91*, 598–604. [CrossRef] [PubMed]
21. Cheng, L.; Weir, M.D.; Xu, H.H.; Antonucci, J.M.; Kraigsley, A.M.; Lin, N.J.; Lin-Gibson, S.; Zhou, X. Antibacterial amorphous calcium phosphate nanocomposites with a quaternary ammonium dimethacrylate and silver nanoparticles. *Dent. Mater.* **2012**, *28*, 561–572. [CrossRef] [PubMed]
22. Zhang, K.; Melo, M.A.S.; Cheng, L.; Weir, M.D.; Bai, Y.; Xu, H.H.K. Effect of quaternary ammonium and silver nanoparticle-containing adhesives on dentin bond strength and dental plaque microcosm biofilms. *Dent. Mater.* **2012**, *28*, 842–852. [CrossRef] [PubMed]
23. Cheng, L.; Zhang, K.; Zhou, C.C.; Weir, M.D.; Zhou, X.D.; Xu, H.H. One-year water-ageing of calcium phosphate composite containing nano-silver and quaternary ammonium to inhibit biofilms. *Int. J. Oral Sci.* **2016**, *29*, 172–181. [CrossRef] [PubMed]
24. Feng, J.; Cheng, L.; Zhou, X.; Xu, H.H.; Weir, M.D.; Meyer, M.; Maurer, H.; Li, Q.; Hannig, M.; Rupf, S. In situ antibiofilm effect of glass-ionomer cement containing dimethylaminododecyl methacrylate. *Dent. Mater.* **2015**, *31*, 992–1002. [CrossRef] [PubMed]
25. Beyth, N.; Yudovin-Farber, I.; Perez-Davidi, M.; Domb, A.J.; Weiss, E.I. Polyethyleneimine nanoparticles incorporated into resin composite cause cell death and trigger biofilm stress in vivo. *Proc. Natl. Acad. Sci. USA* **2010**, *107*, 22038–22043. [CrossRef] [PubMed]
26. Marsh, P.D. Microbiology of dental plaque biofilms and their role in oral health and caries. *Dent. Clin. N. Am.* **2010**, *54*, 441–454. [CrossRef] [PubMed]
27. Chen, C.; Weir, M.D.; Wang, L.; Zhou, X.; Xu, H.H.K.; Melo, M.A. Dental Composite Formulation Design with Bioactivity on Protein Adsorption Combined with Crack-Healing Capability. *J. Funct. Biomater.* **2017**, *8*, 40. [CrossRef] [PubMed]
28. Melo, M.A.; Codes, B.M.; Passos, V.F.; Lima, J.P.M.; Rodrigues, L.K. In Situ Response of Nanostructured Hybrid Fluoridated Restorative Composites on Enamel Demineralization, Surface Roughness, and Ion Release. *Eur. J. Prosthodont. Restor. Dent.* **2014**, *22*, 185–190. [PubMed]
29. Chatzistavrou, X.; Lefkelidou, A.; Papadopoulou, L.; Pavlidou, E.; Paraskevopoulos, K.M.; Fenno, J.C.; Flannagan, S.; González-Cabezas, C.; Kotsanos, N.; Papagerakis, P. Bactericidal and Bioactive Dental Composites. *Front. Physiol.* **2018**, *16*, 99–103. [CrossRef] [PubMed]
30. Sjollema, J.; Zaat, S.A.J.; Fontaine, V.; Ramstedt, M.; Luginbuehl, R.; Thevissen, K.; Li, J.; van der Mei, H.C.; Busscher, H.J. In vitro methods for the evaluation of antimicrobial surface designs. *Acta Biomater.* **2018**, *70*, 12–24. [CrossRef] [PubMed]
31. Khvostenko, D.; Hilton, T.J.; Ferracane, J.L.; Mitchell, J.C.; Kruzic, J.J. Bioactive glass fillers reduce bacterial penetration into marginal gaps for composite restorations. *Dent. Mater. Off. Publ. Acad. Dent. Mater.* **2016**, *32*, 73–81. [CrossRef] [PubMed]
32. Stencel, R.; Kasperski, J.; Pakieła, W.; Mertas, A.; Bobela, E.; Barszczewska-Rybarek, I.; Chladek, G. Properties of Experimental Dental Composites Containing Antibacterial Silver-Releasing Filler. *Materials* **2018**, *11*, 1031. [CrossRef] [PubMed]
33. Kasraei, S.; Sami, L.; Hendi, S.; AliKhani, M.-Y.; Rezaei-Soufi, L.; Khamverdi, Z. Antibacterial properties of composite resins incorporating silver and zinc oxide nanoparticles on Streptococcus mutans and Lactobacillus. *Restor. Dent. Endod.* **2014**, *39*, 109–114. [CrossRef] [PubMed]
34. Hu, X.; Lin, X.; Zhao, H.; Chen, Z.; Yang, J.; Li, F.; Liu, C.; Tian, F. Surface Functionalization of Polyethersulfone Membrane with Quaternary Ammonium Salts for Contact-Active Antibacterial and Anti-Biofouling Properties. *Materials* **2016**, *17*, 376. [CrossRef] [PubMed]
35. Bowen, W.H.; Koo, H. Biology of Streptococcus mutans-derived glucosyltransferases: Role in extracellular matrix formation of cariogenic biofilms. *Caries Res.* **2011**, *45*, 69–86. [CrossRef] [PubMed]
36. Hanada, N.; Kuramitsu, H.K. Isolation and characterization of the Streptococcus mutans gtfD gene, coding for primer-dependent soluble glucan synthesis. *Infect. Immun.* **1989**, *57*, 2079–2085. [PubMed]
37. Xiao, J.; Hara, A.T.; Kim, D.; Zero, D.T.; Koo, H.; Hwang, G. Biofilm three-dimensional architecture influences in situ pH distribution pattern on the human enamel surface. *Int. J. Oral Sci.* **2017**, *9*, 74–79. [CrossRef] [PubMed]

38. Zhou, H.; Weir, M.D.; Antonucci, J.M.; Schumacher, G.E.; Zhou, X.D.; Xu, H.H. Evaluation of three-dimensional biofilms on antibacterial bonding agents containing novel quaternary ammonium methacrylates. *Int. J. Oral Sci.* **2014**, *6*, 77–86. [CrossRef] [PubMed]
39. Zhou, H.; Liu, H.; Weir, M.D.; Reynolds, M.A.; Zhang, K.; Xu, H.H. Three-dimensional biofilm properties on dental bonding agent with varying quaternary ammonium charge densities. *J. Dent.* **2016**, *53*, 73–81. [CrossRef] [PubMed]
40. Beyth, N.; Yudovin-Farber, I.; Bahir, R.; Domb, A.J.; Weiss, E.I. Antibacterial activity of dental composites containing quaternary ammonium polyethylenimine nanoparticles against Streptococcus mutans. *Biomate* **2006**, *27*, 995–4002. [CrossRef] [PubMed]
41. Auschill, T.M.; Arweiler, N.B.; Netuschil, L.; Brecx, M.; Reich, E.; Sculean, A. Spatial distribution of vital and dead microorganisms in dental biofilms. *Arch. Oral Biol.* **2001**, *46*, 471–476. [CrossRef]
42. Tawakoli, P.N.; Al-Ahmad, A.; Hoth-Hannig, W.; Hannig, M.; Hannig, C. Comparison of different live/dead stainings for detection and quantification of adherent microorganisms in the initial oral biofilm. *Clin. Oral Investig.* **2013**, *17*, 841–850. [CrossRef] [PubMed]
43. Liu, Y.; Naha, P.C.; Hwang, G.; Kim, D.; Huang, Y.; Simon-Soro, A.; Jung, H.I.; Ren, Z.; Li, Y.; Gubara, S.; et al. Topical ferumoxytol nanoparticles disrupt biofilms and prevent tooth decay in vivo via intrinsic catalytic activity. *Nat. Commun.* **2018**, *9*, 2920. [CrossRef] [PubMed]
44. Li, F.; Weir, M.D.; Xu, H.H. Effects of Quaternary Ammonium Chain Length on Antibacterial Bonding Agents. *J. Dent. Res.* **2013**, *92*, 932–938. [CrossRef] [PubMed]
45. Li, F.; Weir, M.D.; Chen, J.; Xu, H.H. Effect of charge density of bonding agent containing a new quaternary ammonium methacrylate on antibacterial and bonding properties. *Dent. Mater.* **2014**, *30*, 433–441. [CrossRef] [PubMed]
46. Melo, M.A.S.; Weir, M.D.; Rodrigues, L.K.A.; Xu, H.H.K. Novel calcium phosphate nanocomposite with caries-inhibition in a human in situ model. *Dent. Mater.* **2013**, *29*, 231–240. [CrossRef] [PubMed]
47. Hara, A.T.; Turssi, C.P.; Ando, M.; González-Cabezas, C.; Zero, D.T.; Rodrigues, A.L., Jr.; Serra, M.C.; Cury, J.A. Influence of fluoride-releasing restorative material on root dentine secondary caries in situ. *Caries Res.* **2006**, *40*, 435–439. [CrossRef] [PubMed]
48. Melo, M.A.; Morais, W.A.; Passos, V.F.; Lima, J.P.M.; Rodrigues, L.K. Fluoride releasing and enamel demineralization around orthodontic brackets by fluoride-releasing composite containing nanoparticles. *Clin. Oral Investig.* **2013**, *18*, 1343–1350. [CrossRef] [PubMed]

12

Covalently-Linked Hyaluronan versus Acid Etched Titanium Dental Implants: A Crossover RCT in Humans

Saturnino Marco Lupi [1,*], Arianna Rodriguez y Baena [1], Clara Cassinelli [2], Giorgio Iviglia [2], Marco Tallarico [3], Marco Morra [2] and Ruggero Rodriguez y Baena [1]

1 Department of Clinico-Surgical, Diagnostic and Pediatric Sciences, Dental Clinic, University of Pavia, P.le Golgi 2, 27100 Pavia, Italy; arianna_rodriguez@hotmail.it (A.R.yB.); ruggero.rodriguez@unipv.it (R.R.yB.)

2 Nobil Bio Ricerche srl, V. Valcastellana 26, 14037 Portacomaro, Italy; ccassinelli@nobilbio.it (C.C.); giviglia@nobilbio.it (G.I.); mmorra@nobilbio.it (M.M.)

3 Private Practice, V. Vincenzo Ussani 86, 00151 Roma, Italy; me@studiomarcotallarico.it

* Correspondence: saturninomarco.lupi@unipv.it

Abstract: Biochemical modification of titanium surfaces (BMTiS) entails immobilization of biomolecules to implant surfaces in order to induce specific host responses. This crossover randomized clinical trial assesses clinical success and marginal bone resorption of dental implants bearing a surface molecular layer of covalently-linked hyaluronan in comparison with control implants up to 36 months after loading. Patients requiring bilateral implant rehabilitation received hyaluronan covered implants in one side of the mouth and traditional implants in the other side. Two months after the first surgery, a second surgery was undergone to uncover the screw and to place a healing abutment. After two weeks, the operator proceeded with prosthetic procedures. Implants were evaluated by periapical radiographs and the crestal bone level was recorded at mesial and distal sites—at baseline and up to 36 months. One hundred and six implants were positioned, 52 HY-coated, and 48 controls were followed up. No differences were observed in terms of insertion and stability, wound healing, implant success, and crestal bone resorption at any time considered. All interventions had an optimal healing, and no adverse events were recorded. This trial shows, for the first time, a successful use in humans of biochemical-modified implants in routine clinical practice and in healthy patients and tissues with satisfactory outcomes.

Keywords: dental implants; surface modification; hyaluronan; clinical trial

---

1. Introduction

Ever since the pioneering studies of Professor Brånemark, osseointegration of titanium implant fixtures has been recognized as an interfacial event [1]. The clinical practice of implant dentistry has been based on the intimate apposition of newly formed bone tissue to the titanium surface. A great deal of literature has been devoted to the relationship between titanium surface properties and new bone formation [2–4]. The primary physical-chemical variables, titanium oxide surface chemistry, and implant surface topography dictate relevant surface parameters—such as surface charge and wettability—and have been deeply investigated in relation to cellular events leading to peri-implant bone regeneration [5–11]. The understanding of such relationships prompted the clinical evolution of titanium implants from the original turned to present day micro- and nano-rough surfaces [12–14].

Parallel to the growth and widespread acceptance of dental implantology, rising knowledge framed relevant interfacial biological events within a broader picture [15–18]. Cellular mechanisms leading to new bone formation and soft tissue healing, as well as inflammatory response leading to loss of supporting soft and hard tissue, are mediated by biological molecules and relevant signaling. The presentation of biomolecular cues, rather than the comparatively rough inorganic chemistry of titanium, seems a reasonable highway towards the evolution of better and innovative implant surfaces [19]. Accordingly, surface engineering of medical devices has long since been involved with the immobilization of a wide range of biomolecules to medical materials surfaces [20,21]. Biochemical modification of titanium surfaces (BMTiS) was defined by Puleo and Nancy [22] as the immobilization of proteins, enzymes, or peptides with the purpose of inducing specific cell and tissue responses using critical organic components of bone to affect tissue response. BMTiS are generally based on surface modification either by peptides, ECM proteins, or polysaccharides, all from animal and vegetal sources [23–34]. Despite a huge number of studies and promising in vitro and pre-clinical results [35], no practical application exists so far, and clinical performances of present-day dental implants are still dictated by the titanium/host tissue interface and mostly based on stimulation of cell behavior by surface topography.

This work presents the results of the first clinical trial involving bio-molecular modification of titanium implant surfaces. Implant fixtures used in the present trial bear a surface nano-layer (a few nm thick) of covalently-linked hyaluronic acid or hyaluronan [while its common acronym is HA, it is indicated as HY in the present paper to avoid any risk of confusion with the widely used inorganic HA (hydroxyapatite)-coatings]. This means that they present a complex macromolecular chemistry and not the relatively simple inorganic chemistry of titanium surfaces at the implant/tissue interface.

HY (Figure 1) is a linear polysaccharide consisting of the repeating disaccharide unit *N*-acetyl-D-glucosamine-D-glucuronate linked by β1-4 and β1-3 linkages. It is involved with a huge number of cellular processes [36–39].

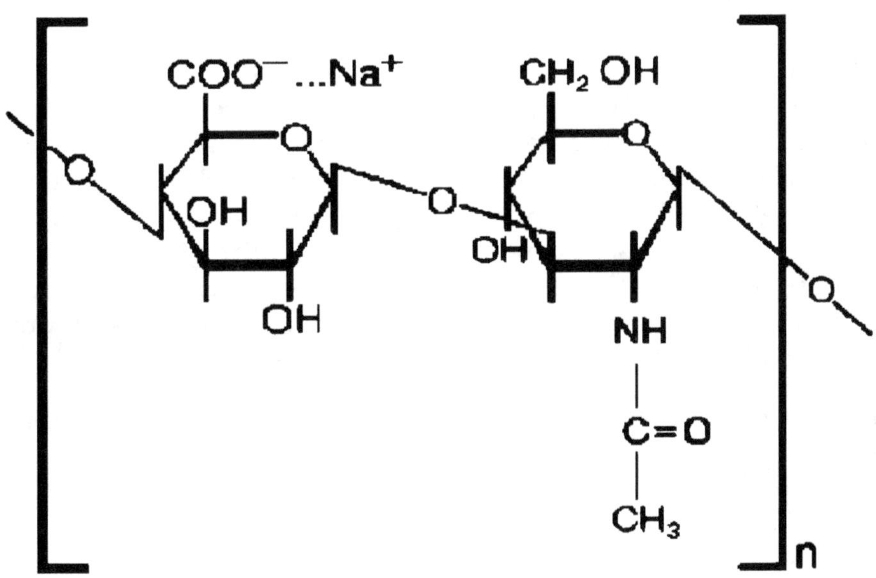

Figure 1. The repeating unit of Hyaluronan (HY).

Contrary to more complex glycosaminoglycans, HY is not sulfated, and it does not occur as part of a proteoglycan linked to a protein carrier. Significant interest in HY as a biomaterial and in biomaterials surface modification exists [40]. HY in medicine is mostly exploited because of its physical properties (hydration, viscosity, space filling), or by taking advantage of the hydration-promoted ability to reduce non-specific adhesion. Growing knowledge on HY as a key molecule in the regulation of many cellular processes involved with wound healing and tissue regeneration suggests that even more opportunities lie in the exploitation of its specific biological and bioactive properties [41–43].

Several literature reports indicate the potential interest of HY in BMTiS. Concerning bone regeneration, since the fifties it has been known that considerable HY is synthesized in the early stages of callus formation during the repair of fractured long bones [44]. Iwata and Urist [45] found that large amounts of HY were secreted when implants of decalcified bone underwent remineralization as bone. Bernard and coworkers presented studies aimed at developing "a foundation for the use of HY as a superior carrier for osteotropic substrates, even as HY acts to enhance osteogenesis due to its own molecular structure" [46]. Their in vitro studies using fetal calvarial cells and bone marrow osteogenic stem cells show that osteogenesis in vitro is significantly enhanced by HY 30–160 kDa, while high Mw HY (550–1300 kDa) shows weak inhibitory effects compared to the control. Zou and coworkers reported that 800 kDa HY added to bone marrow stromal cells cultured in vitro accelerates cell proliferation, increases alkaline phosphatase activity and osteocalcin gene expression, and that HY interacts with BMP-2 to generate direct and specific cellular effects [47]. Ito and coworkers showed that locally applied 900 kDa HY has a positive effect in bone ingrowth in Titanium fiber mesh implant in rats [48]. According to Cho, HY shows a positive effect in early bone consolidation in distraction osteogenesis [49]. HY based scaffolds aid in the regeneration of cartilage and bone defects in tissue engineering applications. The hypothesis of an active role played by local HY delivery upon scaffold degradation was suggested [50]. Zhao et al. [51] investigated the role of molecular weight and concentration of HY on the proliferation and osteogenic differentiation of rabbit bone marrow-derived stem cells in vitro. Factorial analysis indicated that molecular weight (MW) and concentration had an interactive effect on alkaline phosphatase mRNA expression ($p < 0.05$). HY of higher MW and higher concentration promoted bone formation. Regarding the in vivo studies on HY-coated implants, Aebli et al. [52] did not find bone growth increase in tests involving a sheep model. It should be noted that in the quoted study, the water-soluble HY was simply applied from solution to hydroxyapatite-coated implants without any intervening chemical bond to prevent rapid wash off [40]. An in vivo study on surface-engineered titanium implants bearing instead of a covalently-linked HY molecular surface layer in a four week rabbit model showed improvement of both bone to implant contact and bone ingrowth by hystomorphometry, while mechanical testing and evaluation of interfacial bone micro-hardness confirmed a faster bone maturation around HY coated implants [53]. Based on these and other encouraging pre-clinical results, the present study was conducted to investigate the clinical potential of HY covalently-linked implants and to set a starting point for future developments. The main goal was to confirm, in clinical practice and adopting objective clinical evaluation criteria, that "it is possible to do without the titanium surface chemistry". Once this point is set in routine clinics, pathways to actual exploitation of biomolecular signaling properties in compromised or challenging cases can be explored.

The paper presents first a detailed investigation of HY-coated titanium implants surfaces and relevant uncoated controls by SEM, energy dispersive X-ray spectroscopy (EDX), and X-ray photoelectron spectroscopy (XPS). Results of the clinical trial are then presented and discussed.

This split-mouth randomized clinical trial is aimed at assessing the clinical success and marginal bone resorption of dental implants bearing a surface molecular layer of covalently-linked hyaluronan in comparison with traditional sand-blasted and etched titanium implants up to 36 months after loading.

2. Results

2.1. Scanning Electron Microscopy/EDX Analysis

The surface topography of control and HY-coated implants was evaluated by SEM. Figures 2 and 3 show obtained results at 3000× and 10,000×.

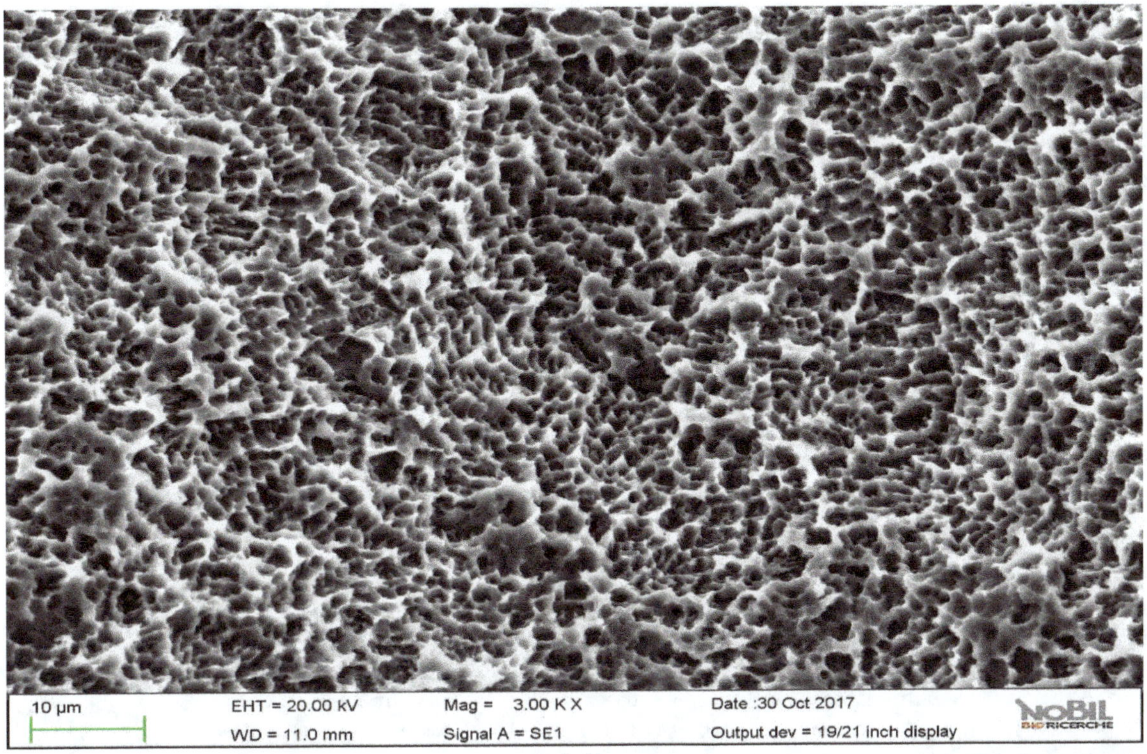

(a)

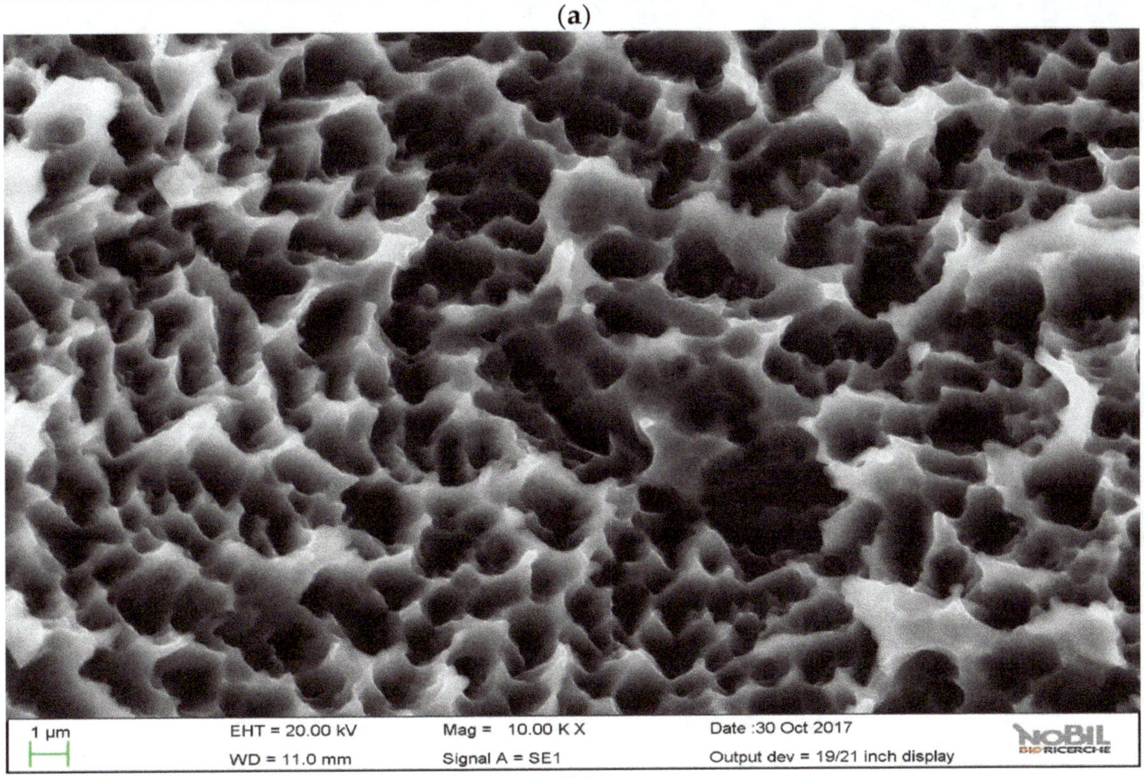

(b)

Figure 2. SEM images of the control implant surface, (**a**) 3000×; (**b**) 10,000×.

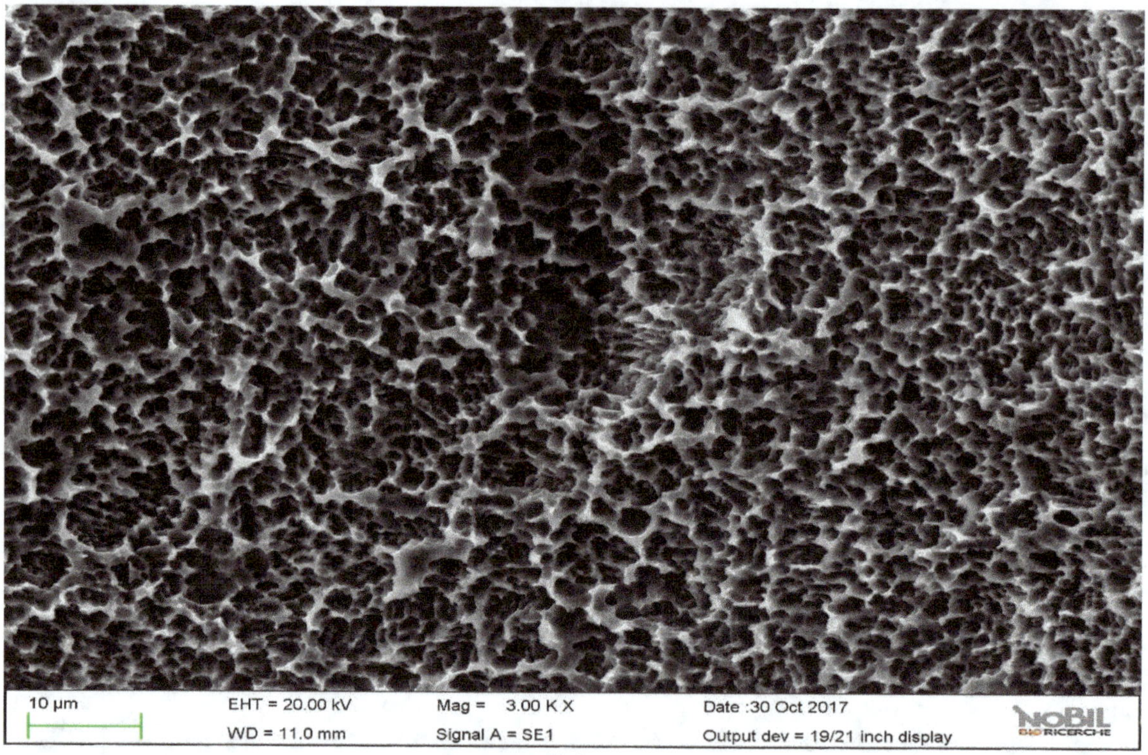

(a)

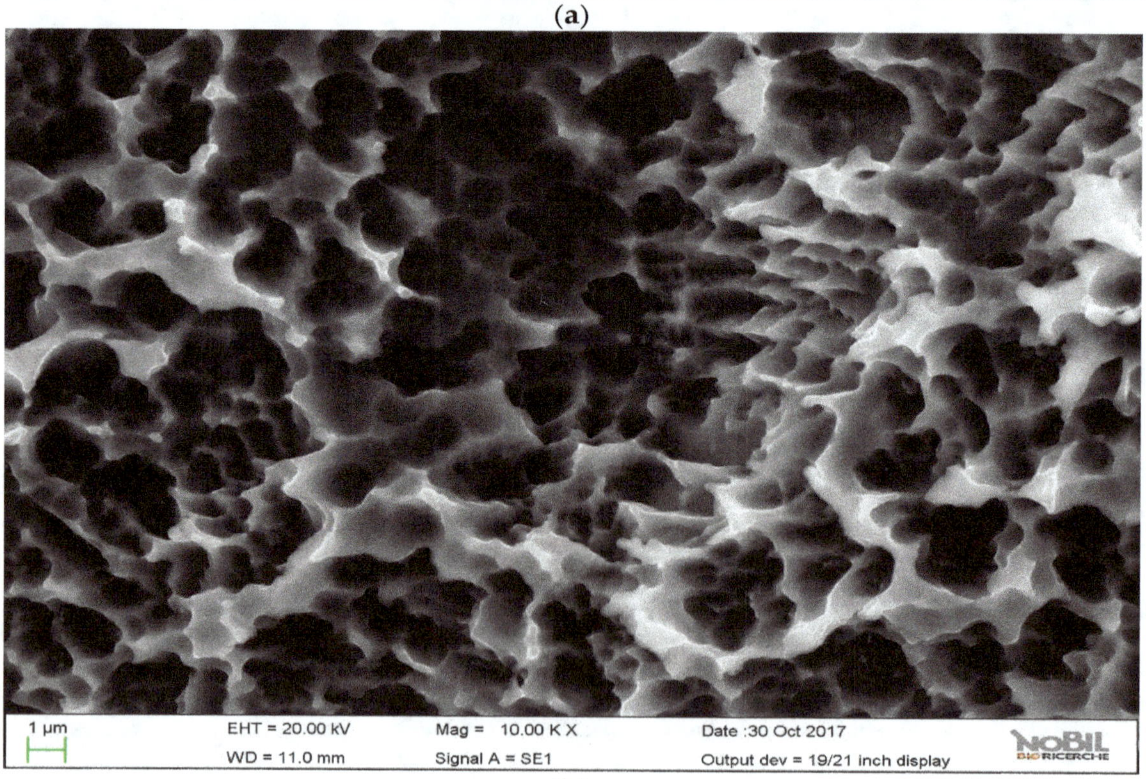

(b)

Figure 3. SEM images of the hyaluronan- (HY) coated implant surface, (**a**) 3000×; (**b**) 10,000×.

Both samples showed the typical microtopography of doubly acid etched surfaces—a microrough surface where the distance between peaks was of the order of the micrometer. As reported in the literature, a peak distance lower than the typical cell length can stimulate cell behavior, thus promoting accelerated osteogenesis [54,55]. No evidence of the HY coating was observed, even at 10,000×.

Surface linking of HY involved just molecular layers, whose thicknesses were approximately a few nanometers at most [40]. At this level of magnification, it was not detected over the microrough landscape provided by the doubly acid etched titanium surface. Table 1 reports the roughness parameters according to ISO 4287 that were obtained by the stereo-SEM reconstruction of the surface topography obtained from 2000× images, as described in the Materials section. A 900 μm path length and an 80 μm cut-off wavelength were used. No significant difference between samples was observed.

Table 1. Roughness parameters obtained by stereo-SEM. Data are expressed in μm as average and standard deviation of three measurements.

Parameter	Control		HY-Coated		Description
	Mean	Std	Mean	Std	
Ra	0.97	0.19	0.93	0.24	Average roughness of profile
Rq	1.26	0.29	1.23	0.34	Root-Mean-Square roughness of profile
Rt	7.96	0.77	6.87	1.13	Maximum peak to valley height of roughness profile
Rz	5.67	1.23	5.77	1.15	Mean peak to valley height of roughness profile
Rmax	7.93	0.75	6.41	0.99	Maximum peak to valley height of roughness profile within a sampling length
Rp	4.33	0.63	3.93	0.73	Maximum peak height of roughness profile
Rv	3.63	0.14	2.93	0.45	Maximum valley height of roughness profile
Rc	3.69	0.64	3.62	1.03	Mean height of profile irregularities of roughness profile
Rsm	43.22	9.69	53.77	19.90	Mean spacing of profile irregularities of roughness profile

Figure 4 shows the energy dispersive X-ray spectroscopy (EDX) spectra obtained from the two samples. Both of them showed a very strong signal from titanium. In the case of the HY-coated implant, small but significant peaks due to carbon and oxygen were detected as well, suggesting the presence of an organic surface layer.

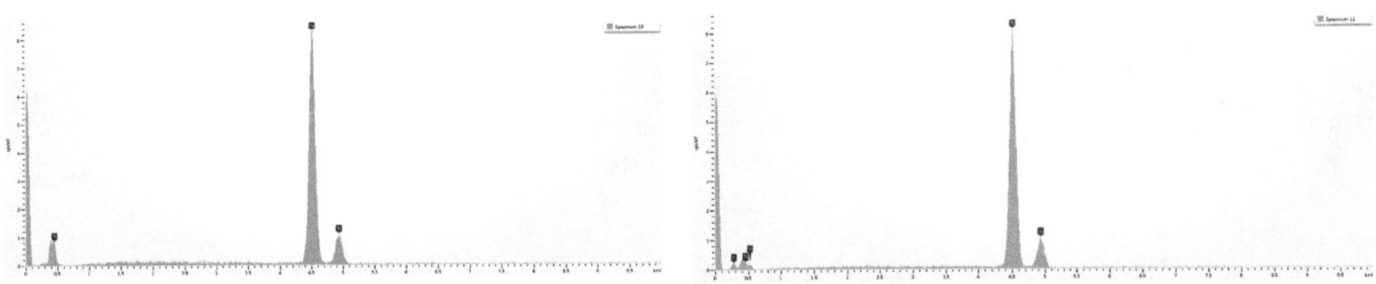

(a) (b)

Figure 4. EDX spectra of control (**a**) and HY-coated (**b**) titanium implant.

2.2. *X-Ray Photoelectron Spectroscopy*

XPS wide-scan spectra of control and HY-coated dental implants used in the present clinical trial are shown in Figure 5.

The control implant showed the typical composition of titanium surfaces, yielding signals due to photoemitted electrons from core levels of the expected elements: titanium, oxygen (because of the native titanium oxide surface layer), and carbon (due to surface adsorption of ubiquitous carbon-containing compounds from the atmosphere and nitrogen). The overall surface composition, reported in Table 2, was in good quantitative agreement with data from the literature. It showed no unexpected elements or contamination, and its C/Ti ratio was indicative of excellent surface cleanliness [7,56].

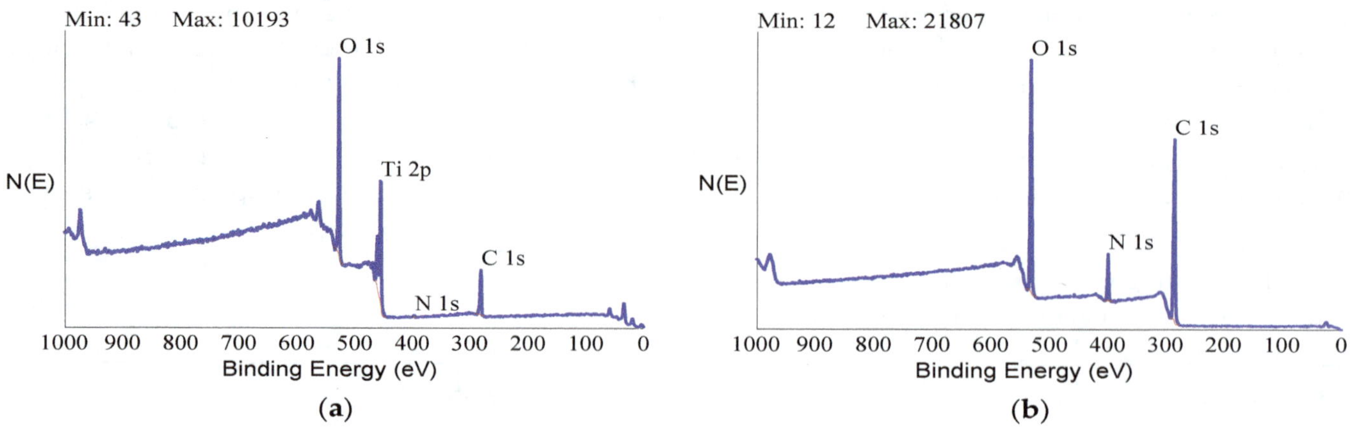

Figure 5. X-ray photoelectron spectroscopy (XPS) wide-scan spectra of control (**a**) and HY-coated (**b**) titanium implant.

Table 2. Surface composition (% at.) of Control and HY-coated implants.

Sample	O	Ti	N	C
Control	51.4	17.1	1.0	30.5
HY-coated	28.7	-	7.9	63.4

The XPS spectrum of the HY-coated implant, on the other hand, showed a completely different picture. First and foremost, there was no signal from titanium at all. The only elements detected in the nanometer-thick sampling depth probed by XPS were the basic elements of organic chemistry—oxygen, carbon, and nitrogen. The elemental ratio reported in Table 2 was consistent with typical polysaccharides stoichiometry, showing a high O/C ratio. Perusal of the literature confirmed that the detected surface stoichiometry was consistent with the reported composition of covalently-linked HY through aminated spacers [57]. Further clues were offered by the sensitivity to the carbon chemical environment provided by the high-resolution peak of C1s photoelectrons. Figure 6 shows C1s peaks of the tested control and HY-coated dental implants.

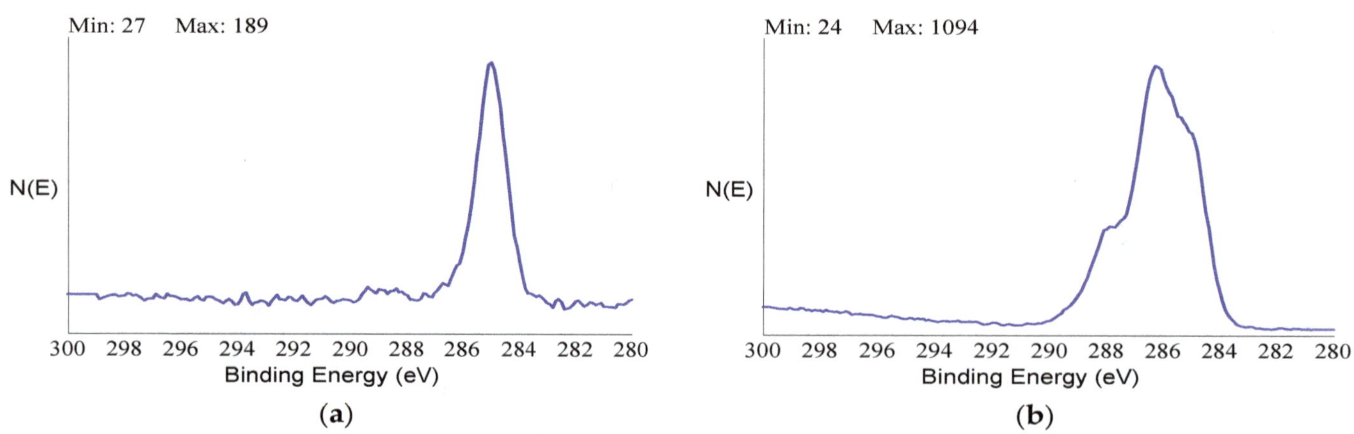

Figure 6. XPS high-resolution C1s peak of control (**a**) and HY-coated (**b**) titanium implant.

In the former case, the peak was relatively simple and symmetrical, confirming that it was mostly due to C-C and C-H functionalities from adventitious hydrocarbons. The C1s peak of the HY-coated implant was much broader and clearly contained different components. De-convolution of the C1s peak of the HY-coated implant following general XPS practice [58] is shown in Figure 7.

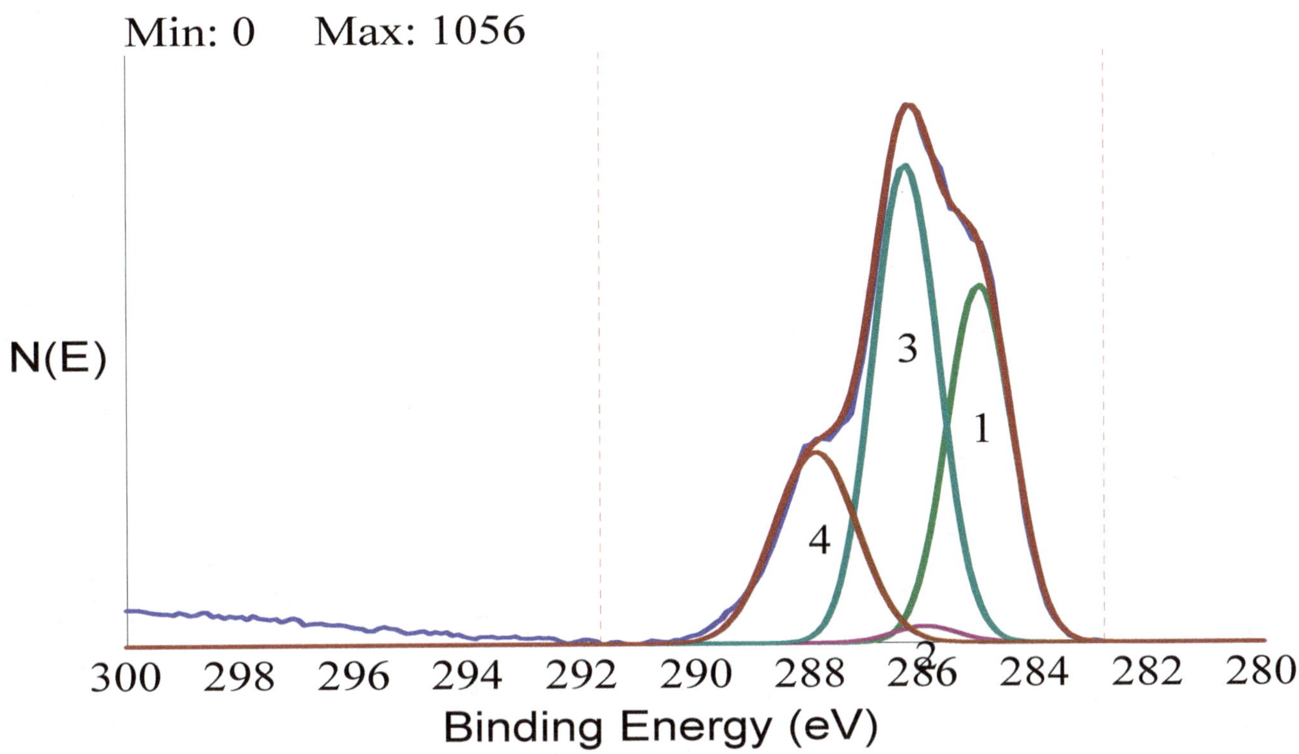

Figure 7. Curve fitting of high-resolution C1s peak of the HY-coated titanium implant by the four components expected from the molecular structure of hyaluronan.

The experimental curve was fitted according to literature indication [59] by four components located at 285.00 eV (C-C, C-H), 286.15 eV (C-N), 286.50 eV (C-O), and 288.10 eV (C=O, N-C=O, and O-C=O functionalities). Peak de-convolution showed that the carbon chemical environment at the HY-coated titanium implant surface was dominated by the carbon single bond oxygen functionality typical of polysaccharides, and that the experimental C1s peak contained all features expected from the molecular structure of HY. Taken together, these data convincingly showed that the outermost nanometers of the HY-coated implant surface presented to the external environment the molecular cues stemming from the HY repeating unit, which was a completely different chemical nature when compared to the titanium oxide surface of the conventional control implant.

2.3. Clinical Trial

From 8 April 2013 to 17 October 2014, 106 implants were positioned in 30 patients (demographic data in Table 3).

Table 3. Demographic data and implant location. Data in absolute values and (%).

Demographic Data	Total	HY	C
Males	21 (70)		
Females	9 (30)		
Patients mean age	59.8 ± 10.6		
Implant location			
Anterior maxilla	18 (17.0)	9 (16.4)	9 (17.6)
Posterior maxilla	41 (38.7)	24 (43.6)	17 (33.3)
Anterior mandibula	10 (9.4)	5 (9.0)	5 (9.8)
Posterior mandibula	37 (34.9)	17 (30.9)	20 (39.2)

During surgery, no differences were observed in regards to the insertion and stability between the two types of implants (test and control), nor were differences observed in the post-operative visits in regards to the indices of inflammation and wound healing. The healing was uneventful in all of the patients in the variability of the surgical situation, and no adverse events whatsoever were recorded. Only 102 implants in 29 subjects out of the 106 implanted were loaded and taken as baselines for X-ray values (mesial and distal). Two implants (one control and one HY coated) in two different patients failed and were removed. In both cases, the mucosa appeared edematous and bleeding, indicating signs of an infection. In one case, the implant was not replaced, and since no matching controls were available, the subject (Subject N°34) was excluded from the efficacy analysis. In the second subject, the failed implant was relocated in the same place after two months, reaching healing and tissue stabilization. Therefore, the subject was maintained in the statistics. One subject with two implants (one control and one HA) dropped out between the 12 months and the 18 months follow up visits due to a desire for pregnancy and therefore the unethical use of X-ray procedures. Results are summarized in Table 4.

Table 4. Bone resorption.

Time Points	HY		C		p (between-Group)	95% Confidence Interval	
	n	Mean ± sd	n	Mean ± sd		Min	Max
Mesial							
3	51	0.55 ± 0.46	47	0.51 ± 0.65	0.64	−0.24	0.55
6	24	0.72 ± 0.38	20	0.65 ± 0.39	0.58	−0.30	0.17
12	35	0.83 ± 0.61	35	0.66 ± 0.58	0.25	−0.45	0.12
18	16	0.65 ± 0.63	17	0.36 ± 0.43	0.14	−0.67	0.10
24	34	0.80 ± 0.87	32	0.50 ± 0.57	0.10	−0.66	0.06
36	21	0.55 ± 0.40	19	0.32 ± 0.36	0.06	−0.47	0.01
Distal							
3	51	0.71 ± 0.60	47	0.70 ± 0.62	0.97	−0.25	0.24
6	24	0.77 ± 0.60	20	0.93 ± 0.46	0.30	−0.15	0.49
12	35	0.83 ± 0.63	35	0.85 ± 0.60	0.90	−0.28	0.31
18	16	0.72 ± 0.53	17	0.47 ± 0.45	0.16	−0.59	0.11
24	34	0.76 ± 0.42	32	0.63 ± 0.62	0.33	−0.39	0.14
36	21	0.62 ± 0.53	19	0.55 ± 0.62	0.70	−0.44	0.30

Time points: months; n: number of implants; mean ± standard deviation (sd) expressed in mm.

The non-inferiority analysis did not show any significant differences between the HY- and the control- in terms of mesial and distal bone resorption at any time point.

3. Discussion

In the present clinical trial, a widely adopted microrough titanium surface and the same surface further modified by a covalently-linked nanolayer of hyaluronan were compared in terms of clinical success in routine clinical practice.

Analytical data confirmed the exquisitely superficial nature of the surface modification process that was adopted. The analytical signal captured in EDX analysis stemmed from a surface volume that was a few micrometers deep [60]. Thus, within the EDX sampling depth, the signal by the nanometers-thick HY surface layer was diluted within the micrometer-thick analytical layer, and the resulting spectrum contained convoluted contributions from the underlying Ti implant and the overlying HY molecules in roughly a 1000:1 ratio. As a consequence, the elements composing the surface layer were barely detectable. For this reason, a more surface-sensitive analytical technique, namely XPS, was conducted to fully appreciate the biomolecular modification of the HY-coated implants. Contrary to EDX analysis, the physics of photoelectrons escaped from solids endowed XPS with just a few nanometers of sampling depth, consequently providing chemical information on the outermost atomic layers of materials [58]. For this reason, XPS was extensively used in the surface analysis of dental implants [7,61–63].

Despite the widely different surface chemistry, objective optimal healing was observed for both groups, and no differences were detected in the clinical outcome for all tested parameters. Far from being uneventful, the described results suggested some important reflections. From a chemical-physical point of view, it would be difficult to imagine two more different surface structures—the titanium surface (in particular, the outermost few nanometers of oxidized titanium) presented a hard, impervious interface to the host tissue, whose chemical behavior was controlled by titanium oxide interfacial chemistry, as widely described in many scientific papers [7,8,61]. On the contrary, the HY-coated implant aqueous interface was diffuse, soft, and hydrated [64]. Its chemistry stemmed from the molecular details of the *N*-acetyl-D-glucosamine-D-glucuronate repeating unit. Shortly, one of them (the control arm) belonged to inorganic chemistry. The HY-coated surface belonged instead to organic biomacromolecular chemistry. Despite being two worlds apart, no significant difference was detected in the tested clinical variables, and both of them led to successful osseointegration and clinical success. The first significant reflection from the data of the present work is that the titanium surface chemistry is not necessary to achieve a clinically satisfactory load-bearing capacity by a titanium dental implant.

The previous point could be interpreted as a no-effect of surface chemistry on osseointegration. As long as the implant surface is inert and no disturbance is introduced in the bone healing mechanism—that is, as long as no toxic or irritating compounds are released in the evolving new bone matrix independent from specific details of surface chemistry—clinically effective osseointegration will occur. If this is the case, no advancement is expected by BMTiS over conventional surfaces, and the sole opportunity to direct tissue response is through surface topography.

The last sentence falls short when compared to existing scientific evidence gathered from animal data, which shows direct effects of interfacial chemistry on bone healing in terms of peri-implant bone volume, bone to implant contact, or gene expression by peri-implant bone cells [35,53,65,66]. In the present clinical trial, a patient's selection and surgery addressed comparatively routine clinical practice. The control arm, involving a state-of-the-art doubly acid etched microrough surface, obviously provided optimal healing and clinical success. Endpoint variables aimed at general clinical evidence expectedly confirmed that both the well-known titanium interfacial chemistry and the biologically relevant HY molecular cued direct cellular events involved with peri-implant tissue healing towards proper clinical response.

HY is a key molecule in many tissue regeneration processes; it is involved with most of the mammalian cells' healing mechanisms [67–69] in a concentration and size-dependent way. The permanent linking of HY to materials surfaces avoids quick wash-off of the water soluble HY and aims at providing these regenerative properties at the peri-implant interface, as confirmed by several in vivo evidences. It is not clear yet how surface-immobilized HY compares with HY in solution in terms of the effect of the hindered conformational freedom on the multiple ligand-receptor interactions required to trigger a biological response [40]. It would be of interest to check the stimulation of bone tissue regeneration at machined interfaces of hybrid implants, the effect on soft tissue healing in the transmucosal section of tissue level implants, or the control of inflammatory responses of periodontal patients [70] and relevant clinical implications. The positive evidence supplied by the present clinical trial in standard practice opens the path to comprehensive investigation of the merits of BMTiS in clinical implantology by further finely-targeted clinical trials.

A last observation involves the relationship of present results with in vitro investigation of dental implant surfaces. A widely adopted approach involves the "adhesion and growth" paradigm, meaning that prospective surface structures are screened in terms of effects on adhesion and growth of osteoblast cells—the faster and more extensive the surface colonization by cells, the better the properties. Against this view, HY-coated surfaces are notoriously anti-adhesive in vitro [64,71], meaning that they prevent cell adhesion of a number of cell lines, including osteoblasts. Several applications of HY-coated surfaces are based on tissue-anti-adhesive properties. In vitro tests of present clinically successful HY-coated implants would provide unsatisfactory results if judged according to the "adhesion and growth" paradigm. Yet, clinical evidence as supplied by the present trial indicates that they are fit for the intended use. Far from being inconsistent, this evidence simply indicates the complexity of the peri-implant environment as opposed to the comparatively simple biological environment of in vitro tests. In clinics, osteoblasts do not adhere and grow onto the implant surface. Rather, they come to a complex peri-implant milieu after the blood clot and relevant blood cells, inflammatory cells, and the sequela of cytokine and growth factors are released in the initial stage of inflammation and healing [72]. Rather than the direct effect of the interfacial HY (or of any surface-linked biomolecular layer) on osteoblasts, it is the effect of molecular signaling on the evolution of the peri-implant biochemical environment that directs clinical outcome and that holds the potential merits of BMTiS in clinics.

In summary, the clinical trial did not record any significant difference between the HY- and the C-group in terms of clinical success and marginal bone resorption. In the present study, for the first time in clinics (to the author's knowledge), dental implants with a biomolecular nanolayer on the surface showed a behavior similar to the commercial pure titanium one. This study presents the limits to having a follow up limited to 36 months. The duration of the follow up was chosen because in this span of time, the HY layer should be completely integrated within the newly formed interfacial tissue. Further studies should be conducted to evaluate the long-term success of HY-implants. Present data build up the ethical basis for the investigation into the merits of HY-coated implants in more challenging and compromised cases where signaling and regenerative properties encoded within the HY molecular structure could play a role that is presently not supplied by the comparatively rough titanium surface chemistry.

4. Materials and Methods

4.1. Titanium Implant

The fixture used in the clinical trial was a CE marked titanium grade 4, internal hexagon, doubly acid etched implant (Ornaghi Luigi & C, Brugherio, Italy). The implant fixture was further coated by covalently-linked HY by Nobil Bio Ricerche (Nobil Bio Ricerche srl, Portacomaro, Italy) through a proprietary process, as described in the Results section. Covalent-linking prevented the rapid wash-off of the water-soluble HY molecules, degradation by hyaluronidase, and release. The thickness of the coating, as discussed in the following sections, was a few nanometers and did not modify the nominal dimensions. The control was the same implant not coated with covalently-linked HY.

4.2. Surface Characterization

4.2.1. Scanning Electron Microscopy

The surface topography of the implants was evaluated by SEM. Analysis was conducted using an EVO MA 10 SEM (Carl Zeiss Microscopy GmbH, Jena, Germany). The electron acceleration voltage was maintained at 20 kV with the working distance between 10 and 12.5 mm. These parameters are reported in the images, along with level of magnification (MAG) and the kind of detector utilized (Signal A = SE1 or CZ BSD).

Images were acquired in both conventional mode (Signal A = SE1) and in backscattered electron mode (Signal A = CZ BSD), allowing improved contrast between different chemical elements.

Roughness was evaluated quantitatively by stereo-SEM (SSEM) using dedicated software to convert conventional SEM images into three-dimensional data (Mex 6.0, Alicona Imaging, Raaba/Graz, Austria). A stereo-pair was built by the acquisition of the same field of view at zero and after five degrees of eccentric tilting. Following the principles of stereoscopic vision, the stereo pair was transformed into a three-dimensional reconstruction of the surface by the quoted software, providing height profiles values used as input data for the calculation of roughness parameters according to ISO 4287. The stereo-pairs were built from 2000× images taken from three randomly selected areas for each implant.

4.2.2. X-ray Photoelectron Spectroscopy (XPS)

XPS analysis was performed using a Perkin Elmer PHI 5600 ESCA system (PerkinElmer Inc., Waltham, MA, USA). The instrument was equipped with a monochromatized Al anode operating at 10 kV and 200 W. The diameter of the analyzed spot was approximately 500 micrometers, and the analyzed depth was about 5 nanometers. The base pressure was maintained at 10–8 Pa. The angle between the electron analyzer and the sample surface was 45°. Analysis was performed by acquiring a wide-range survey spectra (0–1000 eV binding energy) and detailed high-resolution peaks of relevant elements. Quantification of elements was accomplished using the software and sensitivity factors supplied by the manufacturer. High-resolution C1s peaks were acquired using pass energy of 11.75 eV and a resolution of 0.100 eV/step.

4.3. Clinical Trial

The study "Blind Comparison of Covalently-Linked Hyaluronan versus Control-Dental Implants in a Randomized Crossover Clinical Investigation" is a post market clinical follow-up according to MEDDEV 2.12-2 rev 2 January 2012 conducted at the Dental Service, Department of Clinical, Surgical, Diagnostic, and Pediatric Sciences, University of Pavia, Pavia, Italy. The clinical trial was conducted according to the ISO 14155-11 and the Good Clinical Practice Guidelines (GCP). The study was carried out following the rules of the Declaration of Helsinki, as revised in 2013 and approved by the Ethical Committee of the University of Pavia on 13 December 2012. On 28 February 2013, the initiation of the study was communicated to the Italian Ministry of Health with the reference number 000017. All subjects gave their informed consent for inclusion before they participated in the study. The primary objective of this non-inferiority, crossover, fixed-size, and single-center trial was to assess the dental implant success (survival rate) of HA coating implants in comparison with control implants at one year. The secondary objective was to assess marginal bone resorption of HA coating implants in respect to traditional titanium implants measured at 3, 6, 12, 18, 24, and 36 months. To test the non-inferiority hypothesis of the HY-coated implant in respect to control implants, the null hypothesis was that the HY-coated implant resulted in a lower survival rate and a higher marginal bone loss in respect to the control implant. The P level of significance was set at 0.05. Patients with bilateral partial or full edentulism requiring implant rehabilitation were enrolled; inclusion and exclusion criteria are shown in Tables 5 and 6.

Table 5. Criteria for inclusion in the clinical trial.

Inclusion Criteria
Over 18 years of age;
Bilateral loss of one or more molars and bicuspids and/or bilateral loss of anterior teeth and the need for more than one implant in the same rehabilitation;
Edentulousness of both upper or lower jaw with need of at least 2 bilateral implants to stabilize a denture or to support a fixed prosthesis;
In general good health condition and with physical ability to tolerate surgical and prosthetic procedure (ASA 1 and 2);
Good plaque control and oral hygiene;
The subject who agree to return to the center for follow-up.

Table 6. Criteria for exclusion from the clinical trial.

Exclusion Criteria
Active infection or severe inflammation or suspected lesions in the areas intended for implant installation;
Diabetes (regardless of control);
Need for concomitant bone grafting and/or having less than 1 mm bone available at the buccal, lingual, and apical aspects of the implant. Less than 3 mm distance between implant and other dentition;
Under treatment and/or within the past 12 months with radiotherapy to the head or chemotherapy;
Suspected hypersensitivity and/or contraindication to any ingredients of the Investigational Device (ID)/Control ID;
Subjects under any study medication treatment in the last 30 days;
Pregnancy, breast feeding, oocyte donation, or oocyte implantation planned during the study;
Subjects not able to follow study procedures, e.g., language problems, psychological disorders;
Clinically relevant abnormal laboratory values suggesting an unknown disease and requiring further clinical evaluation (as assessed by the investigators);
Female subjects of childbearing potential, not using and not willing to continue using a medically reliable method of contraception for the entire study duration;
Any other untoward medical condition that could interfere with the participation of the subject in the trial.

In this study, concealment and randomization were implemented centrally by an operator (G.O.) unrelated to the surgical team, to the clinical examiner, and to the statistician. After manufacturing, implants were packaged in consecutively numbered boxes. Each box contained six implants, three with the HY surface (marked with A or B) and three with the control surface (marked with B if the HY implants were marked with A, or marked with A on the contrary). All of the implants were 4 mm in diameter and were 8, 10, and 12 mm long. The two surfaces were macroscopically indistinguishable. The assignation of the label (A or B) to the surfaces was randomly assigned in each box by a computer random number generator. Data were communicated to the statistician, omitting the surface characteristic. The list of randomization was concealed until after statistical analysis was concluded. Due to the split-mouth design of the study and the randomization process, the allocation ratio was 1:1. No block restrictions were applied.

4.3.1. Surgical Procedure

During surgery, implant(s) with one surface were placed in one side of the mouth and implant(s) with the other surface were placed in the other side of the mouth. When a patient required placement of the number of implants equal in both sides of the mouth, each couple of implants came out from a different box. When the number of implants required in one side of the mouth was greater than the other side, implants were chosen among those available in the opened boxes. If the odd implants were not available in the opened boxes, no experimental implants were positioned. This procedure was implemented after protocol approval because the surgical team signaled the problem of re-operating in patients with a different number of edentulous sites in the two sides of the mouth. Even though it was not necessary because randomization was implemented before surgery, the implant label choice for the sides of the mouth was randomized by a coin toss. The surgical protocol of installing the implants was well documented and consisted of a full thickness mucosal flap elevation, the preparation of the implant site, the installation of the implant with the prosthetic platform (that is, the edge of the collar) at the level of the bone crest, the positioning of the surgical cover screw, and the closing of the flap with sutures [73–80]. The surgery was done under coverage of antibiotics (2 g of amoxicillin and clavulanic acid per os one hour before surgery, followed by administration of 1 g after 6 and 18 h). The post-operative instructions indicated rinses with chlorhexidine 0.12% × three times a day from the day after surgery and for 30 days and control of the pain with anti-inflammatory drugs as needed. The removal of the sutures was carried out from the tenth to the fourteenth day.

The second stage of surgery was conducted after two months, both in the mandibular and in the maxillary arch. After about two weeks, the operator proceeded with the prosthesis installation. During follow-up visits, normal hygienic procedures were carried out when needed [81].

4.3.2. Investigation Hypothesis or Pass/Fall Criteria

The primary objective of the present study was to assess the success of HY coated implants in comparison with control implants after one year. The implant is considered successful (primary endpoints) if: (A) the implant is still present without any sign of mobility and (B) there is no evidence of radiolucency by means of periapical X-rays and (C) there is no clinical sign of peri-implantitis. The secondary objective of the present study was to demonstrate a non-inferiority of the HY-coated implants compared to the control implants considering the marginal bone resorption parameter. To do this, the null hypothesis is that control implants demonstrate an inferior crestal bone resorption in respect to HY coated implants.

Sample Size Calculation

The sample size was estimated based on the crestal bone level at 12 months post implant.

Since the objective of this study was the non-inferiority of the investigational device (ID) compared to the Control ID in a crossover design from data published by Mumcu [82], inferior limits for the Control ID were estimated.

Practically, from pooling data reported in Table 1 of Mumcu and Coll., an inferior limit of 0.7 mm was estimated and considered clinically appropriate. This implies that if the lower bond of the 95% confidence interval for the estimated difference in crestal bone level between implants is above −0.7 mm, then the ID is considered non-inferior to the Control ID.

Sample size was calculated under the following assumptions:

- Lower limits in difference between implants: −0.70 mm (Δ)
- Hypothesis testing:
- H0: μControl ID- μID ≤ Δ
- H1: μControl ID- μID > Δ (ID implant is non-inferior with respect to the mean response)
- α level of probability: 0.025 for one-sided test
- 1-β (power) level: 90% for a conservative approach
- Standard deviation for mean difference: 0.66, which corresponded to 80% of the pooled mean calculated from Mumcu (0.83 mm). In this estimate, it was considered that the ID presented on the crestal bone level a greater variability in respect to the Control ID and that reported in the publication.

By applying the formula reported in Julius [83] for non-inferiority trials in crossover design:

$$n = \frac{2\sigma^2\left(Z_{(1-\beta)} + Z_{(1-\alpha)}\right)^2}{((\mu_{Control\ ID} - \mu_{ID}) - d)^2}$$

18 evaluable subjects are needed to demonstrate the non-inferiority of the ID in respect to the Control ID. Considering that a couple of devices are implanted into each subject, we need to have at least 18 implant pairs in order to reach the trial primary objective.

5. Conclusions

The clinical trial "Blind Comparison of Covalently-Linked Hyaluronan versus Control-Dental Implants in a Randomized Crossover Clinical Investigation" evaluated clinical success up to 36 months with HY-coated dental implants compared to the control—uncoated microrough Ti grade 4 implants. Results showed a lack of differences between the two arms of the study. Both of them provided optimal healing.

Substitution of the clinically accepted and consolidated titanium surface chemistry with the molecular structure of HY and ensuing interfacial interactions results in a satisfactory clinical outcome.

Author Contributions: Conceptualization: S.M.L., A.R.yB., C.C., G.I., M.T., M.M. and R.R.yB.; methodology: S.M.L., C.C., M.M. and R.R.yB.; validation: A.R.yB., G.I., M.T. and R.R.yB.; formal analysis, S.M.L., C.C., M.M. and R.R.yB.; investigation, A.R.yB., G.I., M.T. and R.R.yB.; resources, A.R.yB.; data curation, S.M.L., M.M. and R.R.yB.; writing—original draft preparation, S.M.L. and M.M.; writing—review and editing, S.M.L., A.R.yB., C.C., G.I., M.T., M.M. and R.R.yB.; supervision, R.R.yB.; project administration, M.M.; funding acquisition, C.C., M.M. and R.R.yB.

Acknowledgments: The authors thank: BSDpharma srl, under the responsibility of Claudio F. Omini, for the role in CRO duties and for monitoring of the study; Gabriele Omini for randomization list and labels and for monitoring of the study; Guido Fedele for statistical support; Giuseppe Zuccari for Quality Assurance; AA Gandolfi for monitoring of the study.

Abbreviations

BMTiS	Biochemical modification of titanium surfaces
ECM	Extra Cellular Matrix
EDX	Energy Dispersive X-ray Analysis
GCP	Good Clinical Practice
HY	hyaluronic acid or hyaluronan
ID	Investigational Device
MAG	level of magnification
RCT	Randomized Clinical Trial
SEM	Scanning Electron Microscopy
XPS	X-ray Photoelectron Spectroscopy

References

1. Branemark, P.I. Osseointegration and its experimental background. *J. Prosthet. Dent.* **1983**, *50*, 399–410. [CrossRef]
2. Brunette, D.M.; Tengvall, P.; Textor, M.; Thomsen, P. *Titanium in Medicine: Material Science, Surface Science, Engineering, Biological Responses and Medical Applications*; Springer: Berlin, Germany, 2001.
3. Davies, J.E. *The Bone-Biomaterial Interface*; University of Toronto Press: Toronto, ON, Canada, 1991.
4. Ellingsen, J.E.; Lyngstadaas, S.P. *Bio-Implant Interface: Improving Biomaterials and Tissue Reactions*; CRC Press: London, UK, 2003.
5. Kasemo, B.; Lausmaa, J. Biomaterial and implant surfaces: A surface science approach. *Int. J. Oral Maxillofac. Implants* **1988**, *3*, 247–259. [PubMed]
6. Kasemo, B.; Lausmaa, J. Biomaterial and implant surfaces: On the role of cleanliness, contamination, and preparation procedures. *J. Biomed. Mater. Res.* **1988**, *22*, 145–158. [CrossRef] [PubMed]
7. Kasemo, B.; Lausmaa, J. Material-tissue interfaces: The role of surface properties and processes. *Environ. Health Perspect.* **1994**, *102*, 41–45. [PubMed]
8. Larsson Wexell, C.; Thomsen, P.; Aronsson, B.O.; Tengvall, P.; Rodahl, M.; Lausmaa, J.; Kasemo, B.; Ericson, L.E. Bone response to surface-modified titanium implants: Studies on the early tissue response to implants with different surface characteristics. *Int. J. Biomater.* **2013**, *2013*, 412482. [CrossRef] [PubMed]
9. Thomsen, P.; Larsson, C.; Ericson, L.E.; Sennerby, L.; Lausmaa, J.; Kasemo, B. Structure of the interface between rabbit cortical bone and implants of gold, zirconium and titanium. *J. Mater. Sci. Mater. Med.* **1997**, *8*, 653–665. [CrossRef] [PubMed]
10. Rupp, F.; Gittens, R.A.; Scheideler, L.; Marmur, A.; Boyan, B.D.; Schwartz, Z.; Geis-Gerstorfer, J. A review on the wettability of dental implant surfaces i: Theoretical and experimental aspects. *Acta Biomater.* **2014**, *10*, 2894–2906. [CrossRef] [PubMed]
11. Rupp, F.; Scheideler, L.; Olshanska, N.; de Wild, M.; Wieland, M.; Geis-Gerstorfer, J. Enhancing surface free energy and hydrophilicity through chemical modification of microstructured titanium implant surfaces. *J. Biomed. Mater. Res. A* **2006**, *76*, 323–334. [CrossRef]

12. Wennerberg, A.; Albrektsson, T. On implant surfaces: A review of current knowledge and opinions. *Int. J. Oral Maxillofac. Implants* **2010**, *25*, 63–74.
13. Rupp, F.; Liang, L.; Geis-Gerstorfer, J.; Scheideler, L.; Huttig, F. Surface characteristics of dental implants: A review. *Dent. Mater.* **2018**, *34*, 40–57. [CrossRef]
14. Rodriguez y Baena, R.; Rizzo, S.; Manzo, L.; Lupi, S.M. Nanofeatured titanium surfaces for dental implantology: Biological effects, biocompatibility, and safety. *J. Nanomater.* **2017**. [CrossRef]
15. Nishimura, I. Genetic networks in osseointegration. *J. Dent. Res.* **2013**, *92*, 109S–118S. [CrossRef] [PubMed]
16. Smeets, R.; Stadlinger, B.; Schwarz, F.; Beck-Broichsitter, B.; Jung, O.; Precht, C.; Kloss, F.; Grobe, A.; Heiland, M.; Ebker, T. Impact of dental implant surface modifications on osseointegration. *Biomed. Res. Int.* **2016**, *2016*, 6285620. [CrossRef] [PubMed]
17. Brett, E.; Flacco, J.; Blackshear, C.; Longaker, M.T.; Wan, D.C. Biomimetics of bone implants: The regenerative road. *Biores. Open Access* **2017**, *6*, 1–6. [CrossRef] [PubMed]
18. Insua, A.; Monje, A.; Wang, H.L.; Miron, R.J. Basis of bone metabolism around dental implants during osseointegration and peri-implant bone loss. *J. Biomed. Mater. Res. A* **2017**, *105*, 2075–2089. [CrossRef] [PubMed]
19. Bryers, J.D.; Giachelli, C.M.; Ratner, B.D. Engineering biomaterials to integrate and heal: The biocompatibility paradigm shifts. *Biotechnol. Bioeng.* **2012**, *109*, 1898–1911. [CrossRef]
20. Morra, M. Biochemical modification of titanium surfaces: Peptides and ecm proteins. *Eur. Cell. Mater.* **2006**, *12*, 1–15. [CrossRef]
21. Morra, M. Biomolecular modification of implant surfaces. *Expert Rev. Med. Devices* **2007**, *4*, 361–372. [CrossRef]
22. Puleo, D.A.; Nanci, A. Understanding and controlling the bone-implant interface. *Biomaterials* **1999**, *20*, 2311–2321. [CrossRef]
23. Morra, M.; Cassinelli, C.; Cascardo, G.; Cahalan, P.; Cahalan, L.; Fini, M.; Giardino, R. Surface engineering of titanium by collagen immobilization. Surface characterization and in vitro and in vivo studies. *Biomaterials* **2003**, *24*, 4639–4654. [CrossRef]
24. Morra, M.; Cassinelli, C.; Cascardo, G.; Mazzucco, L.; Borzini, P.; Fini, M.; Giavaresi, G.; Giardino, R. Collagen i-coated titanium surfaces: Mesenchymal cell adhesion and in vivo evaluation in trabecular bone implants. *J. Biomed. Mater. Res. A* **2006**, *78*, 449–458. [CrossRef] [PubMed]
25. Morra, M.; Cassinelli, C.; Cascardo, G.; Nagel, M.D.; Della Volpe, C.; Siboni, S.; Maniglio, D.; Brugnara, M.; Ceccone, G.; Schols, H.A.; et al. Effects on interfacial properties and cell adhesion of surface modification by pectic hairy regions. *Biomacromolecules* **2004**, *5*, 2094–2104. [CrossRef] [PubMed]
26. Kim, H.W.; Li, L.H.; Lee, E.J.; Lee, S.H.; Kim, H.E. Fibrillar assembly and stability of collagen coating on titanium for improved osteoblast responses. *J. Biomed. Mater. Res. A* **2005**, *75*, 629–638. [CrossRef] [PubMed]
27. Rammelt, S.; Heck, C.; Bernhardt, R.; Bierbaum, S.; Scharnweber, D.; Goebbels, J.; Ziegler, J.; Biewener, A.; Zwipp, H. In vivo effects of coating loaded and unloaded ti implants with collagen, chondroitin sulfate, and hydroxyapatite in the sheep tibia. *J. Orthop. Res.* **2007**, *25*, 1052–1061. [CrossRef] [PubMed]
28. Rammelt, S.; Illert, T.; Bierbaum, S.; Scharnweber, D.; Zwipp, H.; Schneiders, W. Coating of titanium implants with collagen, rgd peptide and chondroitin sulfate. *Biomaterials* **2006**, *27*, 5561–5571. [CrossRef] [PubMed]
29. Stadlinger, B.; Pilling, E.; Huhle, M.; Mai, R.; Bierbaum, S.; Bernhardt, R.; Scharnweber, D.; Kuhlisch, E.; Hempel, U.; Eckelt, U. Influence of extracellular matrix coatings on implant stability and osseointegration: An animal study. *J. Biomed. Mater. Res. B Appl. Biomater.* **2007**, *83*, 222–231. [CrossRef] [PubMed]
30. Stadlinger, B.; Pilling, E.; Mai, R.; Bierbaum, S.; Berhardt, R.; Scharnweber, D.; Eckelt, U. Effect of biological implant surface coatings on bone formation, applying collagen, proteoglycans, glycosaminoglycans and growth factors. *J. Mater. Sci. Mater. Med.* **2008**, *19*, 1043–1049. [CrossRef] [PubMed]
31. Stadlinger, B.; Pilling, E.; Huhle, M.; Mai, R.; Bierbaum, S.; Scharnweber, D.; Kuhlisch, E.; Loukota, R.; Eckelt, U. Evaluation of osseointegration of dental implants coated with collagen, chondroitin sulphate and bmp-4: An animal study. *Int. J. Oral Maxillofac. Surg.* **2008**, *37*, 54–59. [CrossRef]
32. Kokkonen, H.; Verhoef, R.; Kauppinen, K.; Muhonen, V.; Jorgensen, B.; Damager, I.; Schols, H.A.; Morra, M.; Ulvskov, P.; Tuukkanen, J. Affecting osteoblastic responses with in vivo engineered potato pectin fragments. *J. Biomed. Mater. Res. A* **2012**, *100*, 111–119. [CrossRef]

33. Gurzawska, K.; Svava, R.; Jorgensen, N.R.; Gotfredsen, K. Nanocoating of titanium implant surfaces with organic molecules. Polysaccharides including glycosaminoglycans. *J. Biomed. Nanotechnol.* **2012**, *8*, 1012–1024. [CrossRef]
34. Gurzawska, K.; Svava, R.; Syberg, S.; Yihua, Y.; Haugshoj, K.B.; Damager, I.; Ulvskov, P.; Christensen, L.H.; Gotfredsen, K.; Jorgensen, N.R. Effect of nanocoating with rhamnogalacturonan-i on surface properties and osteoblasts response. *J. Biomed. Mater. Res. A* **2012**, *100*, 654–664. [CrossRef] [PubMed]
35. Kellesarian, S.; Malignaggi, V.; Kellesarian, T.; Bashir Ahmed, H.; Javed, F. Does incorporating collagen and chondroitin sulfate matrix in implant surfaces enhance osseointegration? A systematic review and meta-analysis. *IJOMS* **2018**, *47*, 241–251. [CrossRef] [PubMed]
36. Evered, D.E.; Whelan, J.E. *The Biology of Hyaluronan*; Wiley: Chichester, UK, 1989.
37. Laurent, T.C. *The Chemistry, Biology and Medical Applications of Hyaluronan and Its Derivative*; Portland Press: London, UK, 1998.
38. Abatangelo, G.; Weigel, P.H. New Frontiers in Medical Sciences: Redefining Hyaluronan. In Proceedings of the Symposium on New Frontiers in Medical Sciences, Padua, Italy, 17–19 June 1999; Elsevier: Oxford, UK, 2000.
39. Kennedy, J.F.; Balazs, E.A.F.; Phillips, G.O.E.; Williams, P.A.E. *Hyaluronan 2000: An International Meeting Celebrating the 80th Birthday of Endre a Balazs*; Woodhead: Cambridge, CA, USA, 2002.
40. Morra, M. Engineering of biomaterials surfaces by hyaluronan. *Biomacromolecules* **2005**, *6*, 1205–1223. [CrossRef] [PubMed]
41. Valachova, K.; Volpi, N.; Stern, R.; Soltes, L. Hyaluronan in medical practice. *Curr. Med. Chem.* **2016**, *23*, 3607–3617. [CrossRef] [PubMed]
42. Salwowska, N.M.; Bebenek, K.A.; Zadlo, D.A.; Wcislo-Dziadecka, D.L. Physiochemical properties and application of hyaluronic acid: A systematic review. *J. Cosmet. Dermatol.* **2016**, *15*, 520–526. [CrossRef] [PubMed]
43. Casale, M.; Moffa, A.; Vella, P.; Sabatino, L.; Capuano, F.; Salvinelli, B.; Lopez, M.A.; Carinci, F.; Salvinelli, F. Hyaluronic acid: Perspectives in dentistry. A systematic review. *Int. J. Immunopathol. Pharmacol.* **2016**, *29*, 572–582. [CrossRef] [PubMed]
44. Maurer, P.H.; Hudack, S.S. The isolation of hyaluronic acid from callus tissue of early healing. *Arch. Biochem. Biophys.* **1952**, *38*, 49–53. [CrossRef]
45. Iwata, H.; Urist, M.R. Hyaluronic acid production and removal during bone morphogenesis in implants of bone matrix in rats. *Clin. Orthop. Relat. Res.* **1973**, 236–245.
46. Bernard, G.W.; Pilloni, A.; Kang, M.; Sison, J.; Hunt, D.; Jovanovic, S. Osteogenesis in vitro and in vivo with hyaluronan and bone morphogenetic protein-2. In *New Frontiers in Medical Sciences: Redefining Hyaluronan*; Abatangelo, G., Weigel, P.H., Eds.; Elsevier: New York, NY, USA, 2000; pp. 215–231.
47. Zou, X.; Li, H.; Chen, L.; Baatrup, A.; Bunger, C.; Lind, M. Stimulation of porcine bone marrow stromal cells by hyaluronan, dexamethasone and rhbmp-2. *Biomaterials* **2004**, *25*, 5375–5385. [CrossRef]
48. Itoh, S.; Matubara, M.; Kawauchi, T.; Nakamura, H.; Yukitake, S.; Ichinose, S.; Shinomiya, K. Enhancement of bone ingrowth in a titanium fiber mesh implant by rhbmp-2 and hyaluronic acid. *J. Mater. Sci. Mater. Med.* **2001**, *12*, 575–581. [CrossRef]
49. Cho, B.C.; Park, J.W.; Baik, B.S.; Kwon, I.C.; Kim, I.S. The role of hyaluronic acid, chitosan, and calcium sulfate and their combined effect on early bony consolidation in distraction osteogenesis of a canine model. *J. Craniofac. Surg.* **2002**, *13*, 783–793. [CrossRef] [PubMed]
50. Solchaga, L.A.; Temenoff, J.S.; Gao, J.; Mikos, A.G.; Caplan, A.I.; Goldberg, V.M. Repair of osteochondral defects with hyaluronan- and polyester-based scaffolds. *Osteoarthr. Cartilage* **2005**, *13*, 297–309. [CrossRef]
51. Zhao, N.; Wang, X.; Qin, L.; Guo, Z.; Li, D. Effect of molecular weight and concentration of hyaluronan on cell proliferation and osteogenic differentiation in vitro. *Biochem. Biophys. Res. Commun.* **2015**, *465*, 569–574. [CrossRef] [PubMed]
52. Aebli, N.; Stich, H.; Schawalder, P.; Theis, J.C.; Krebs, J. Effects of bone morphogenetic protein-2 and hyaluronic acid on the osseointegration of hydroxyapatite-coated implants: An experimental study in sheep. *J. Biomed. Mater. Res. A* **2005**, *73*, 295–302. [CrossRef] [PubMed]
53. Morra, M.; Cassinelli, C.; Cascardo, G.; Fini, M.; Giavaresi, G.; Giardino, R. Covalently-linked hyaluronan promotes bone formation around ti implants in a rabbit model. *J. Orthop. Res.* **2009**, *27*, 657–663. [CrossRef]

54. Gomi, K.; Davies, J.E. Guided bone tissue elaboration by osteogenic cells in vitro. *J. Biomed. Mater. Res.* **1993**, *27*, 429–431. [CrossRef] [PubMed]
55. Lossdorfer, S.; Schwartz, Z.; Wang, L.; Lohmann, C.H.; Turner, J.D.; Wieland, M.; Cochran, D.L.; Boyan, B.D. Microrough implant surface topographies increase osteogenesis by reducing osteoclast formation and activity. *J. Biomed. Mater. Res. A* **2004**, *70*, 361–369. [CrossRef]
56. Morra, M.; Cassinelli, C.; Bruzzone, G.; Carpi, A.; Di Santi, G.; Giardino, R.; Fini, M. Surface chemistry effects of topographic modification of titanium dental implant surfaces: 1. Surface analysis. *Int. J. Oral Maxillofac. Implants* **2003**, *18*, 40–45.
57. Morra, M.; Cassinelli, C. Simple model for the xps analysis of polysaccharides coated surface. *Surf. Interface Anal.* **1998**, *26*, 742–747. [CrossRef]
58. Briggs, D.; Seah, M.P. Practical surface analysis. In *Auger and X-ray Photoelectron Spectroscopy*; Wiley: Chichester, UK, 1996.
59. Shard, A.; Davies, M.; Tendler, S.; Bennedetti, L.; Purbrick, M.; Paul, A.; Beamson, G. X-ray photoelectron spectroscopy and time-of-flight sims investigations of hyaluronic acid derivatives. *Langmuir* **1997**, *13*, 2808–2814. [CrossRef]
60. Goldstein, J. *Scanning Electron Microscopy and X-ray Microanalysis*; Plenum Press: New York, NY, USA, 2003.
61. Lausmaa, J. Surface spectroscopic characterization of titanium implant materials. *J. Electron. Spectros. Relat. Phenomena* **1996**, *81*, 343–361. [CrossRef]
62. Sawase, T.; Hai, K.; Yoshida, K.; Baba, K.; Hatada, R.; Atsuta, M. Spectroscopic studies of three osseointegrated implants. *J. Dent.* **1998**, *26*, 119–124. [CrossRef]
63. Kang, B.S.; Sul, Y.T.; Oh, S.J.; Lee, H.J.; Albrektsson, T. Xps, aes and sem analysis of recent dental implants. *Acta Biomater.* **2009**, *5*, 2222–2229. [CrossRef] [PubMed]
64. Cassinelli, C.; Morra, M.; Pavesio, A.; Renier, D. Evaluation of interfacial properties of hyaluronan coated poly(methylmethacrylate) intraocular lenses. *J. Biomater. Sci. Polym. Ed.* **2000**, *11*, 961–977. [CrossRef]
65. Sverzut, A.T.; Crippa, G.E.; Morra, M.; de Oliveira, P.T.; Beloti, M.M.; Rosa, A.L. Effects of type i collagen coating on titanium osseointegration: Histomorphometric, cellular and molecular analyses. *Biomed. Mater.* **2012**, *7*, 035007. [CrossRef] [PubMed]
66. Sartori, M.; Giavaresi, G.; Parrilli, A.; Ferrari, A.; Aldini, N.N.; Morra, M.; Cassinelli, C.; Bollati, D.; Fini, M. Collagen type i coating stimulates bone regeneration and osteointegration of titanium implants in the osteopenic rat. *Int. Orthop.* **2015**, *39*, 2041–2052. [CrossRef]
67. Litwiniuk, M.; Krejner, A.; Speyrer, M.S.; Gauto, A.R.; Grzela, T. Hyaluronic acid in inflammation and tissue regeneration. *Wounds* **2016**, *28*, 78–88.
68. Maytin, E.V. Hyaluronan: More than just a wrinkle filler. *Glycobiology* **2016**, *26*, 553–559. [CrossRef]
69. Zhao, N.; Wang, X.; Qin, L.; Zhai, M.; Yuan, J.; Chen, J.; Li, D. Effect of hyaluronic acid in bone formation and its applications in dentistry. *J. Biomed. Mater. Res. A* **2016**, *104*, 1560–1569. [CrossRef]
70. Gurgel, B.C.V.; Montenegro, S.C.L.; Dantas, P.M.C.; Pascoal, A.L.B.; Lima, K.C.; Calderon, P.D.S. Frequency of peri-implant diseases and associated factors. *Clin. Oral Implants Res.* **2017**, *28*, 1211–1217. [CrossRef]
71. Morra, M.; Cassineli, C. Non-fouling properties of polysaccharide-coated surfaces. *J. Biomater. Sci. Polym. Ed.* **1999**, *10*, 1107–1124. [CrossRef] [PubMed]
72. Davies, J.E. *Bone Engineering*; University of Toronto Press: Toronto, ON, Canada, 2000.
73. Rizzo, S.; Zampetti, P.; Rodriguez, Y.B.R.; Svanosio, D.; Lupi, S.M. Retrospective analysis of 521 endosseous implants placed under antibiotic prophylaxis and review of literature. *Minerva. Stomatol.* **2010**, *59*, 75–88. [PubMed]
74. Lupi, S.M.; Rodriguez, Y.B.A.; Cervino, G.; Todaro, C.; Rizzo, S. Long-term effects of acute myeloid leukemia treatment on the oral system in a pediatric patient. *Open Dent. J.* **2018**, *12*, 230–237. [CrossRef] [PubMed]
75. Rodriguez y Baena, R.; Pastorino, R.; Gherlone, E.F.; Perillo, L.; Lupi, S.M.; Lucchese, A. Histomorphometric evaluation of two different bone substitutes in sinus augmentation procedures: A randomized controlled trial in humans. *Int. J. Oral Maxillofac. Implants* **2017**, *32*, 188–194. [CrossRef] [PubMed]
76. Lupi, S.M.; Cislaghi, M.; Rizzo, S.; Rodriguez, Y.B.R. Rehabilitation with implant-retained removable dentures and its effects on perioral aesthetics: A prospective cohort study. *Clin. Cosmet. Investig. Dent.* **2016**, *8*, 105–110. [PubMed]

77. RR, Y.B.; Lupi, S.M.; Pastorino, R.; Maiorana, C.; Lucchese, A.; Rizzo, S. Radiographic evaluation of regenerated bone following poly(lactic-co-glycolic) acid/hydroxyapatite and deproteinized bovine bone graft in sinus lifting. *J. Craniofac. Surg.* **2013**, *24*, 845–848.
78. Rodriguez, Y.B.R.; D'Aquino, R.; Graziano, A.; Trovato, L.; Aloise, A.C.; Ceccarelli, G.; Cusella, G.; Pelegrine, A.A.; Lupi, S.M. Autologous periosteum-derived micrografts and plga/ha enhance the bone formation in sinus lift augmentation. *Front. Cell Dev. Biol.* **2017**, *5*, 87. [CrossRef] [PubMed]
79. Ceccarelli, G.; Presta, R.; Lupi, S.M.; Giarratana, N.; Bloise, N.; Benedetti, L.; Cusella De Angelis, M.G.; Rodriguez, Y.B.R. Evaluation of poly(lactic-co-glycolic) acid alone or in combination with hydroxyapatite on human-periosteal cells bone differentiation and in sinus lift treatment. *Molecules* **2017**, *22*. [CrossRef] [PubMed]
80. Lupi, S.M.; Rodriguez, Y.B.A.; Todaro, C.; Ceccarelli, G.; Rodriguez, Y.B.R. Maxillary sinus lift using autologous periosteal micrografts: A new regenerative approach and a case report of a 3-year follow-up. *Case Rep. Dent.* **2018**, *2018*, 3023096. [CrossRef]
81. Lupi, S.M.; Granati, M.; Butera, A.; Collesano, V.; Rodriguez, Y.B.R. Air-abrasive debridement with glycine powder versus manual debridement and chlorhexidine administration for the maintenance of peri-implant health status: A six-month randomized clinical trial. *Int. J. Dent. Hyg.* **2017**, *15*, 287–294. [CrossRef]
82. Mumcu, E.; Bilhan, H.; Cekici, A. Marginal bone loss around implants supporting fixed restorations. *J. Oral Implantol.* **2011**, *37*, 549–558. [CrossRef] [PubMed]
83. Julious, S.A. Sample sizes for clinical trials with normal data. *Stat. Med.* **2004**, *23*, 1921–1986. [CrossRef] [PubMed]

13

Bone Healing in Rabbit Calvaria Defects Using a Synthetic Bone Substitute: A Histological and Micro-CT Comparative Study

Minas Leventis [1,*], Peter Fairbairn [2], Chas Mangham [3], Antonios Galanos [4], Orestis Vasiliadis [1], Danai Papavasileiou [1] and Robert Horowitz [5]

1 Laboratory of Experimental Surgery and Surgical Research N. S. Christeas, Medical School, University of Athens, 75 M. Assias Street, Athens 115 27, Greece; orestis@vasiliadis.net (O.V.); d.pap.mes@gmail.com (D.P.)
2 Department of Periodontology and Implant Dentistry, School of Dentistry, University of Detroit Mercy, 2700 Martin Luther King Jr Boulevard, Detroit, MI 48208, USA; peterdent66@aol.com
3 Manchester Molecular Pathology Innovation Centre, The University of Manchester, Nelson Street, Manchester M13 9NQ, UK; D.C.Mangham@manchester.ac.uk
4 Laboratory of Research of the Musculoskeletal System, Medical School, University of Athens, 2 Nikis Street, Athens 145 61, Greece; galanostat@yahoo.gr
5 Departments of Periodontics, Implant Dentistry, and Oral Surgery, New York University College of Dentistry, 345 E 24th Street, New York, NY 10010, USA; rah7@nyu.edu
* Correspondence: mlevent@dent.uoa.gr

Abstract: Bioactive alloplastic materials, like beta-tricalcium phosphate (β-TCP) and calcium sulfate (CS), have been extensively researched and are currently used in orthopedic and dental bone regenerative procedures. The purpose of this study was to compare the performance of EthOss versus a bovine xenograft and spontaneous healing. The grafting materials were implanted in standardized 8 mm circular bicortical bone defects in rabbit calvariae. A third similar defect in each animal was left empty for natural healing. Six male rabbits were used. After eight weeks of healing, the animals were euthanized and the bone tissue was analyzed using histology and micro-computed tomography (micro-CT). Defects treated with β-TCP/CS showed the greatest bone regeneration and graft resorption, although differences between groups were not statistically significant. At sites that healed spontaneously, the trabecular number was lower ($p < 0.05$) and trabecular separation was higher ($p < 0.05$), compared to sites treated with β-TCP/CS or xenograft. Trabecular thickness was higher at sites treated with the bovine xenograft ($p < 0.05$) compared to sites filled with β-TCP/CS or sites that healed spontaneously. In conclusion, the novel β-TCP/CS grafting material performed well as a bioactive and biomimetic alloplastic bone substitute when used in cranial defects in this animal model.

Keywords: bone regeneration; β-tricalcium phosphate; calcium sulfate; bone substitutes; animal study

---

1. Introduction

Bone grafting procedures are performed to manage osseous defects of the jaw due to pathological processes or trauma, to preserve the alveolar ridge after extraction, and to augment the bone around dental implants. For this purpose, a wide variety of bone substitutes, barrier membranes, and growth-factor preparations are routinely used, and several different surgical methods have been proposed [1,2]. Autogenous bone is still considered the gold standard among bone grafting materials as it possess osteoconductive, osteoinductive, and osteogenetic properties; it neither transmits diseases nor triggers immunologic reactions; and is gradually absorbed and replaced by newly-formed high quality osseous tissue. The disadvantages of using autogenous bone include restricted availability, the need for additional surgical site, increased morbidity, and extended operating time [3,4]. As an alternative solution, bone graft substitutes are widely used in bone reconstructive surgeries, and the science of biomaterials has become one of the fastest growing scientific fields in recent years [5]. By definition, bone substitutes are any "synthetic, inorganic or biologically organic combination which can be inserted for the treatment of a bone defect instead of autogenous or allogenous bone" [6]. This definition applies to a wide variety of materials of different origins, composition, and biological mechanisms of function regarding graft resorption and new bone formation. Thus, the selection of biomaterials in clinical practice must be based on their biocompatibility, biodegradability, bioactivity, and mechanical properties, as well as the resulting cell behavior [7–11]. Parameters like the physicochemical characteristics, hydrophilicity and hydrophobicity, and molecular weight may influence the handling and performance of bone substitutes [12,13]. In general, the ideal grafting material should act as a substrate for bone ingrowth into the defect, to be ultimately fully replaced by host bone with an appropriate degradation rate in relation to new bone development for complete regeneration up to the condition of *restitutio ad integrum* [1,14]. The grafting material should also be able to retain the volume stability of the augmented area [1].

Bioactivity is a characteristic of chemical bonding between bone grafts and host biological tissues. Calcium phosphate ceramics and calcium sulfates are considered bioactive materials as they have the ability to evoke a controlled action and reaction to the host tissue environment with a controlled chemical dissolution and resorption, to ultimately be fully replaced by regenerated bone [5,15].

Among bioactive ceramics, β-TCP and hydroxyapatite (Ca10(PO4)6(OH)2) are frequently utilized in dental bone regenerative procedures [13]. Their composition is similar to that of natural bone, they are biocompatible and osteoconductive materials, can osseointegrate with the defect site, and due to their non-biologic origin, their use does not involve any risk of transmitting infections or diseases [16–22]. The degradation process of these biomaterials produces and releases ions that can create an alkaline environment that seems to enhance cell activity and accelerate bone reconstruction [13]. Recent in vitro and in vivo experimental studies have shown that such alloplastic bone substitutes can stimulate stem cells to differentiate to osteogenic differentiation of stem cells, as well as ectopic bone induction [23–27]. β-TCP may promote the proliferation and differentiation of endothelial cells and improve neovascularization in the grafted site, having clear benefits for osteogenic processes [13,28].

The ability of the bacteriostatic CS to set is well documented. Adding CS to β-TCP produces a compound alloplastic biomaterial that hardens in situ and binds directly to the host bone, helping maintain the space and shape of the grafted site, and acts as a stable scaffold [29–35]. The improved mechanical stability of the graft is a crucial factor for bone healing and differentiation of mesenchymal cells to osteoblasts [36], thus contributing to enhanced regeneration of high quality hard tissue [37,38]. The in situ hardening CS element may act as a cell occlusive barrier membrane, halting soft connective tissue proliferation into the graft during the first stages of healing [39–41].

Both CS and β-TCP are fully resorbable bone substitutes, leading to the regeneration of high quality vital host bone without the long-term presence of graft remnants. The CS element resorbs over a three- to six-week period, depending on patient physiology, creating a vascular porosity in the β-TCP scaffold for improved vascular ingrowth and angiogenesis. The β-TCP element resorbs by hydrolysis and enzymatic and phagocytic processes, usually over a period of 9–16 months. Although evaluating these resorptive mechanisms is difficult, it seems that cell-based degradation might be more important than dissolution, and macrophages and osteoclasts may be involved in phagocytosis, again largely dependent on host physiology [22,41–43].

As recent studies in bone reconstruction are gradually shifting their focus to biodegradable and bioactive materials, resorbable alloplastic bone substitutes might be a potential alternative to autogenous bone or bovine xenografts in dental bone reconstructive procedures. However, limited information is available in the recent literature. Therefore, the aim of this study was to compare the performance of a novel alloplastic bone substitute composed of β-TCP and CS, versus a bovine xenograft and spontaneous healing, in cranial bone defects in rabbits.

2. Experimental Section

2.1. Animals

Six adult male New Zealand White rabbits, each weighing 3 kg (±250 g), were used in this study with the approval of the Institutional Animal Care and Use Committee of the Veterinary Department, Greek Ministry of Rural Development and Veterinary, Attica Prefecture, Greece (project identification code: 5176/10-10-2017). Animals were provided with an appropriate balanced dry diet and water ad libitum, and caged individually in a standard manner at the N. S. Christeas animal research facility, Medical School, University of Athens, Greece. All animals were allowed seven days from their arrival to the facility in order to acclimatize to their new environment.

2.2. Surgical Procedures

Surgical procedures are shown in Figure 1. Under general anesthesia by orotracheal intubation, a longitudinal midline linear incision was made in the skin over the top of the cranial vault to expose the skull. The overlying periosteum was then excised, and three separate and identical 8-mm-diameter bicortical cranial round defects were created in the calvaria of each animal using a trephine drill with an internal diameter of 8 mm (Komet Inc., Lemgo, Germany) on a slow-speed electric handpiece by applying 0.9% physiologic saline irrigation. During the osteotomy, care was taken not to injure the dura mater under the bone. Then, using a thin periotome, the circular bicortical bone segment was mobilized and luxated.

Following a randomization technique using cards, the three resultant bone defects in each animal were randomly assigned treatment: (1) one defect was filled with 150 mg of the test alloplastic biomaterial (group 1), (2) one defect was filled with 150 mg of bovine xenograft (group 2), and (3) one sham defect remained unfilled (group 3).

The test bone graft substitute used in group 1 (EthOss, Ethoss Regeneration Ltd., Silsden, UK) is a self-hardening biomaterial consisting of β-TCP (65%) and CS (35%), preloaded in a sterile plastic syringe. In accordance with the manufacturer's instructions, prior to applying the alloplastic graft into the bone defect, the particles of the biomaterial were mixed in the syringe with sterile saline.

After application, a bone plunger was used to gently condense the moldable graft particles in order to occupy the entire volume of the site up to the level of the surrounding host bone. A saline-wet gauze was used to further compact the graft particles and accelerate the in situ hardening of the CS element of the graft. As a result, after a few minutes, the alloplastic bone substitute formed a stable, porous scaffold for host osseous regeneration.

As a xenograft, a bovine deproteinized cancellous bone graft with a particle size of 0.25–1 mm (Bio-Oss, Geistleich Pharmaceutical, Wollhausen, Switzerland) was used in group 2. Bio-Oss consists of loose particles. According to the manufacturer's instructions, before application, the material was mixed with sterile saline and then placed into the bone defect, avoiding excessive compression.

Interrupted resorbable 4-0 sutures (Vicryl, Ethicon, Johnson & Johnson, Somerville, NJ, USA) were used to close the overlying soft tissues in layers.

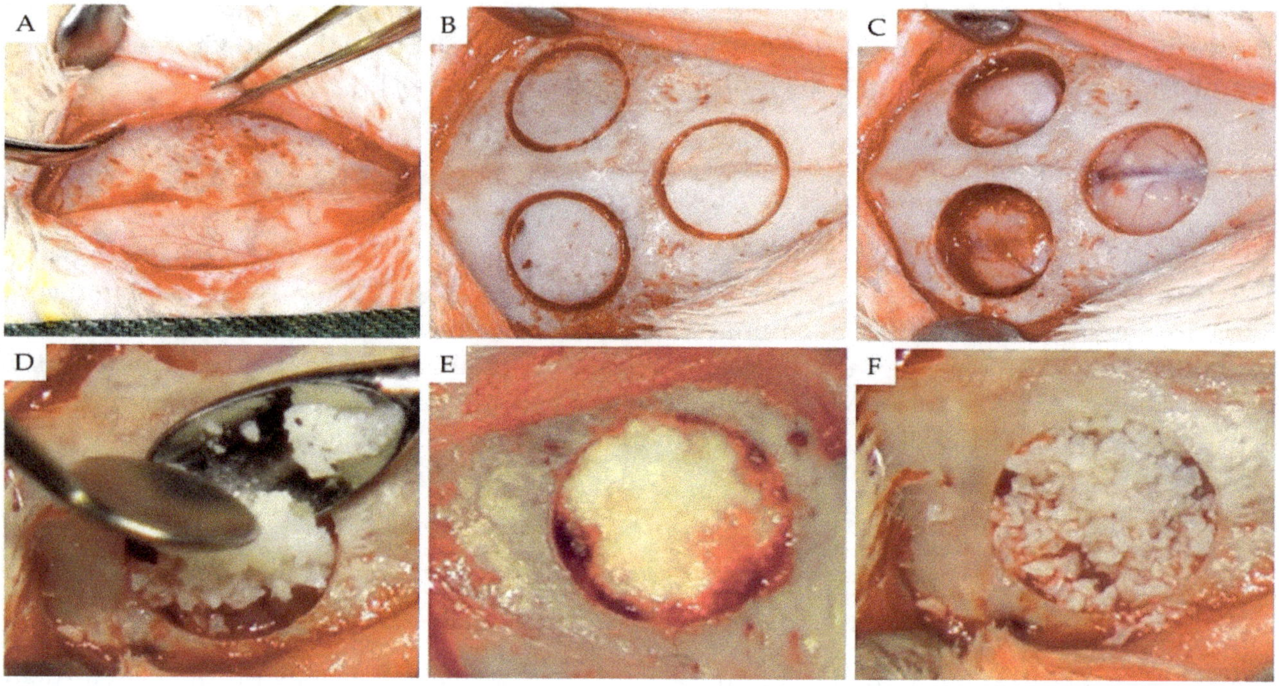

Figure 1. The surgical process. (**A**) Surgical exposure of the rabbit calvaria; (**B**) using a trephine burr, three identical circular osteotomies were performed; and (**C**) after removing the bicortical bone segments. The circular three-defect model was utilized with a frontal bone defect affecting the inter-frontal suture plus two bilateral defects affecting the parietal bones. (**D**) Two sites were treated with bone substitutes and the third left unfilled. (**E**) EthOss and (**F**) Bio-Oss.

Each experimental animal received antibiotics (30 mg/kg of Zinadol, GlaxoWellcome, Athens, Greece) every 24 h and analgesics (15 mg/kg of Depon; Bristol-Myers Squibb, Athens, Greece) for 2 days postoperatively. An intravenous injection of sodium thiopental (100 mg/kg of Pentothal; Abbott Hellas, Athens, Greece) was used to euthanize all animals after an 8-week healing period. The calvaria bones containing the healed sites were surgically harvested and immediately fixed in neutral buffered formalin (10%) for 24 h.

2.3. Micro-CT Evaluation

Each calvaria was scanned using a micro-CT scanner (Skyscan 1076, Bruker, Belgium) at 50 kV, 200 μA, and a 0.5 mm aluminum filter. The pixel size was 18.26 μm. Two images were captured every 0.7° through 180° rotation of the sample; the exposure time per image was 420 ms. The X-ray images were reconstructed using the NRecon software (Skyscan, Bruker, Belgium) and analyzed using Skyscan CT analysis software. Specific thresholds were set on segmenting the micro-CT images in order to distinguish the newly-formed bone from the connective tissue and the grafting materials. A lower threshold (level 60) was used for all groups to segment the bone tissue, whereas higher threshold levels were used to segment the Bio-Oss and the EthOss particles (level 90 and level 120, respectively). Analysis was performed using an 8-mm-diameter circular region that was placed in the center of the initial defect area. Trabecular bone analysis was performed, and based on the micro-CT results several parameters regarding new bone formation, residual graft, and the microarchitecture of the regenerated bone were calculated (Table 1).

Table 1. Parameters assessed by analysis of the micro-computed tomography (CT) data.

Parameter	Abbreviation	Description	Standard Unit
Bone volume fraction	BV/TV	Ratio of the segmented newly-formed bone volume to the total volume of the region of interest	%
Residual material volume fraction	RMVF	Ratio of the residual grafting material volume to the total volume of the region of interest	%
Trabecular number	Tb.N	Measure of the average number of trabeculae per unit length	1/mm
Trabecular thickness	Tb.Th	Mean thickness of trabeculae, assessed using direct 3D methods	mm
Trabecular separation	Tb.Sp	Mean distance between trabeculae, assessed using direct 3D methods	mm

2.4. Histology

After micro-CT analysis, bone specimens were decalcified in bone decalcification solution (Diapath S.p.a., Martinengo, Italy) for 14 days. After routine processing, slices were obtained from the central part of each healed bone defect using a saw (Exakt saw 312, Exakt Apparatebau GmbH, Norderstedt, Germany), embedded in paraffin, sectioned longitudinally into multiple 3-μm-thick sections and stained with Hematoxylin and Eosin stain. For qualitative analysis of the bone regenerative process, the stained preparations were examined under a light microscope (Nikon Eclipse 80, Nikon, Tokyo, Japan) and the entire section was evaluated. Images of each section were acquired with a digital camera microscope unit (Nikon DS-2MW, Nikon, Tokyo, Japan).

2.5. Statistics

Statistical analysis was performed using SPSS software (v. 17, SPSS Inc., Chicago, IL, USA). Data are expressed as mean ± standard deviation (SD). The Shapiro-Wilk test was utilized for normality analysis of the parameters. The comparison of variables among the 3 groups was performed using the one-way ANOVA model. Pairwise comparisons were performed using the Bonferroni test. All tests were two-sided, and statistical significance was set at $p < 0.05$.

3. Results

3.1. Overall

All animals survived for the duration of the study without complications. At eight weeks, there were no clinical signs of infection, hematoma, or necrosis at the defect sites. The dura mater and brain tissues under all bone defect sites exhibited no clinical evidence of inflammation, scar formation, or an adverse tissue reaction to the bone grafting materials (Figure 2A). Closure of the cortical window and filling of the defects with new bone were macroscopically observed at all defect sites. At bone defect sites grafted with bovine xenograft (Bio-Oss), graft particles embedded in newly formed hard tissue were clinically observed, whereas the newly-formed hard tissue occupying the sites treated with the alloplastic biomaterial (EthOss) was macroscopically homogeneous, without clear clinical distinction of residual graft particles. Clinical observation of sites left empty revealed that the spontaneously healed circular bone defects were bridged by a thin layer of newly-formed hard tissue (Figure 2B, Video S1).

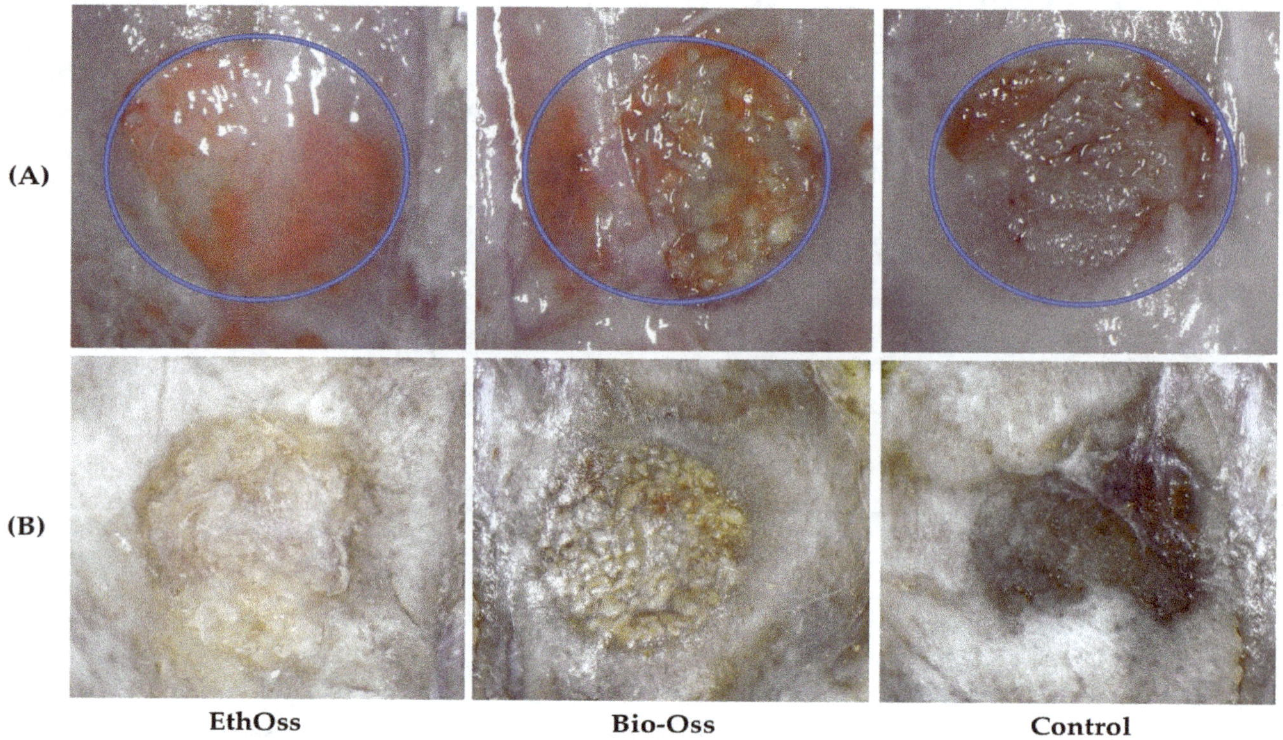

Figure 2. Gross observations of the 8-mm-diameter calvaria bone defect sites after eight weeks of healing: (**A**) fresh harvested rabbit calvaria and (**B**) after removing the dura mater and fixed in neutral buffered formalin (10%) for 24 h. Clinical observation revealed a different pattern of healing of the osseous defect between groups.

3.2. Micro-CT Evaluation

The radiological imaging results acquired from the micro-CT after eight weeks of healing are shown in Figure 3.

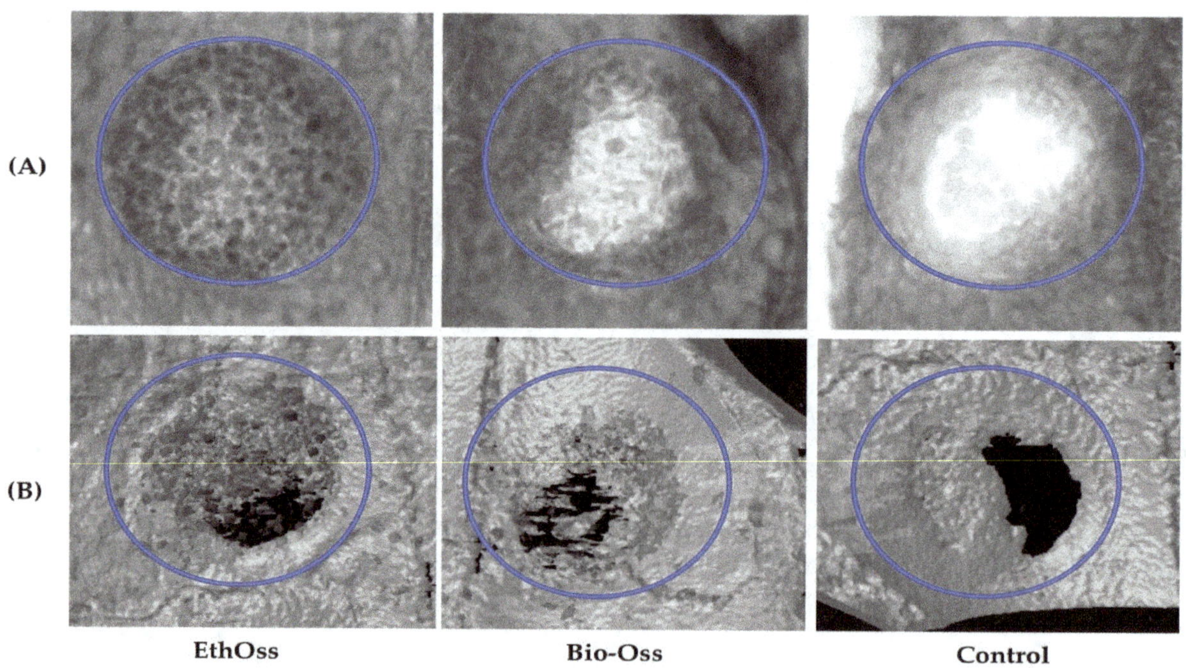

Figure 3. (**A**) Axial sections and (**B**) reconstructed three-dimensional (3D) micro-computed tomography (CT) images of the 8-mm-diameter defect sites after eight weeks of healing.

There were no significant differences between parameters that expressed new bone regeneration (BV/TV), between the three groups. At this time point, there were no statistically significant differences regarding the percentage of the residual graft material (RMVF) between groups 1 and 2, where EthOss and Bio-Oss were used as bone substitutes, respectively (Figure 4 and Table 2).

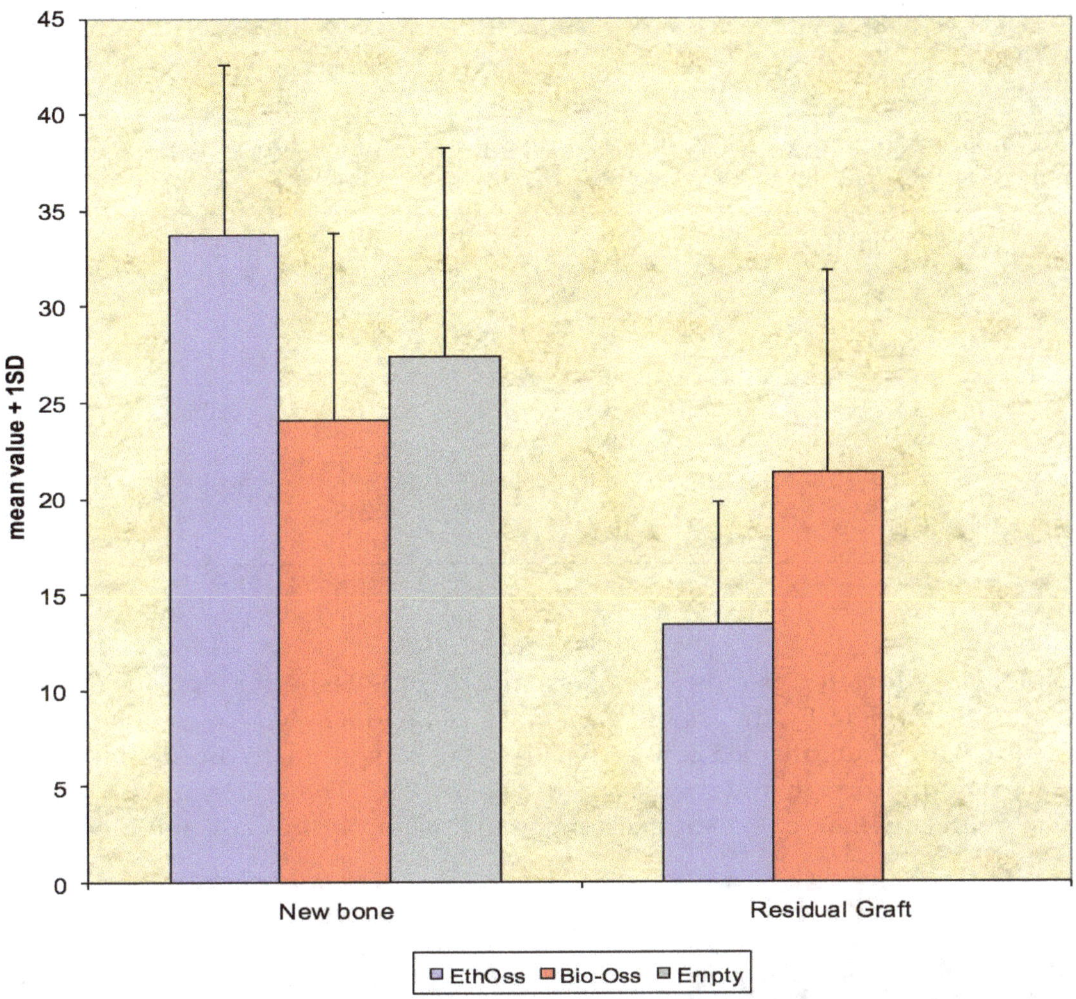

Figure 4. The percentage of new bone (BV/TV) between the three groups, and the percentage of residual graft (RMVF) in sites treated with EthOss and Bio-Oss, after eight weeks of healing. Data are presented as means. The differences between groups were not statistically significant ($p > 0.05$).

Table 2. Comparison of parameters associate with the newly-formed bone (BV/TV) and the residual grafting material (RMVF). The differences between groups were not statistically significant ($p > 0.05$).

Parameter	Site	N	Mean	SD	*p*-Value
BV/TV	EthOss	6	33.70	8.94	0.525
	Bio-Oss	6	24.07	9.69	
	Control	6	27.36	10.95	
RMVF	EthOss	6	13.41	6.43	0.070
	Bio-Oss	6	21.36	10.05	
	Control	6	-	-	-

At eight weeks, there were statistically significant differences between the three groups in the parameters associated with the microarchitecture of the newly-formed hard tissue (Table 3). Regarding the parameter Tb.N, pairwise comparisons indicated statistically significant difference between group 3 (Empty) and group 1 (EthOss) ($p < 0.001$), and group 2 (Bio-Oss) ($p < 0.001$), whereas there was no difference between group 1 (EthOss) and group 2 (Bio-Oss) ($p = 0.126$). Regarding the parameter Tb.Th, pairwise comparisons indicated statistically significant difference between group 2 (Bio-Oss) and group1 (EthOss) ($p = 0.001$), and Empty ($p < 0.001$), whereas there was no difference between group 1 (EthOss) and group 3 (Empty) ($p = 1.000$). For parameter Tb.S, pairwise comparisons indicated statistically significant difference between group 3 (Empty) and group 1 (EthOss) ($p = 0.001$), and group 2 (Bio-Oss) ($p < 0.001$), whereas there was no difference between group 1 (EthOss) and group 2 (Bio-Oss) ($p = 0.662$).

Table 3. Comparison of parameters associated with the microarchitecture of the newly-formed hard tissue in the three groups (a: $p < 0.05$ vs. control; b: $p < 0.05$ vs. Bio-Oss).

Parameter	Site	N	Mean	SD	*p*-Value
Tb.N	EthOss	6	1.511 [a]	0.255 [a]	<0.001
	Bio-Oss	6	1.213 [a]	0.198 [a]	
	Control	6	0.541	0.239	
Tb.Th	EthOss	6	0.219 [b]	0.018 [b]	<0.001
	Bio-Oss	6	0.291	0.029	
	Control	6	0.210 [b]	0.028 [b]	
Tb.S	EthOss	6	0.486 [a]	0.136 [a]	<0.001
	Bio-Oss	6	0.713 [a]	0.238 [a]	
	Control	6	1.686	0.455	

3.3. Histology

The histological slides for groups 1 (EthOss) and 2 (Bio-Oss) after eight weeks of healing are shown in Figure 5. Histologically, the analyzed biopsy contained newly-formed bone, residual grafting material, and vascularized uninflamed connective tissue. In all specimens, no significant inflammatory response, no necrosis, or foreign body reactions were observed. The graft particles were surrounded by or in contact with lamellar bone, demonstrating good osteoconductivity and biocompatibility.

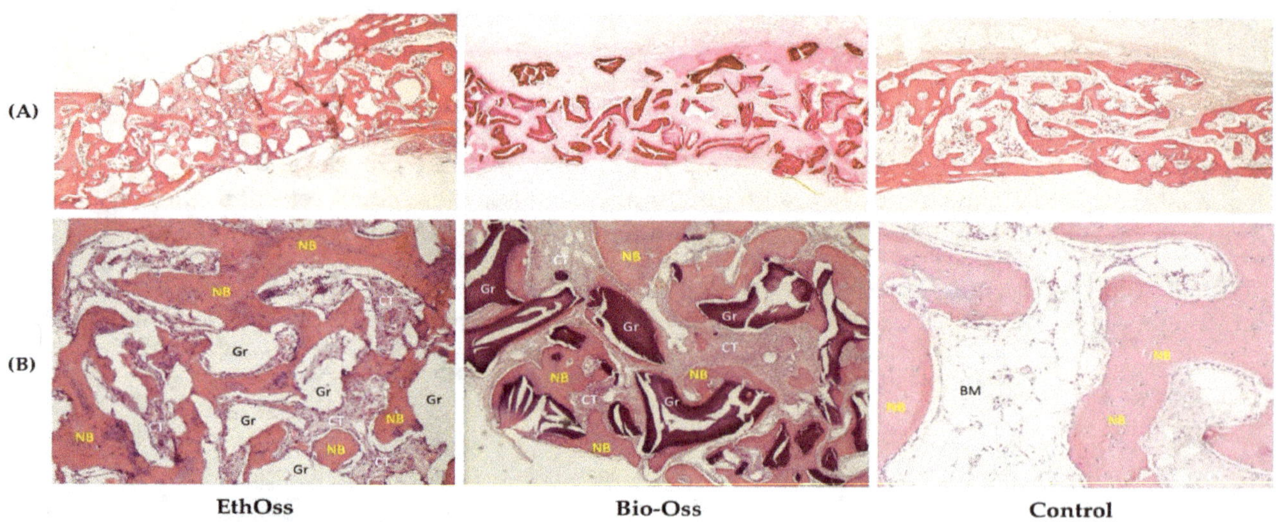

Figure 5. Histological specimens at eight weeks of healing (Hematoxylin and Eosin staining). (**A**) Cross-sections of the grafted and nongrafted sites (original magnification 5×); (**B**) EthOss and Bio-Oss particles (Gr) are embedded in well-perfused connective tissue (CT) and newly-formed bone (NB). Control group showing newly-formed bone trabeculae, bone marrow, and connective tissue (original magnification 50×).

4. Discussion

The aim of this animal study was to evaluate the host response after implantation of a novel bioactive and fully resorbable alloplastic grafting material in comparison to the effect of a bovine xenograft or spontaneous natural healing, in surgically-created calvaria bone defects in rabbits.

The β-TCP/CS material was compared to a bovine xenograft. Anorganic bovine bone substitutes have been extensively studied and used in oral surgery and implantology. Numerous pre-clinical studies and clinical trials in dentistry have shown and described in detail their osteoconductive properties and their ability to maintain the volume of the augmented site in the long-term [44–50]. However, controversy still remains as to whether this graft source is truly resorbable [51,52]. Mordenfeld et al. [51] performed histological and histomorphometrical analyses of human biopsies that were harvested 11 years after sinus floor augmentation with deproteinized bovine and autogenous bone. They found that the xenograft particles were not resorbed but were well-integrated in lamellar bone with no significant changes in particle size. Another important issue is that there are still significant concerns that bone grafts of bovine origin may carry a possible risk of transmitting prions to patients [53]. According to Kim et al. [54], screening prions within the animal genome is difficult. Moreover, there is a long latency period to manifestation of bovine spongiform encephalopathy (from one year to over 50 years) in infected patients. These factors provide a framework for the discussion of possible long-term risks of the xenografts that are used so extensively in dentistry. Thus, the authors suggested abolishing the use of bovine bone. They also highlighted that patient counseling should always include a clear description of the bone grafting material origin in bone reconstructive procedures.

In our study, no fibrosis developed between the particles of the biomaterial and the regenerated bone, nor was an inflammatory response observed, confirming the biocompatibility of EthOss. Our results indicate that β-TCP/CS can support new bone formation in parallel with biomaterial dissolution. The test alloplastic graft (β-TCP/CS = 65/35) presented in this study showed pronounced new bone formation (BV/TV = 33.70%) at eight weeks after implantation in circular calvaria bone defects in rabbits. Previous experimental animal studies using similar β-TCP/CS materials reported new bone fractions varying from 26% to 49% after a healing period of three weeks to four months [32,33]. Yang et al. [55], using micro-CT analysis to study the performance of a β-TCP/CS bone substitute in a sheep vertebral bone defect model, reported a 59% hard tissue volume at 36 weeks.

The degradation of β-TCP/CS biomaterials has been demonstrated in other pre-clinical studies. Using histomorphometry, Leventis et al. [33] found a statistically significant decrease in the percentage of residual material between three and six weeks (4.54% and 1.67%, respectively) in grafted rabbit calvaria defects. Podaropoulos et al. [32] reported 21.62% of residual β-TCP/CS four months after implantation of the material in surgically created bone defects on the iliac crest of Beagle dogs, whereas complete biodegradation of the β-TCP/CS graft after 36 weeks of implantation was documented in a previous animal study [55]. In accordance with the above findings, the present study demonstrated the degradation of the β-TCP/CS test biomaterial, showing a mean graft fraction area of 13.41% at eight weeks post-implantation.

In a clinical report, Fairbairn et al. [35] used β-TCP/CS for alveolar ridge preservation. Twelve weeks after socket grafting, a trephine biopsy was performed before the placement of the implant, and the authors histologically and histomorphometrically analyzed the sample of the regenerated bone, revealing 50.28% newly-formed bone and 12.27% remnant biomaterial.

In this study, we used micro-CT to three-dimensionally observe the structure of the newly-formed bone and to analyze important parameters of bone architecture. Micro-CT is a non-invasive, non-destructive analytical method that allows a significantly larger region of interest in the sample to be directly analyzed in three dimensions, compared to traditional histological methods. In combination with the histological findings, a comprehensive image of the regenerated bone can be surveyed to provide a representative and complete description of the healing outcome in the defect site [56].

The analysis of the micro-CT data in the present study revealed statistically significant differences regarding parameters associated with the microarchitecture of the healed sites at eight weeks post-operation. At sites that healed spontaneously, the trabecular number was lower and trabecular separation was higher. These findings in the control group indicate that the grafting materials used for filling the bone defects in the other groups acted as an osteoconductive scaffold, which facilitated the development of a larger number of trabeculae in a denser three-dimensional arrangement. In parallel, defects treated with β-TCP/CS showed the greatest bone regeneration and graft resorption, although differences between groups were not statistically significant.

The use of grafting materials to treat bone defects might have an important effect on the amount of regenerated bone tissue, and the presence of the graft particles may alter the microarchitecture of the newly-formed tissue. The resorption rate and the ability of a given grafting material to assist bone reconstruction seem to affect the bone healing mechanism and the geometry of the newly-formed tissue. Such differences might affect the overall quality of the newly-formed bone [7]. The capacity of the regenerated bone to remodel and adapt to the transmitted occlusal forces, thus minimizing the risk of failure under load, depends on the amount of bone, as well as its shape and microarchitecture (spatial distribution of the bone mass) and the intrinsic properties of the materials that comprise this hard tissue. Although a moderate to strong correlation between trabecular bone volume/architecture and biomechanical properties of trabecular bone has been shown [57], it is still unclear how the long-term presence of remnant non-resorbable or slowly resorbable particles of the graft, and the associated differences in structural parameters of trabecular bone and bone microarchitecture, might interfere with the remodeling and the strength of the new tissue when regenerating bone around dental implants. In a systematic review of the alterations in bone quality after alveolar ridge preservation with different bone graft substitutes, Chan et al. [7] reported significant variations in vital bone formation utilizing different grafting materials and discussed the concern that the presence of residual biomaterial might interfere with normal bone healing and remodeling, reducing the bone-to-implant contacts, and possibly negative affecting the overall quality and architecture of the bone that surrounds the implants. However, whether changes in bone quality influence implant success and peri-implant tissue stability remains unknown.

The outcomes of the present study revealed the highest vital bone content for defects grafted with the test alloplastic material (33.70%), followed by sockets with no graft material (27.36%), and the bovine xenograft (24.07%), whereas the amount of residual graft was higher (21.36%) for the bovine xenograft compared to the alloplast (13.41%). Our findings, although not statistically significant, are in accordance with results from human clinical studies on flapless socket grafting. In a recent systematic review, Jambhekar et al. [10] analyzed the outcomes of randomized controlled trials that reported that, after a minimum healing period of 12 weeks, sockets filled with alloplastic biomaterials had the highest amount of newly-formed bone (45.53%) compared to sites subjected to spontaneous healing with no graft material (41.07%) and xenografts (35.72%). The amount of remnant biomaterial was highest for sites treated with xenografts (19.3%) compared to alloplastic materials (13.67%).

5. Conclusions

The present histological and micro-CT investigation of rabbit cranial bone defects treated with the test resorbable alloplastic β-TCP/CS graft demonstrated excellent biocompatibility of the biomaterial and pronounced new bone formation after a healing period of eight weeks.

Author Contributions: All of the named authors were involved in the work leading to the publication of this paper and have read the paper before this submission. M.L., P.F., O.V. and D.P. performed the whole in vivo experiment; C.M. made the histological slides and performed the histological analysis; A.G. performed the statistical analysis; and M.L., P.F. and R.H. designed the experiment and have given final approval of the version to be published with full management of this manuscript.

Acknowledgments: The authors wish to thank Les A. Coulton, MD for performing the micro-CT examination and analysis, and the animal care team at the Laboratory of Experimental Surgery and Surgical Research, N.S. Christeas, Athens, Greece, for assistance during surgery.

References

1. Yip, I.; Ma, L.; Mattheos, N.; Dard, M.; Lang, N.P. Defect healing with various bone substitutes. *Clin. Oral Implants Res.* **2015**, *26*, 606–614. [CrossRef] [PubMed]
2. Wang, R.E.; Lang, N.P. Ridge preservation after tooth extraction. *Clin. Oral Implants Res.* **2012**, *23* (Suppl. 6), 147–156. [CrossRef]
3. Misch, C.M. Autogenous bone: Is it still the gold standard? *Implant Dent.* **2010**, *19*, 361. [CrossRef] [PubMed]
4. Le, B.Q.; Nurcombe, V.; Cool, S.M.; van Blitterswijk, C.A.; de Boer, J.; La Pointe, V.L.S. The Components of Bone and What They Can Teach Us about Regeneration. *Materials* **2017**, *11*, E14. [CrossRef] [PubMed]
5. Henkel, J.; Woodruff, M.A.; Epari, D.R.; Steck, R.; Glatt, V.; Dickinson, I.C.; Choong, P.F.; Schuetz, M.A.; Hutmacher, D.W. Bone regeneration based on tissue engineering conceptions—A 21st century perspective. *Bone Res.* **2013**, *1*, 216–248. [CrossRef] [PubMed]
6. Schlickewei, W.; Schlickewei, C. The Use of Bone Substitutes in the Treatment of Bone Defects-the Clinical View and History. *Macromol. Symp.* **2007**, *253*, 10–23. [CrossRef]
7. Chan, H.L.; Lin, G.H.; Fu, J.H.; Wang, H.L. Alterations in bone quality after socket preservation with grafting materials: A systematic review. *Int. J. Oral Maxillofac. Implants* **2013**, *28*, 710–720. [CrossRef] [PubMed]
8. Iocca, O.; Farcomeni, A.; Pardiñas Lopez, S.; Talib, H.S. Alveolar ridge preservation after tooth extraction: A Bayesian Network meta-analysis of grafting materials efficacy on prevention of bone height and width reduction. *J. Clin. Periodontol.* **2017**, *44*, 104–114. [CrossRef] [PubMed]
9. Danesh-Sani, S.A.; Engebretson, S.P.; Janal, M.N. Histomorphometric results of different grafting materials and effect of healing time on bone maturation after sinus floor augmentation: A systematic review and meta-analysis. *J. Periodontal Res.* **2017**, *52*, 301–312. [CrossRef] [PubMed]
10. Jambhekar, S.; Kernen, F.; Bidra, A.S. Clinical and histologic outcomes of socket grafting after flapless tooth extraction: A systematic review of randomized controlled clinical trials. *J. Prosthet. Dent.* **2015**, *113*, 371–382. [CrossRef] [PubMed]
11. Horowitz, R.A.; Leventis, M.D.; Rohrer, M.D.; Prasad, H.S. Bone grafting: History, rationale, and selection of materials and techniques. *Compend. Contin. Educ. Dent.* **2014**, *35* (Suppl. 4), 1–6.
12. Pryor, L.S.; Gage, E.; Langevin, C.J.; Herrera, F.; Breithaupt, A.D.; Gordon, C.R.; Afifi, A.M.; Zins, J.E.; Meltzer, H.; Gosman, A.; et al. Review of bone substitutes. *Craniomaxillofac. Trauma Reconstr.* **2009**, *2*, 151–160. [CrossRef] [PubMed]
13. Gao, C.; Peng, S.; Feng, P.; Shuai, C. Bone biomaterials and interactions with stem cells. *Bone Res.* **2017**, *5*, 17059. [CrossRef] [PubMed]
14. Glenske, K.; Donkiewicz, P.; Köwitsch, A.; Milosevic-Oljaca, N.; Rider, P.; Rofall, S.; Franke, J.; Jung, O.; Smeets, R.; Schnettler, R.; et al. Applications of Metals for Bone Regeneration. *Int. J. Mol. Sci.* **2018**, *19*, E826. [CrossRef] [PubMed]
15. Dorozhkin, S.V. Calcium orthophosphates in nature, biology and medicine. *Materials* **2009**, *2*, 399–498. [CrossRef]
16. Araújo, M.G.; Liljenberg, B.; Lindhe, J. β-tricalcium phosphate in the early phase of socket healing: An experimental study in the dog. *Clin. Oral Implants Res.* **2010**, *21*, 445–454. [CrossRef] [PubMed]
17. Trisi, P.; Rao, W.; Rebaudi, A.; Fiore, P. Histologic effect of pure-phase beta-tricalcium phosphate on bone regeneration in human artificial jawbone defects. *Int. J. Periodontics Restorative Dent.* **2003**, *23*, 69–78. [PubMed]
18. Roh, J.; Kim, J.Y.; Choi, Y.M.; Ha, S.M.; Kim, K.N.; Kim, K.M. Bone Regeneration Using a Mixture of Silicon-Substituted Coral HA and β-TCP in a Rat Calvarial Bone Defect Model. *Materials* **2016**, *9*, E97. [CrossRef] [PubMed]

19. Gregori, G.; Kleebe, H.J.; Mayr, H.; Ziegler, G. EELS characterisation of β-tricalcium phosphate and hydroxyapatite. *J. Eur. Ceram. Soc.* **2006**, *26*, 1473–1479. [CrossRef]
20. Daculsi, G.; Laboux, O.; Malard, O.; Weiss, P. Current state of the art of biphasic calcium phosphate bioceramics. *J. Mater. Sci. Mater. Med.* **2003**, *14*, 195–200. [CrossRef] [PubMed]
21. Harel, N.; Moses, O.; Palti, A.; Ormianer, Z. Long-term results of implants immediately placed into extraction sockets grafted with β-tricalcium phosphate: A retrospective study. *J. Oral Maxillofac. Surg.* **2013**, *71*, E63–E68. [CrossRef] [PubMed]
22. Kucera, T.; Sponer, P.; Urban, K.; Kohout, A. Histological assessment of tissue from large human bone defects repaired with β-tricalcium phosphate. *Eur. J. Orthop. Surg. Traumatol.* **2014**, *24*, 1357–1365. [CrossRef] [PubMed]
23. Yuan, H.; Fernandes, H.; Habibovic, P.; de Boer, J.; Barradas, A.M.; de Ruiter, A.; Walsh, W.R.; van Blitterswijk, C.A.; de Bruijn, J.D. Osteoinductive ceramics as a synthetic alternative to autologous bone grafting. *Proc. Natl. Acad. Sci. USA* **2010**, *107*, 13614–13619. [CrossRef] [PubMed]
24. Tang, Z.; Li, X.; Tan, Y.; Fan, H.; Zhang, X. The material and biological characteristics of osteoinductive calcium phosphate ceramics. *Regen. Biomater.* **2018**, *5*, 43–59. [CrossRef] [PubMed]
25. Miron, R.J.; Zhang, Q.; Sculean, A.; Buser, D.; Pippenger, B.E.; Dard, M.; Shirakata, Y.; Chandad, F.; Zhang, Y. Osteoinductive potential of 4 commonly employed bone grafts. *Clin. Oral Investig.* **2016**, *20*, 2259–2265. [CrossRef] [PubMed]
26. Barradas, A.M.; Yuan, H.; van Blitterswijk, C.; Habibovic, P. Osteoinductive biomaterials: Current knowledge of properties, experimental models and biological mechanisms. *Eur. Cell. Mater.* **2010**, *21*, 407–429. [CrossRef]
27. Cheng, L.; Shi, Y.; Ye, F.; Bu, H. Osteoinduction of calcium phosphate biomaterials in small animals. *Mater. Sci. Eng. C Mater. Biol. Appl.* **2013**, *33*, 1254–1260. [CrossRef] [PubMed]
28. Malhotra, A.; Habibovic, P. Calcium phosphates and angiogenesis: Implications and advances for bone regeneration. *Trends Biotechnol.* **2016**, *34*, 983–992. [CrossRef] [PubMed]
29. Ruga, E.; Gallesio, C.; Chiusa, L.; Boffano, P. Clinical and histologic outcomes of calcium sulfate in the treatment of postextraction sockets. *J. Craniofac. Surg.* **2011**, *22*, 494–498. [CrossRef] [PubMed]
30. Anson, D. Using calcium sulfate in guided tissue regeneration: A recipe for success. *Compend. Contin. Educ. Dent.* **2000**, *21*, 365–370. [PubMed]
31. Eleftheriadis, E.; Leventis, M.D.; Tosios, K.I.; Faratzis, G.; Titsinidis, S.; Eleftheriadi, I.; Dontas, I. Osteogenic activity of β-tricalcium phosphate in a hydroxyl sulphate matrix and demineralized bone matrix: A histological study in rabbit mandible. *J. Oral Sci.* **2010**, *52*, 377–384. [CrossRef] [PubMed]
32. Podaropoulos, L.; Veis, A.A.; Papadimitriou, S.; Alexandridis, C.; Kalyvas, D. Bone regeneration using b-tricalcium phosphate in a calcium sulfate matrix. *J. Oral Implantol.* **2009**, *35*, 28–36. [CrossRef] [PubMed]
33. Leventis, M.D.; Fairbairn, P.; Dontas, I.; Faratzis, G.; Valavanis, K.D.; Khaldi, L.; Kostakis, G.; Eleftheriadis, E. Biological response to β-tricalcium phosphate/calcium sulfate synthetic graft material: An experimental study. *Implant Dent.* **2014**, *23*, 37–43. [CrossRef] [PubMed]
34. Fairbairn, P.; Leventis, M. Protocol for Bone Augmentation with Simultaneous Early Implant Placement: A Retrospective Multicenter Clinical Study. *Int. J. Dent.* **2015**, *2015*, 589135. [CrossRef] [PubMed]
35. Fairbairn, P.; Leventis, M.; Mangham, C.; Horowitz, R. Alveolar Ridge Preservation Using a Novel Synthetic Grafting Material: A Case with Two-Year Follow-Up. *Case Rep. Dent.* **2018**, *2018*, 6412806. [CrossRef] [PubMed]
36. Giannoudis, P.V.; Einhorn, T.A.; Marsh, D. Fracture healing: The diamond concept. *Injury* **2007**, *38*, S3–S6. [CrossRef]
37. Troedhan, A.; Schlichting, I.; Kurrek, A.; Wainwright, M. Primary implant stability in augmented sinuslift-sites after completed bone regeneration: A randomized controlled clinical study comparing four subantrally inserted biomaterials. *Sci. Rep.* **2014**, *4*, 5877. [CrossRef] [PubMed]
38. Dimitriou, R.; Mataliotakis, G.I.; Calori, G.M.; Giannoudis, P.V. The role of barrier membranes for guided bone regeneration and restoration of large bone defects: Current experimental and clinical evidence. *BMC Med.* **2012**, *10*, 81. [CrossRef] [PubMed]
39. Pecora, G.; Andreana, S.; Margarone, J.E.; Covani, U.; Sottosanti, J.S. Bone regeneration with a calcium sulfate barrier. *Oral Surg. Oral Med. Oral Pathol. Oral Radiol. Endod.* **1997**, *84*, 424–429. [CrossRef]

40. Mazor, Z.; Mamidwar, S.; Ricci, J.L.; Tovar, N.M. Bone repair in periodontal defect using a composite of allograft and calcium sulfate (DentoGen) and a calcium sulfate barrier. *J. Oral Implantol.* **2011**, *37*, 287–292. [CrossRef] [PubMed]
41. Strocchi, R.; Orsini, G.; Iezzi, G.; Scarano, A.; Rubini, C.; Pecora, G.; Piattelli, A. Bone regeneration with calcium sulfate: Evidence for increased angiogenesis in rabbits. *J. Oral Implantol.* **2002**, *28*, 273–278. [CrossRef]
42. Artzi, Z.; Weinreb, M.; Givol, N.; Rohrer, M.D.; Nemcovsky, C.E.; Prasad, H.S.; Tal, H. Biomaterial Resorption Rate and Healing Site Morphology of Inorganic Bovine Bone and β-Tricalcium Phosphate in the Canine: A 24-month Longitudinal Histologic Study and Morphometric Analysis. *Int. J. Oral Maxillofac. Implants* **2004**, *19*, 357–368. [PubMed]
43. Palti, A.; Hoch, T. A concept for the treatment of various dental bone defects. *Implant Dent.* **2002**, *11*, 73–78. [CrossRef] [PubMed]
44. Artzi, Z.; Tal, H.; Dayan, D. Porous bovine bone mineral in healing of human extraction sockets. Part 1: Histomorphometric evaluations at 9 months. *J. Periodontol.* **2000**, *71*, 1015–1023. [CrossRef] [PubMed]
45. Artzi, Z.; Tal, H.; Dayan, D. Porous bovine bone mineral in healing of human extraction sockets: 2. Histochemical observations at 9 months. *J. Periodontol.* **2001**, *72*, 152–159. [CrossRef] [PubMed]
46. Pang, C.; Ding, Y.; Zhou, H.; Qin, R.; Hou, R.; Zhang, G.; Hu, K. Alveolar ridge preservation with deproteinized bovine bone graft and collagen membrane and delayed implants. *J. Craniofac. Surg.* **2014**, *25*, 1698–1702. [CrossRef] [PubMed]
47. Aludden, H.C.; Mordenfeld, A.; Hallman, M.; Dahlin, C.; Jensen, T. Lateral ridge augmentation with Bio-Oss alone or Bio-Oss mixed with particulate autogenous bone graft: A systematic review. *Int. J. Oral Maxillofac. Surg.* **2017**, *46*, 1030–1038. [CrossRef] [PubMed]
48. Jensen, T.; Schou, S.; Stavropoulos, A.; Terheyden, H.; Holmstrup, P. Maxillary sinus floor augmentation with Bio-Oss or Bio-Oss mixed with autogenous bone as graft: A systematic review. *Clin. Oral Implants Res.* **2012**, *23*, 263–273. [CrossRef] [PubMed]
49. Scheyer, E.T.; Velasquez-Plata, D.; Brunsvold, M.A.; Lasho, D.J.; Mellonig, J.T. A clinical comparison of a bovine-derived xenograft used alone and in combination with enamel matrix derivative for the treatment of periodontal osseous defects in humans. *J. Periodontol.* **2002**, *73*, 423–432. [CrossRef] [PubMed]
50. Chappuis, V.; Rahman, L.; Buser, R.; Janner, S.F.M.; Belser, U.C.; Buser, D. Effectiveness of contour augmentation with guided bone regeneration: 10-year results. *J. Dent. Res.* **2018**, *97*, 266–274. [CrossRef] [PubMed]
51. Mordenfeld, A.; Hallman, M.; Johansson, C.B.; Albrektsson, T. Histological and histomorphometrical analyses of biopsies harvested 11 years after maxillary sinus floor augmentation with deproteinized bovine and autogenous bone. *Clin. Oral Implants Res.* **2010**, *21*, 961–970. [CrossRef] [PubMed]
52. Heberer, S.; Al-Chawaf, B.; Hildebrand, D.; Nelson, J.J.; Nelson, K. Histomorphometric analysis of extraction sockets augmented with Bio-Oss Collagen after a 6-week healing period: A prospective study. *Clin. Oral Implants Res.* **2008**, *19*, 1219–1225. [CrossRef] [PubMed]
53. Kim, Y.; Nowzari, H.; Rich, S.K. Risk of Prion Disease Transmission through Bovine-Derived Bone Substitutes: A Systematic Review. *Clin. Implant Dent. Relat. Res.* **2013**, *15*, 645–653. [CrossRef] [PubMed]
54. Kim, Y.; Rodriguez, A.E.; Nowzari, H. The risk of prion infection through bovine grafting materials. *Clin. Implant Dent. Relat. Res.* **2016**, *18*, 1095–1102. [CrossRef] [PubMed]
55. Yang, H.L.; Zhu, X.S.; Chen, L.; Chen, C.M.; Mangham, D.C.; Coulton, L.A.; Aiken, S.S. Bone healing response to a synthetic calcium sulfate/β-tricalcium phosphate graft material in a sheep vertebral body defect model. *J. Biomed. Mater. Res. B Appl. Biomater.* **2012**, *100*, 1911–1921. [CrossRef] [PubMed]
56. Bouxsein, M.L.; Boyd, S.K.; Christiansen, B.A.; Guldberg, R.E.; Jepsen, K.J.; Müller, R. Guidelines for assessment of bone microstructure in rodents using micro–computed tomography. *J. Bone Miner. Res.* **2010**, *25*, 1468–1486. [CrossRef] [PubMed]
57. Bouxsein, M.L. Determinants of skeletal fragility. *Best Pract. Res. Clin. Rheumatol.* **2005**, *19*, 897–911. [CrossRef] [PubMed]

14

Calcium Charge and Release of Conventional Glass-Ionomer Cement Containing Nanoporous Silica

Koichi Nakamura [1,*], Shigeaki Abe [2], Hajime Minamikawa [3] and Yasutaka Yawaka [1]

[1] Department of Dentistry for Children and Disabled Person, Graduate School of Dental Medicine, Hokkaido University, Kita 13 Nishi 7, Kita-ku, Sapporo 060-8586, Hokkaido, Japan; yawaka@den.hokudai.ac.jp

[2] Department of Biomaterials and Bioengineering, Graduate School of Dental Medicine, Hokkaido University, Sapporo 060-8586, Hokkaido, Japan; sabe@den.hokudai.ac.jp

[3] Department of Dentistry for Molecular Cell Pharmacology, Graduate School of Dental Medicine, Hokkaido University, Sapporo 060-8586, Hokkaido, Japan; minami@den.hokudai.ac.jp

* Correspondence: pika@den.hokudai.ac.jp

Abstract: The aim of this study was to evaluate calcium charge and release of conventional glass-ionomer cement (GIC) containing nanoporous silica (NPS). Experimental specimens were divided into two groups: the control (GIC containing no NPS) and GIC-NPS (GIC containing 10 wt % NPS). The specimens were immersed in calcium chloride solutions of 5 wt % calcium concentration for 24 h at 37 °C, whereupon the calcium ion release of the specimens was measured. The calcium ion release behavior of GIC-NPS after immersion in the calcium solution was significantly greater than that of the control. Scanning electron microscopy and electron-dispersive X-ray spectroscopy results indicated that calcium penetrated inside the GIC-NPS specimen, while the calcium was primarily localized on the surface of the control specimen. It was demonstrated that NPS markedly improved the calcium charge and release property of GIC.

Keywords: nanoporous silica; glass-ionomer cement; calcium

---

1. Introduction

The overall incidence of dental caries has gradually decreased, but it still occurs quite frequently [1]. In the case of small dental carious lesions, the tooth is typically restored by a coronal restoration material, which often requires a retreatment owing to circumstances such as the progress of the dental caries around the restoration or the dental restoration falling out [2,3]. The main cause of coronal restoration treatment failure is secondary caries, which requires coronal restoration or pulp treatment [4,5]. To avoid tooth loss, therefore, it is necessary to prevent secondary caries, for which fluoride takes an important role [6,7]. Fluoride ions are included in dental items such as toothpaste and glass-ionomer cement (GIC) [8,9], and GIC is often used to prevent secondary caries in children [10,11]. GIC is widely used in dentistry such as the luting cement [12], temporary restoration [13], and adhering orthodontic band [14]. The GIC supplemented with TiO_2 nanoparticles also have the effect of antibacterial properties [15].

Calcium is an important component of the tooth. It is essential for the tooth mineralization that the calcium ion exists around the tooth. As one of the methods to supply calcium for teeth, some studies proposed the addition of casein phosphopeptide amorphous calcium phosphate (CPP-ACP) to GIC [16–18]. Addition of CPP-ACP to GIC increased the release of calcium ions. However, CPP-ACP is an ingredient derived from milk, and clinicians should consider potential side effects from ingestion of casein derivative protein in people with immunoglobulin E allergies to milk proteins [19].

Nanoporous silica (NPS) has a structure that possesses a uniform pore size of about 1 nm with a large specific surface area and is attractive in applications such as a sustained drug release carrier and catalyst support [20]. It is believed that NPS can adsorb formaldehyde gas and methylene blue pigments, and it has been confirmed that one of the properties of NPS is its ability to adsorb various ions and substances [21–23]. However, there are few studies on the application of NPS in dentistry.

The purpose of this study was to determine whether conventional GIC containing NPS was able to charge and release calcium ions. Furthermore, the cross-section of the GIC-NPS specimen was observed by scanning electron microscopy (SEM) and the compressive strength was measured. Our null hypotheses were that GIC containing the NPS did not charge and release calcium ions, and that there was no difference in the compressive strength of the GIC control and the GIC-NPS.

2. Materials and Methods

2.1. NPS Synthesis

The NPS was synthesized in accordance with the protocol described by Tagaya et al. [20]. In this process, 1.37 mmol of cetyltrimethylammonium bromide (CTAB: Wako, Osaka, Japan) was added to 120 mL of distilled water, to which 1.75 mL of 2.0 M sodium hydroxide (Wako) solution was added. The mixture was stirred for 30 min at 80 °C, whereupon 12.4 mmol of tetraethoxysilane (Wako) was added and the mixture stirred for 2 h at 80 °C. The resulting suspension was filtered and dried and, to remove the CTAB, the obtained particles were calcined at 550 °C for 4 h. The obtained white particles were subsequently observed using an SEM (S-4800, HITACHI, Tokyo, Japan) and a transmission electron microscope (TEM: JEM-2010, JEOL, Tokyo, Japan).

2.2. Preparation of Test Specimens

The obtained NPS was added to the powder component of the GIC (GC Fuji II, GC, Tokyo, Japan; lot 1606141) at 10 wt % concentration, whereupon the test specimens were prepared by mixing the powder component (with or without NPS) and the liquid component of the GIC (GC Fuji II, GC, Tokyo, Japan; lot 1607041) in accordance with the manufacturer specifications. The specimens were set in two patterns, where the first was 10 mm in diameter and 1 mm in height for the calcium ion release measurement and the SEM and electron-dispersive X-ray spectroscopy analysis, and the second was 4 mm in diameter and 6 mm in height for the compressive testing. The experimental specimens were divided into two groups comprising the control (no NPS) and the GIC-NPS (containing 10 wt % NPS). The specimens were wet ground via hand lapping using P400 grit silicon carbide abrasive papers (SANKYO, Saitama, Japan).

2.3. Calcium Charge and Release

Three 10 mm-diameter, 1 mm-height specimens were immersed in a calcium chloride solution with a 5 wt % calcium concentration (calcium 150 mg/3mL) for 24 h at 37 °C. After removal from the calcium solution, the specimens were rinsed with distilled water and subsequently immersed in 5 mL of distilled water at 37 °C for 7 d. The distilled water was changed every day and was further analyzed daily to determine the calcium ion concentration in the water. N = 6 samples (18 specimens) per group were used. The calcium ion concentration was measured using inductively coupled plasma atomic emission spectroscopy (ICPE-9000, SHIMADZU, Tokyo, Japan). The total weights of the calcium releasing from the specimens were calculated from the calcium concentration. The preparation of specimens was carried out according to Bando's conditions [24], but slightly modified.

2.4. Scanning Electron Microscopy (SEM) and Energy-Dispersive X-ray Spectroscopy (EDS)

Specimens containing calcium were analyzed using SEM and EDS (Genesis, EDAX Japan, Tokyo, Japan). The specimens were immersed in the 5 wt % calcium solution and dried. The specimens were cut perpendicularly, then the specimen surface and cross-section were observed after carbon coating.

2.5. Compressive Strength Test

The 4 mm-diameter, 6 mm-height test specimens were placed in a universal testing machine (Model 4204, Instron, Canton, OH, USA) with a cross-head speed of 1.0 mm/min. N = 12 specimens per group were used for this test. This procedure has been described in detail elsewhere [25].

2.6. Statistical Analysis

Statistical analysis was performed using IBM SPSS Statistics Version 21 (IBM Japan, Tokyo, Japan), and the results were analyzed statistically using the Mann-Whitney U test. The level of significance was set at $p < 0.05$.

3. Results

3.1. Morphological Characteristics of NPS

The SEM and TEM images of NPS particles are shown in Figure 1. The NPS particles were spherical and approximately 200–300 nm in diameter, exhibiting pores a few nanometers in diameter.

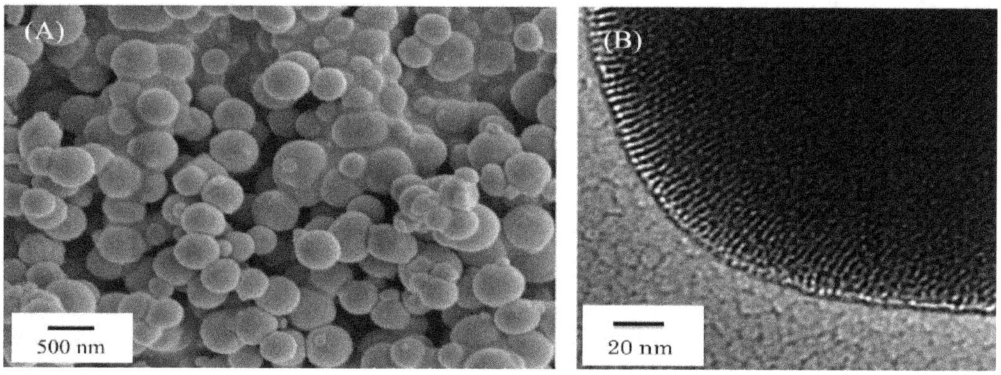

Figure 1. Typical (**A**) SEM and (**B**) TEM images of nanoporous silica particles. The nanoporous silica particles showed sizes approximately 200–300 nm in diameter (**A**), exhibiting pores a few nanometers in diameter (**B**).

3.2. Calcium Charge and Release

Figure 2 shows the time-profile of the release of calcium from the specimens after immersion in the 5 wt % calcium chloride solution. The calcium release behavior of GIC-NPS was significantly greater than that of the control ($p < 0.05$).

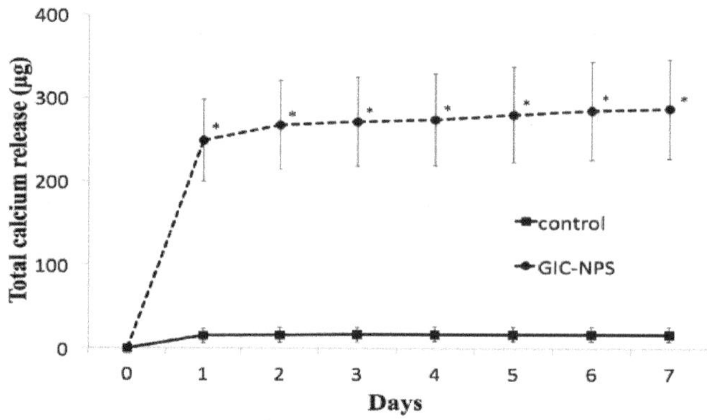

Figure 2. Time-profile of calcium release from the specimens after immersion in 5 wt % calcium chloride solution. Significance was determined using the Mann-Whitney U test ($p < 0.05$).

3.3. EDS Analysis

Figure 3A–C show the results of SEM and EDS for the surface and the cross-section of the specimens. As shown in Figure 3A, calcium was detected on the surfaces of both the control and GIC-NPS specimens; however, the specimen cross-sections exhibited significant amounts of calcium only for the GIC-NPS specimen. Although calcium was localized primarily on the surface of the control specimen, it was observed on the surface and throughout the inside of the GIC-NPS specimen (Figure 3B,C). In the surface of the control specimen (Figure 3B right and 3C right), calcium was distributed uniformly.

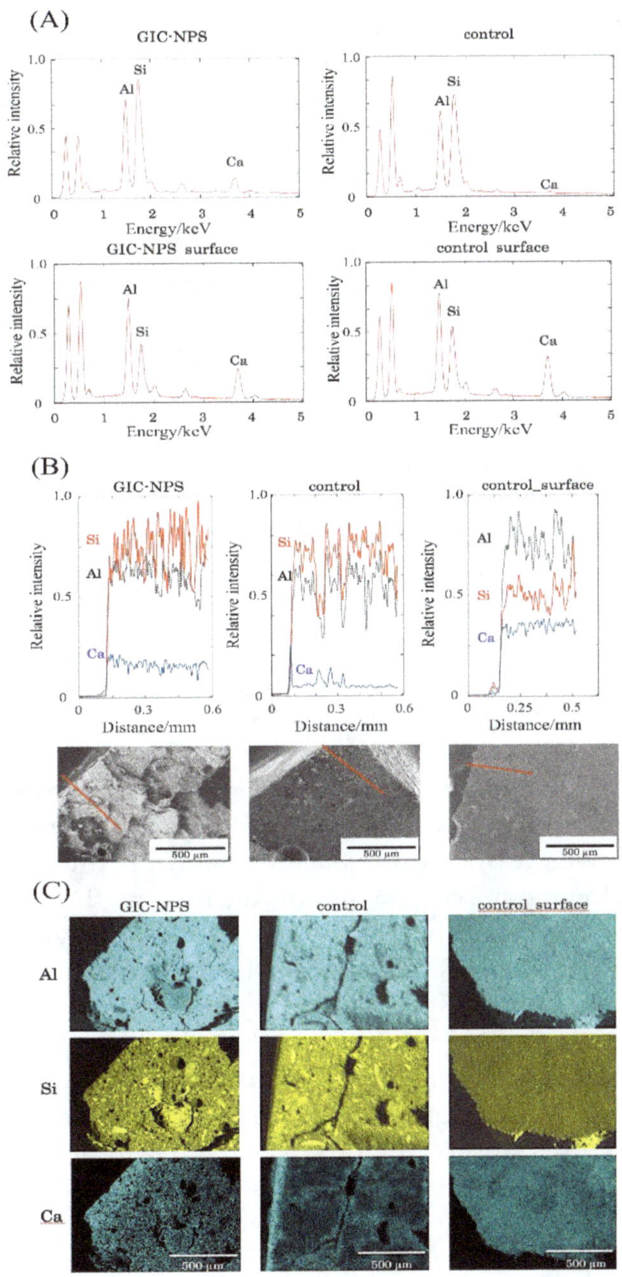

Figure 3. (**A**) Typical EDS spectra from the cross-section (upper) and surface (lower) of the GIC-NPS (left) and control (right) specimens, displaying the constitutive elements. (**B**) SEM images (lower) and EDS line analysis (upper) for the GIC-NPS cross-section (left), control cross-section (center), and control surface (right). (**C**) EDS element mapping of the Al (upper), Si (center), and Ca (lower) in the GIC-NPS cross-section (left), control cross-section (center), and control surface (right).

3.4. Compressive Strength

The compressive strength of the control and GIC-NPS were 111.37 ± 28.75 MPa and 100.32 ± 20.73 MPa (Mean ± SD, N = 12). There was no significant difference between the compressive strength of the control and GIC-NPS ($p = 0.319$).

4. Discussion

In the present study, the amount of the calcium release from the glass-ionomer cement containing nanoporous silica (GIC-NPS) specimen was determined. The results suggested the existence of an NPS-induced calcium ion charge and release property of the GIC-NPS. Even when a concentration of 10 wt % NPS was included in the GIC, the obtained specimens exhibited compressive strength, comparable to that of conventional GIC without NPS. It has been suggested that the possibility exists of NPS being used in dental materials as a calcium source, and it is therefore important that NPS did not reduce significantly the strength properties of the dental materials in the present study. However, other properties (solubility, adhesive strength, etc.) of GIC-NPS still have not been clarified, and so it is necessary for those concerned to hold further studies.

The nanopores in the NPS were approximately the size through which a calcium ion can pass [26]. The EDS images of the GIC-NPS specimens indicated that calcium ions penetrated into the GIC-NPS after immersion in the calcium solution. The NPS is well known as an adsorbent particle, and calcium might be adsorbed in the NPS pores in the same way other substances are adsorbed. It was not confirmed, however, which component of the NPS combined with the calcium, but this should be the subject of future research.

There were 150 mg of calcium in the immersed solution; nevertheless, the total amounts of the calcium released from specimen of control and GIC-NPS were 17.21 ± 8.66 µg and 287.71 ± 56.60 µg, respectively. Almost all of the calcium remained in the immersed solution or was washed away by rinsing with water. The percentage of total calcium released from the specimen in GIC-NPS on the first day, the second day, and the third day were 86.6%, 6.5%, and 1.5%, respectively. In contrast, those percentages for the control on the first day, the second day, and the third day were 87.7%, 6.6%, and 3.3%, respectively. Though the total amount of calcium was different for both, the percentage of calcium released had a similar tendency in both.

In this study, NPS was found to not only adsorb calcium ion but also to release adsorbed calcium ions when placed in an aqueous medium. The GIC-NPS could be expected to function as a source of calcium, and it was suggested that it could be useful to facilitate remineralization. Furthermore, the GIC used in this study was a fluoride-releasing material; thus, GIC-NPS may be useful for producing fluoroapatite by allowing the coexistence of calcium and fluoride ions [27]. This is significant because fluoroapatite possesses a higher acid resistance than hydroxyapatite, the main component of teeth. The amount of fluoride ions released from the GIC depends on the fluoroaluminosilicate glass composition included in the powder [28]. In this study, the inclusion of NPS decreases the relative amount of the GIC powder, so it is likely that the amount of fluoride ions released may be slightly decreased. This reduction may be negligible with a 10 wt % concentration of NPS, however, because of the amount of fluoride ions released from the GIC [29]. Furthermore, the specimens were immersed in calcium chloride solution in this study. Previous research has indicated that the surface hardness of GIC increases with immersion in the calcium chloride solution [30]. The surface property of GIC may have changed by immersion of the solution.

The SEM/EDS analysis indicated that calcium penetrated to the interior of the GIC-NPS specimen. After immersion in the calcium solution, calcium was distributed homogenously on the surfaces of the control specimen similar to the distribution of aluminum and silicon, which are the major constituents of GIC (Figure 3C, right column). However, the distribution behavior in the depth direction was clearly different in the two specimens. In the case of the control, calcium was localized on the surface of specimen (Figure 3C, middle column), while calcium was detected even inside of the GIC-NPS (Figure 3C, left column). The highest concentration of calcium was determined to be on the surface of the GIC-NPS specimen, similar to that found for the control specimen. The EDS mapping suggests that the calcium concentration slightly decreased as a function of depth but persisted throughout the interior of the GIC-NPS specimen.

The EDS spectral line analysis (Figure 3B) also revealed that the calcium concentration profile of the GIC-NPS specimen was clearly different than that of the control specimen. The latter exhibited a sharp peak only around the specimen surface, while the former exhibited a calcium concentration that slightly decreased in a path from the surface to a depth of 0.1 mm, then remained approximately constant up to 0.5 mm of depth.

Nanoporous silica is often applied as a film on the material surface and is rarely contained inside the material [31]. Nevertheless, it was found herein that NPS was capable of the charge and release of calcium ions through the matrix even when the NPS was incorporated throughout the material.

Previous studies of powdered inorganic additives have shown the compressive strength increase and decrease [25,32,33]. In this study, compressive strength has slightly decreased. It may be due to interference of the NPS with the normal GIC reaction. By increasing of NPS component, compressive strength might significantly decrease. However, under the conditions of the present study, there were no significant differences between the two groups.

The appearance of secondary caries requires a certain period time. In the present study, however, the calcium charge and release properties of GIC-NPS were observed over only a week. If it is a repeated charge and release of the calcium, secondary caries were prevented in the long term. To confirm this presumption, further study is needed. We also measured the amount of calcium charge and release; the study of the preventing effect for secondary caries may be needed in the model similar to the oral cavity.

In recent years, many studies of bioactive materials have been conducted [34¯36]. The results of this study may be useful to the development of biomaterials. Firstly, the results herein may be extended to the development of remineralization-inducing materials by the uptake of phosphate ions, which are essential for remineralization, e.g., pit and fissure sealants and restoration materials. Also, this study may inform the drug delivery system by the uptake of antibacterial agents such as Cetylpyridinium Chloride (CPC). Furthermore, the NPS used in this study possesses a negative charge, and therefore cannot adsorb a negatively-charged fluoride ion. However, the NPS may be enabled to adsorb a fluoride ion by also causing it to retain a positive electric charge. This would give the ability of fluoride ion release to the material without also requiring a composite resin that exhibits fluoride ion release characteristics. We believe that it is necessary to study these possibilities in future work.

5. Conclusions

We demonstrated the capacity of GIC-NPS for calcium ion charge/release and contrasted it with that of conventional GIC. The presence of NPS was found to markedly improve the calcium ion charge/release property of GIC. Even for NPS concentrations up to 10 wt % in the GIC, the compressive strength of the GIC was not changed significantly.

Author Contributions: K.N., S.A., and H.M. performed the experiments and analyzed the data; Y.Y. contributed as advisors; and K.N. wrote the paper. All authors read and approved the final manuscript.

References

1. Ramos-Jorge, J.; Alencar, B.M.; Pordeus, I.A.; Soares, M.E.; Marques, L.S.; Ramos-Jorge, M.L.; Paiva, S.M. Impact of dental caries on quality of life among preschool children: Emphasis on the type of tooth and stages of progression. *Eur. J. Oral Sci.* **2015**, *123*, 88–95. [CrossRef] [PubMed]

2. Metz, I.; Rothmaier, K.; Pitchika, V.; Crispin, A.; Hickel, R.; Garcia-Godoy, F.; Bücher, K.; Kühnisch, J. Risk factors for secondary caries in direct composite restorations in primary teeth. *Int. J. Paediatr. Dent.* **2015**, *25*, 451–461. [CrossRef] [PubMed]
3. Pallesen, U.; Van Dijken, J.W. A randomized controlled 27 years follow up of three resin composites in Class II restorations. *J. Dent.* **2015**, *43*, 1547–1558. [CrossRef] [PubMed]
4. Brantley, C.F.; Bader, J.D.; Shugars, D.A.; Nesbit, S.P. Does the cycle of rerestoration lead to larger restorations? *J. Am. Dent. Assoc.* **1995**, *126*, 1407–1413. [CrossRef] [PubMed]
5. Hsu, C.Y.; Donly, K.; Drake, D.; Wefel, J. Effects of aged fluoride-containing restorative materials on recurrent root caries. *J. Dent. Res.* **1998**, *77*, 418–425. [CrossRef] [PubMed]
6. Comar, L.P.; Wiegand, A.; Moron, B.M.; Rios, D.; Buzalaf, M.A.; Buchalla, W.; Magalhães, A.C. In situ effect of sodium fluoride or titanium tetrafluoride varnish and solution on carious demineralization of enamel. *Eur. J. Oral Sci.* **2012**, *120*, 342–348. [CrossRef] [PubMed]
7. Bonetti, D.; Clarkson, J.E. Fluoride Varnish for Caries Prevention: Efficacy and Implementation. *Caries Res.* **2016**, *50*, 45–49. [CrossRef] [PubMed]
8. Kucukyilmaz, E.; Savas, S. Evaluation of shear bond strength, penetration ability, microleakage and remineralisation capacity of glass-ionomer-based fissure sealants. *Eur. J. Paediatr. Dent.* **2016**, *17*, 17–23. [PubMed]
9. Yönel, N.; Bikker, F.J.; Lagerweij, M.D.; Kleverlaan, C.J.; Van Loveren, C.; Özen, B.; Çetiner, S.; Van Strijp, A.J. Anti-erosive effects of fluoride and phytosphingosine: An in vitro study. *Eur. J. Oral Sci.* **2016**, *124*, 396–402. [CrossRef] [PubMed]
10. Goldman, A.S.; Chen, X.; Fan, M.; Frencken, J.E. Cost-effectiveness, in a randomized trial, of glass-ionomer-based and resin sealant materials after 4 yr. *Eur. J. Oral Sci.* **2016**, *124*, 472–479. [CrossRef] [PubMed]
11. Zhao, I.S.; Mei, M.L.; Burrow, M.F.; Lo, E.C.; Chu, C.H. Prevention of secondary caries using silver diamine fluoride treatment and casein phosphopeptide-amorphous calcium phosphate modified glass-ionomer cement. *J. Dent.* **2017**, *57*, 38–44. [CrossRef] [PubMed]
12. Heintze, S.D. Crown pull-off test (crown retention test) to evaluate the bonding effectiveness of luting agents. *Dent. Mater.* **2010**, *26*, 193–206. [CrossRef] [PubMed]
13. Coll, J.A.; Campbell, A.; Chalmers, N.I. Effects of glass ionomer temporary restorations on pulpal diagnosis and treatment outcomes in primary molars. *Pediatr. Dent.* **2013**, *35*, 416–421. [PubMed]
14. Millett, D.T.; Glenny, A.M.; Mattick, R.C.; Hickman, J.; Mandall, N.A. Adhesives for fixed orthodontic bands. *Cochrane Database Syst. Rev.* **2016**, *10*, CD004485. [CrossRef] [PubMed]
15. Garcia-Conreras, R.; Scougall-Vilchis, R.J.; Contreras-Bulner, R.; Sakagami, H.; Morales-Luckie, R.A.; Nakajima, H. Mechanical, antibacterial and bond strength properties of nano-titanium-enriched glass ionomer cement. *J. Appl. Oral Sci.* **2015**, *23*, 321–328. [CrossRef] [PubMed]
16. Mazzaoui, S.A.; Burrow, M.F.; Tyas, M.J.; Dashper, S.G.; Eakins, D.; Reynolds, E.C. Incorporation of casein phosphopeptide–amorphous calcium phosphate into a glass-ionomer cement. *J. Dent. Res.* **2003**, *82*, 914–918. [CrossRef] [PubMed]
17. Al Zraikat, H.; Palamara, J.E.; Messer, H.H.; Burrow, M.F.; Reynolds, E.C. The incorporation of casein phosphopeptide–amorphous calcium phosphate into a glass ionomer cement. *Dent. Mater.* **2011**, *27*, 235–243. [CrossRef] [PubMed]
18. Zalizniak, I.; Palamara, J.E.; Wong, R.H.; Cochrane, N.J.; Burrow, M.F.; Reynolds, E.C. Ion release and physical properties of CPP-ACP modified GIC in acid solutions. *J. Dent.* **2013**, *41*, 449–454. [CrossRef] [PubMed]
19. Azarpazhooh, A.; Limeback, H. Clinical efficacy of casein derivatives: A systematic review of the literature. *J. Am. Dent. Assoc.* **2008**, *139*, 915–924. [CrossRef] [PubMed]
20. Tagaya, M.; Ikoma, T.; Yoshioka, T.; Motozuka, S.; Xu, Z.; Minami, F.; Tanaka, J. Synthesis and luminescence properties of Eu(III)-doped nanoporous silica spheres. *J. Colloid Interface Sci.* **1999**, *218*, 462–467. [CrossRef] [PubMed]
21. Barbé, C.; Bartlett, J.; Kong, L.; Finnie, K.; Lin, H.Q.; Larkin, M.; Calleja, S.; Bush, A.; Calleja, G. Silica Particles: A Novel Drug-Delivery System. *Adv. Mater.* **2004**, *16*, 1959–1966. [CrossRef]

22. Fazaeli, Y.; Feizi, S.; Jalilian, A.R.; Hejrani, A. Grafting of [(64)Cu]-TPPF20 porphyrin complex on Functionalized nano-porous MCM-41 silica as a potential cancer imaging agent. *Appl. Radiat. Isotopes* **2016**, *112*, 13–19. [CrossRef] [PubMed]
23. Wang, L.; Chen, Q.; Li, C.; Fang, F. Nano-Web Cobalt Modified Silica Nanoparticles Catalysts for Water Oxidation and MB Oxidative Degradation. *J. Nanosci. Nanotechnol.* **2016**, *16*, 5364–5368. [CrossRef] [PubMed]
24. Bando, Y.; Nakanishi, K.; Abe, S.; Yamagata, S.; Yoshida, Y.; Iida, J. Electric charge dependence of controlled dye-release behavior in glass ionomer cement containing nano-poruos silica particles. *J. Nanosci. Nanotechnol.* **2018**, *18*, 75–79. [CrossRef] [PubMed]
25. Elsaka, S.E.; Hamouda, I.M.; Swain, M.V. Titanium dioxide nanoparticles addition to a conventional glass-ionomer restorative: Influence on physical and antibacterial properties. *J. Dent.* **2011**, *39*, 589–598. [CrossRef] [PubMed]
26. Hille, B. *Ion Channels of Excitable Membranes*, 3rd ed.; Sinauer Associates: Sunderland, MA, USA, 2001.
27. Wegehaupt, F.J.; Tauböck, T.T.; Sener, B.; Attin, T. Long-term protective effect of surface sealants against erosive wear by intrinsic and extrinsic acids. *J. Dent.* **2012**, *40*, 416–422. [CrossRef] [PubMed]
28. Dennis, C.S. Development of glass-ionomer cement systems. *Biomaterials* **1998**, *19*, 467–478.
29. Okte, Z.; Bayrak, S.; Fidanci, U.R.; Sel, T. Fluoride and aluminum release from restorative materials using ion chromatography. *J. Appl. Oral Sci.* **2012**, *20*, 27–31. [CrossRef] [PubMed]
30. Shiozawa, M.; Takahashi, H.; Iwasaki, N.; Wada, T.; Uo, M. Effect of immersion time of restorative glass ionomer cements and immersion duration in calcium chloride solution on surface hardness. *Dent. Mater.* **2014**, *30*, 377–383. [CrossRef] [PubMed]
31. Song, D.P.; Naik, A.; Li, S.; Ribbe, A.; Watkins, J.J. Rapid, Large-Area Synthesis of Hierarchical Nanoporous Silica Hybrid Films on Flexible Substrates. *J. Am. Chem. Soc.* **2016**, *138*, 13473–13476. [CrossRef] [PubMed]
32. Xie, D.; Weng, Y.; Guo, X.; Zhao, J.; Gregory, R.L.; Zheng, C. Preparation and evaluation of a novel glass-ionomer cement with antibacterial functions. *Dent. Mater.* **2011**, *27*, 487–496. [CrossRef] [PubMed]
33. Bellis, C.A.; Nobbs, A.H.; O'sullivan, D.J.; Holder, J.A.; Barbour, M.E. Glass ionomer cements functionalised with a concentrated paste of chlorhexidine hexametaphosphate provides dose-dependent chlorhexidine release over at least 14 months. *J. Dent.* **2016**, *45*, 53–58. [CrossRef] [PubMed]
34. Lee, J.H.; Seo, S.J.; Kim, H.W. Bioactive glass-based nanocomposites for personalized dental tissue regeneration. *Dent. Mater. J.* **2016**, *35*, 710–720. [CrossRef] [PubMed]
35. Uo, M.; Wada, T.; Asakura, K. Structural analysis of strontium in human teeth treated with surface pre-reacted glass-ionomer filler eluate by using extended X-ray absorption fine structure analysis. *Dent. Mater. J.* **2017**, *36*, 214–221. [CrossRef] [PubMed]
36. Gandolfi, M.G.; Iezzi, G.; Piattelli, A.; Prati, C.; Scarano, A. Osteoinductive potential and bone-bonding ability of ProRoot MTA, MTA Plus and Biodentine in rabbit intramedullary model: Microchemical characterization and histological analysis. *Dent. Mater.* **2017**, *33*, 221–238. [CrossRef] [PubMed]

Permissions

All chapters in this book were first published by MDPI; hereby published with permission under the Creative Commons Attribution License or equivalent. Every chapter published in this book has been scrutinized by our experts. Their significance has been extensively debated. The topics covered herein carry significant findings which will fuel the growth of the discipline. They may even be implemented as practical applications or may be referred to as a beginning point for another development.

The contributors of this book come from diverse backgrounds, making this book a truly international effort. This book will bring forth new frontiers with its revolutionizing research information and detailed analysis of the nascent developments around the world.

We would like to thank all the contributing authors for lending their expertise to make the book truly unique. They have played a crucial role in the development of this book. Without their invaluable contributions this book wouldn't have been possible. They have made vital efforts to compile up to date information on the varied aspects of this subject to make this book a valuable addition to the collection of many professionals and students.

This book was conceptualized with the vision of imparting up-to-date information and advanced data in this field. To ensure the same, a matchless editorial board was set up. Every individual on the board went through rigorous rounds of assessment to prove their worth. After which they invested a large part of their time researching and compiling the most relevant data for our readers.

The editorial board has been involved in producing this book since its inception. They have spent rigorous hours researching and exploring the diverse topics which have resulted in the successful publishing of this book. They have passed on their knowledge of decades through this book. To expedite this challenging task, the publisher supported the team at every step. A small team of assistant editors was also appointed to further simplify the editing procedure and attain best results for the readers.

Apart from the editorial board, the designing team has also invested a significant amount of their time in understanding the subject and creating the most relevant covers. They scrutinized every image to scout for the most suitable representation of the subject and create an appropriate cover for the book.

The publishing team has been an ardent support to the editorial, designing and production team. Their endless efforts to recruit the best for this project, has resulted in the accomplishment of this book. They are a veteran in the field of academics and their pool of knowledge is as vast as their experience in printing. Their expertise and guidance has proved useful at every step. Their uncompromising quality standards have made this book an exceptional effort. Their encouragement from time to time has been an inspiration for everyone.

The publisher and the editorial board hope that this book will prove to be a valuable piece of knowledge for researchers, students, practitioners and scholars across the globe.

List of Contributors

Izabela Zieniewska
Doctoral Studies, Medical University of Bialystok, 24a M. Sklodowskiej-Curie Street, 15-274 Bialystok, Poland

Mateusz Maciejczyk
Department of Hygiene, Epidemiology and Ergonomics, Medical University of Bialystok, 15-022 Bialystok, Poland

Anna Zalewska
Experimental Dentistry Laboratory, Medical University of Bialystok, 24a M. Sklodowskiej-Curie Street, 15-274 Bialystok, Poland

Yu Hao, Xiaoyu Huang, Xuedong Zhou and Lei Cheng
State Key Laboratory of Oral Diseases, Sichuan University, Chengdu 610041, China
Department of Cariology and Endodontics, West China School of Stomatology, Sichuan University, Chengdu 610041, China
National Clinical Research Center for Oral Diseases, Sichuan University, Chengdu 610041, China

Mingyun Li, Biao Ren and Xian Peng
State Key Laboratory of Oral Diseases, Sichuan University, Chengdu 610041, China
National Clinical Research Center for Oral Diseases, Sichuan University, Chengdu 610041, China

Akira Kuroiwa, Hiroyuki Kanzaki, Yoshiki Nakamura and Tomomi Sudo
Department of Orthodontics, Tsurumi University School of Dental Medicine, Yokohama 230-8501, Japan

Yoshiaki Nomura and Nobuhiro Hanada
Department of Translational Research, Tsurumi University School of Dental Medicine, Yokohama 230-8501, Japan

Tsuyoshi Ochiai
Photocatalyst Group, Research and Development Department, Local Independent Administrative Agency Kanagawa Institute of industrial Science and TEChnology (KISTEC), 407 East Wing, Innovation Center Building, KSP, 3-2-1 Sakado, Takatsu-ku, Kawasaki, Kanagawa 213-0012, Japan
Materials Analysis Group, Kawasaki Technical Support Department, KISTEC, Ground Floor East Wing, Innovation Center Building, KSP, 3-2-1 Sakado, Takatsu-ku, Kawasaki, Kanagawa 213-0012, Japan
Photocatalysis International Research Center, Tokyo University of Science, 2641 Yamazaki, Noda, Chiba 278-8510, Japan

Rie Nomoto and Tohru Hayakawa
Department of Dental Engineering, Tsurumi University School of Dental Medicine, Yokohama 230-8501, Japan

Rafael Delgado-Ruiz
Department of Prosthodontics and Digital Technology, School of Dental Medicine, Stony Brook University, New York, NY 11794, USA

Georgios Romanos
Department of Periodontics, School of Dental Medicine, Stony Brook University, New York, NY 11794, USA
Department of Oral Surgery and Implant Dentistry, Dental School, Johann Wolfgang Goethe University, 60323 Frankfurt, Germany

Chung-Min Kang
Department of Pediatric Dentistry, College of Dentistry, Yonsei University, Seoul, 03722, Korea
Department of Pharmacology, College of Medicine, Yonsei University, Seoul 03722, Korea

Jiwon Hwang
Department of Pediatric Dentistry, College of Dentistry, Yonsei University, Seoul, 03722, Korea

Je Seon Song, Jae-Ho Lee and Hyung-Jun Choi
Department of Pediatric Dentistry, College of Dentistry, Yonsei University, Seoul, 03722, Korea
Oral Science Research Center, College of Dentistry, Yonsei University, Seoul 03722, Korea

Yooseok Shin
Oral Science Research Center, College of Dentistry, Yonsei University, Seoul 03722, Korea
Department of Conservative Dentistry, College of Dentistry, Yonsei University, 50-1 Yonseiro, Seodaemun-Gu, Seoul 03722, Korea

Mohammad Zakir Hossain, Shumpei Unno and Junichi Kitagawa
Department of Oral Physiology, School of Dentistry, Matsumoto Dental University, 1780 Gobara Hirooka, Shiojiri, Nagano 399-0781, Japan

Marina Mohd Bakri and Farhana Yahya
Department of Oral and Craniofacial Sciences, Faculty of Dentistry, University of Malaya, Kuala Lumpur 50603, Malaysia

Hiroshi Ando
Department of Biology, School of Dentistry, Matsumoto Dental University, 1780 Gobara, Hirooka, Shiojiri, Nagano 399-0781, Japan

Grzegorz Sokolowski
Department of Prosthetic Dentistry, Medical University of Lodz, 251 Pomorska St., 92-213 Lodz, Poland

Agata Szczesio, Kinga Bociong and Karolina Kaluzinska
University Laboratory of Materials Research, Medical University of Lodz, 251 Pomorska St., 92-213 Lodz, Poland

Barbara Lapinska, Jerzy Sokolowski, Monika Domarecka and Monika Lukomska-Szymanska
Department of General Dentistry, Medical University of Lodz, 251 Pomorska St., 92-213 Lodz, Poland

Edina Lempel and Zoltán Varga
Department of Restorative Dentistry and Periodontology, University of Pécs, 5 Dischka Gy Street, Pécs H-7621, Hungary

Zsuzsanna Czibulya, Bálint Kovács and Sándor Kunsági-Máté
Department of General and Physical Chemistry, University of Pécs, 6 Ifjúság Street, Pécs H-7624, Hungary
János Szentágothai Research Center, University of Pécs, 20 Ifjúság Street, Pécs H-7624, Hungary

József Szalma
Department of Oral and Maxillofacial Surgery, University of Pécs, 5 Dischka Gy Street, Pécs H-7621, Hungary

Ákos Tóth
Faculty of Sciences, University of Pécs, 6 Ifjúság Street, Pécs H-7621, Hungary

Katalin Böddi
Department of Biochemistry and Medical Chemistry, University of Pécs, 12 Szigeti Street, Pécs H-7624, Hungary

Manuel Toledano-Osorio, Raquel Osorio and Manuel Toledano
Dental School, University of Granada, Campus de Cartuja s/n, 18071 Granada, Spain

Jegdish P. Babu and Franklin García-Godoy
College of Dentistry, University of Tennessee Health Science Center, 875 Union Avenue, Memphis, TN 381632110, USA

Antonio L. Medina-Castillo
NanoMyP, Spin-Off Enterprise from University of Granada, Edificio BIC-Granada, Av. Innovación 1, Armilla, 18016 Granada, Spain

Mary Anne S. Melo and Michael D. Weir
Department of Advanced Oral Sciences and Therapeutics, University of Maryland School of Dentistry, Baltimore, MD 21201, USA

Vanara F. Passos and Lidiany K. A. Rodrigues
Postgraduate Program in Dentistry, Faculty of Pharmacy, Dentistry and Nursing, Federal University of Ceara, Fortaleza, CE 60430-355, Brazil

Juliana P. M. Rolim
Faculty of Dentistry UniChristus, Fortaleza, CE 60160-230, Brazil

Christopher D. Lynch
Restorative Dentistry, University Dental School and Hospital, University College Cork, Wilton T12 K8AF, Ireland

Hockin H. K. Xu
Department of Advanced Oral Sciences and Therapeutics, University of Maryland School of Dentistry, Baltimore, MD 21201, USA
Center for Stem Cell Biology & Regenerative Medicine, University of Maryland School of Medicine, Baltimore, MD 21201, USA
Marlene and Stewart Greenebaum Cancer Center, University of Maryland School of Medicine, Baltimore, MD 21201, USA

Saturnino Marco Lupi, Arianna Rodriguez y Baena and Ruggero Rodriguez y Baena
Department of Clinico-Surgical, Diagnostic and Pediatric Sciences, Dental Clinic, University of Pavia, P.le Golgi 2, 27100 Pavia, Italy

Marco Tallarico
Private Practice, V. Vincenzo Ussani 86, 00151 Roma, Italy

Minas Leventis, Orestis Vasiliadis and Danai Papavasileiou
Laboratory of Experimental Surgery and Surgical Research N. S. Christeas, Medical School, University of Athens, 75 M. Assias Street, Athens 115 27, Greece

Antonios Galanos
Laboratory of Research of the Musculoskeletal System, Medical School, University of Athens, 2 Nikis Street, Athens 145 61, Greece

Peter Fairbairn
Department of Periodontology and Implant Dentistry, School of Dentistry, University of Detroit Mercy, 2700 Martin Luther King Jr Boulevard, Detroit, MI 48208, USA

Chas Mangham
Manchester Molecular Pathology Innovation Centre, The University of Manchester, Nelson Street, Manchester M13 9NQ, UK

Clara Cassinelli, Giorgio Iviglia and Marco Morra
Nobil Bio Ricerche srl, V. Valcastellana 26, 14037 Portacomaro, Italy

Robert Horowitz
Departments of Periodontics, Implant Dentistry, and Oral Surgery, New York University College of Dentistry, 345 E 24th Street, New York, NY 10010, USA

Koichi Nakamura and Yasutaka Yawaka
Department of Dentistry for Children and Disabled Person, Graduate School of Dental Medicine, Hokkaido University, Kita 13 Nishi 7, Kita-ku, Sapporo 060-8586, Hokkaido, Japan

Shigeaki Abe
Department of Biomaterials and Bioengineering, Graduate School of Dental Medicine, Hokkaido University, Sapporo 060-8586, Hokkaido, Japan

Hajime Minamikawa
Department of Dentistry for Molecular Cell Pharmacology, Graduate School of Dental Medicine, Hokkaido University, Sapporo 060-8586, Hokkaido, Japan

Index

www.ingramcontent.com/pod-product-compliance
Lightning Source LLC
LaVergne TN
LVHW081034210926
848485LV00004B/1024
9781639276530